This book is dedicated to my late friend and colleague, the psychologist Dr Steve Baldwin (1957–2001), who framed all his work as an ethical undertaking and to Dr Thomas S. Szasz, without doubt, the pre-eminent moral philosopher of psychiatry.

Mental Hea<!-- partially obscured -->

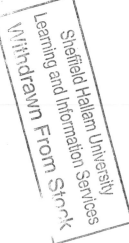

All human behaviour is, ultimately, a moral undertaking, in which each situation must be considered on its own merits. As a result ethical conduct is complex. Despite the proliferation of Codes of Conduct and other forms of professional guidance, there are no easy answers to most human problems. *Mental Health Ethics* encourages readers to heighten their awareness of the key ethical dilemmas found in mainstream contemporary mental health practice.

This text provides an overview of traditional and contemporary ethical perspectives and critically examines a range of ethical and moral challenges present in contemporary 'psychiatric-mental' health services. Offering a comprehensive and interdisciplinary perspective, it includes six parts, each with their own introduction, summary and set of ethical challenges, covering:

- fundamental ethical principles;
- legal issues;
- specific challenges for different professional groups;
- working with different service user groups;
- models of care and treatment;
- recovery and human rights perspectives.

Providing detailed consideration of issues and dilemmas, *Mental Health Ethics* helps all mental health professionals keep people at the centre of the services they offer.

Phil Barker is a psychotherapist in private practice and a Director of Clan Unity International, a mental health recovery consultancy. He is also Honorary Professor in the Faculty of Medicine, Dentistry and Nursing, University of Dundee, UK.

Mental Health Ethics

The human context

Edited by
Phil Barker

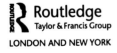

Routledge
Taylor & Francis Group

LONDON AND NEW YORK

First published 2011
by Routledge
2 Park Square, Milton Park, Abingdon, Oxon OX14 4RN

Simultaneously published in the USA and Canada
by Routledge
711 Third Avenue, New York, NY 10017

Routledge is an imprint of the Taylor & Francis Group, an informa business

Typeset in Baskerville by
Book Now Ltd, London

British Library Cataloguing in Publication Data
A catalogue record for this book is available from the British Library

Library of Congress Cataloging-in-Publication Data
A catalog record for this book has been requested

ISBN13: 978-0-415-57099-2 (hbk)
ISBN13: 978-0-415-57100-5 (pbk)
ISBN13: 978-0-203-83905-8 (ebk)

Contents

Contributors

Professor Jacqueline Atkinson is Professor of Mental Health Policy in the Section of Public Health and Health Policy, Faculty of Medicine, University of Glasgow, Scotland.

Professor Phil Barker is Honorary Professor in the Faculty of Medicine, Dentistry and Nursing, University of Dundee, Scotland.

Lesley Brady is Project Leader at Mental Health Services, Crosshouse Hospital, Kilmarnock, Scotland.

Poppy Buchanan-Barker is Director at Clan Unity International, Mental Health Recovery Agency, Fife, Scotland.

Dr Michelle Cleary is Associate Professor (Mental Health Nursing) in the Faculty and Community Health Research Group, School of Nursing and Midwifery, University of Western Sydney, Australia.

Dr Elizabeth Collier is Lecturer in Mental Health at University of Salford, Salford, England.

Professor John Cutcliffe is Acadia Professor of Psychiatric–Mental Health Nursing at the University of Maine, Orono, Maine, USA.

Robert Davidson is (Former) Director of Nursing and First Chair of the Mental Health Nurses Forum (Scotland), NHS Greater Glasgow and Clyde Mental Health Services, Scotland.

Dr Duncan Double is Consultant Psychiatrist for the Norfolk and Waveney Mental Health NHS Trust, England.

Dr Suman Fernando is (Former) Consultant Psychiatrist and Honorary Senior Lecturer in Mental Health at the European Centre for Migration and Social Care (MASC) at the University of Kent, England.

Kevin Franz is Lead Mental Healthcare Chaplain at the Gartnavel Royal Hospital, Glasgow, Scotland.

Dawn Gawthorpe is Senior Lecturer at the University of Salford, Allerton Campus, Salford, England.

Dr Agnes Higgins is Associate Professor in the School of Nursing and Midwifery, Trinity College Dublin, Ireland.

Dr Jan Horsfall is Consultant at the Sydney South West Area Mental Health Service, Australia.

Dr Glenn E. Hunt is Senior Research Fellow, Discipline of Psychological Medicine at the University of Sydney and Research Unit, Sydney South West Area Health Service, Australia.

Dr Lucy Johnstone is Programme Director at the Bristol Clinical Psychology Doctorate, Bristol University, Bristol, England.

Joanne Keeling is Lecturer in Mental Health Nursing at the School of Nursing, University of Salford, England.

Professor Paul Links is Professor of Psychiatry at the University of Toronto and Arthur Sommer Rotenberg Chair in Suicide Studies at St Michael's Hospital, Toronto, Canada.

Dr Sue McAndrew is Lecturer in Mental Health Nursing at the University of Leeds, England.

Tim McDougall is Nurse Consultant and Lead Nurse for CAMHS and Former CAMHS Advisor to the Department of Health at the Cheshire and Wirral Partnership Trust, England.

Professor Tom Mason is Professor of Mental Health and Learning Disability in the Faculty of Health and Social Care at the University of Chester, England.

Vince Mitchell is Mental Health Nurse and Book Review Editor – *Nursing Ethics*, The Retreat, York, England.

Craig Newnes is Consultant Clinical Psychologist and Former Psychological Therapies Director, Shropshire, and Editor of the *Journal of Critical Psychotherapy and Counseling*, England.

Dr Brodie Paterson is Senior Lecturer at the School of Nursing and Midwifery, University of Stirling, Scotland.

Professor Shulamit Ramon works for the Mental Health Recovery Centre, Hertfordshire, England.

Dr Denis Ryan is Senior Lecturer in the Department of Nursing at the University of Applied Science, Utrecht, The Netherlands, and Director of Academic Affairs at the National Counselling Institute of Ireland, Limerick, Ireland.

Dr Jeffrey A. Schaler is the Professor in the Department of Justice, Law and Society School of Public Affairs, American University, Washington DC, USA.

Dr Austyn Snowden is Lecturer in Mental Health Nursing in the School of Health Nursing and Midwifery, University of West of Scotland, Paisley, Scotland.

Professor Garry Walter is Chair of Child and Adolescent Psychiatry at the University of Sydney and Area Clinical Director, Child and Adolescent Mental Health Services, Northern Sydney Central Coast Health, Australia.

Professor Tony Warne is Professor in Mental Health Care at the School of Nursing, University of Salford, England.

Natalie Yates-Bolton is Lecturer in the School of Nursing and Midwifery, University of Salford, England.

Preface

A 7-year-old boy comes home from his Catholic school and declares, excitedly, to his parents that he has become a Celtic[1] supporter. Another pupil had worn the team's colours beneath his school shirt and tie and when the green-and-white hoops were revealed in the playground, the whole class began singing and dancing. The boy didn't know exactly 'who' or 'what' Celtic was or were, but he wanted to be a part of this excitement. The boy's father listened patiently to the story, and then sat down beside him. His voice was soft, his words simple and direct: 'football and religion don't mix'. Suddenly, the playground excitement faded. The sun still streamed in the window but the room felt cool and still. The boy felt uncomfortable. He didn't know what to say.

It may be over 50 years ago but those events haunt my consciousness, as if from yesterday. Life seemed simpler in the 1950s, where a 7-year-old boy could be ignorant of football colours, far less of fashion, and still appear 'normal'. Like many such felt memories, it is easy to slip back into that room; to experience again my introduction to what I now think of as the wide world of ethics. I say think because I am uncertain as to what, exactly, this word 'ethics' means. I have read the many different definitions offered by dictionaries and philosophy primers. I have read most of the major philosophical authorities. I have enrolled in classes taught by eminent ethicists and have debated some of the dominant theories with colleagues, but perhaps most frequently with myself. All this reading and discourse appears only to have heightened my sense of unease and reinforced my uncertainty.

I can talk fluently about ethics and can conjure examples of ethical dilemmas at will. However, if you ask me to offer a definition of ethics, which would be meaningful to the person in the street, I would drop all my books, abandon my preferred theories and turn my back on the disembodied voices of the great philosophers. To satisfy this ordinary person I would need to say, 'football and religion don't mix'.[2]

Doubtless, they would then ask me 'why' and I could begin to talk about what I learned from my father and how his simple, direct message became threaded through almost every human conflict I have experienced personally, or have related to, when experienced by others. Although I did not know it at the time, my father was talking about neither football nor religion, but rather he was talking about how I might conduct my life.[3] Perhaps his simple lecture was an appeal to follow in his philosophical footsteps; to begin to consider some of the lessons he had learned about life from the living of his own life.

Even as I write I still feel something of the conflict that stirred within me that day a half century ago. Since he was my father, I knew he was right, but still I felt uncomfortable. I didn't know how I knew, but I knew all the same. All these years later I wrestle with the same questions. How did he know what was 'right'? What made his sense of 'right' more 'right' than mine? What do I mean by 'right' anyway? And, most importantly, how do I know any of this, anyway?

What seems beyond doubt is that at the age of 7 – that critical age for the Jesuit teacher – my father introduced me to the messy business of morality and the difficult business of making moral choices. I discovered that day that moral dilemmas are found in everyday life – not in books on moral philosophy. Their resolution requires us to exercise 'good sense' and to act – not simply to bury ourselves in more reading and contemplation. I also learned that being 'good' or doing 'right' could be difficult. Decisions need to be taken alone and often result in yet more isolation.

As an only child, I was already an outsider at my Catholic school, where almost every pupil had several brothers and sisters and, of course, where all the family were staunchly Catholic. My father was not a Catholic – indeed he professed no faith, other than in loyalty, sportsmanship and other such values that, today, seem strangely dated. However, he did not influence my mother's practice of her religion, nor influenced her choice of a Catholic school for her son. Looking back, his libertarian stance set him apart from the rest of our small community, where people were religiously territorial, nationalistic or harboured other petty prejudices. However, my father's human qualities served only to isolate me further from the crowd of my classmates, who were cocooned by their Catholic ghetto.

As the sun streamed into the room that day, I knew that I could never be a Celtic supporter – or at least, not without letting down my father's side. That he was advocating not taking sides simply made the realisation all the more confusing. That first moral choice I had to face would bring in its wake the realisation that not only did I have to make this decision alone, but also that by making it, I might become even more isolated from my peers.

I never did 'become a Celtic supporter'. Indeed, increasingly, I found it difficult to support anything (or anyone) without questioning my reasons for offering allegiance. My father's philosophy was a simple one: be your own man. Down the years I may have strayed often from the path my father's words signalled, but even today it remains the only path that stretches out before me. It is not a very busy path. It is not so much the 'path less travelled' as the path one is required to walk alone.

In one sense my father was no philosopher – of ethics, far less of anything else. He left school at 14 and spent his life working in a range of dirty and dangerous occupations: a highly skilled workman with no particular trade – an Everyman. He might have signed his name every so often, but that was the limits to his writing. He read the newspapers and some books, but mainly about sport, especially boxing: again, one man against another in simple, preferably gentlemanly, conflict. However, my father had no need to parade his education. He had been to the 'University of Life': in his case, a far greater form of education than that hackneyed euphemism could ever convey.

A few weeks before he died, we sat on the Esplanade in Kirkcaldy, staring out into the Firth of Forth. I had taken him for one of his last, futile, outpatient appointments. He was dying, stoically, from lung cancer, in much the same way as he had lived, stoically, with all sorts of other insults, injuries and disappointments in life. The man who used to sup several pints on a Saturday night pushed away his half-pint glass, its head barely touched by his quivering lips. Without warning, he began a short story of his wartime experiences, which until that day he had never discussed. His eyes lingered on the horizon and clearly he was in no shape for telling stories. Instead, he set the scene, sketched a few important details, then pulled his glass up to his lips, then put it to one side. Refreshment itself had become a chore. It was time to go home.

I drove him home in silence – the jumbled story buzzing inside me. I was back in that bright, sunlit room of my childhood, where I could only feel coolness and the awareness that, once again, I was at a loss for words.

What he had called, with no trace of irony, the 'bare bones' of his story involved the relief of Belsen concentration camp.[1] Along with some of his regiment he had been assigned to the Allied Forces team. He offered no dramatic descriptions, just a simple, mundane account of the pathetic waste of life: his supervision of the mass burials and the names of some of the more notorious commandants arrested, all of which appeared indelibly fixed in his memory. However, he held no one to account: everyone must account for themselves. His side may have been the victor, but there was dishonour on all sides. No one came out of this war untarnished.

I always knew my father was a 'decorated soldier', although his medals were stuffed away at the back of a drawer at home. He did wear his regimental badge on his blazer pocket when he went to his Ex-Serviceman's Club; but he waited over 25 years to parade in public his part in that war. A couple of years later, he also wore a Campaign for Nuclear Disarmament (CND) badge that my wife gave him, on his lapel, above his army badge. He had been proud to be a soldier, but knew that war was futile – and could be demeaning. War – and all the reasons for war – took the meaning out of life. It might be a necessary evil, but it was evil just the same.

His short story, told that day on the seafront – incoherent, jumbled and unfinished – was my father's legacy. I have no idea why he waited 41 years to tell me, or why it was so close to a deathbed confession. I never thought to ask him, but doubt that he would have answered, even if I had.

I offer these few pages from my life story in an effort to follow my father's footsteps – by being simple and direct. It is important for me to make my part in this book deeply personal. A week before he died my father asked me to bury him. When I asked him what he meant, he said, 'Just say a few words'. He wanted no ministers of religion, or other 'professional mourners', peddling kind words and clichés. Instead, I was to say 'just a few words', about the man, to his few friends and even fewer relatives, but many comrades and workmates. By the time he died I was an accomplished platform speaker, who enjoyed addressing audiences, large or small. More than 20 years later, the call to 'just say a few words' remains the most challenging piece of public speaking I have ever undertaken, for there was no room for insincerity or weasel words, flannel or blarney.

In later chapters I may well tie myself in knots, with long, possibly rambling, 'academic' reflections on different aspects of ethics in mental health. However, here I want to declare the importance of being direct and simple when talking about life and the rules that might guide the living of it. Regrettably, much of our talk about ethics – as with almost everything related to philosophy – is frequently made incomprehensible, as authors parade their obvious intelligence and superlative vocabulary. Ethics is far too important to risk being sidelined as an academic pursuit: something to be engaged in only from the comfort of an armchair. Ethics deals with human nature[5] – how we conduct ourselves in life. My ethics represent what I consider right and fitting. Ultimately, others will judge whether or not they agree with me.

When we come to address the particular situations that are commonly called 'mental health issues or problems or difficulties', we may discover that the promise of a simple, direct form of ethical wisdom, is drowned by a sea of jargon, political correctness and 'legalese'. However, if we are to navigate these potentially muddy waters, we must have a firm sense of our purpose: what is the point of all this reflection and discourse? What are we trying to get at?

Unlike some other writers, I don't believe that everything I ever learned of any significance, I learned at my father's knee – far less in kindergarten. However, much of what I have learned about ethics, and the values embedded within it, takes me back to that childhood experience from 50 years ago. In a very important sense, that was the beginning and end-point of all my ethical striving. I set out that day to discover what my father's message meant, only to find myself, years later, back at the same spot; having toured several ethical empires; returning laden with nuggets of philosophical wisdom; reconciled to the fact that all the great thinkers discovered much the same, simple truths as my father did, especially that religion and football don't mix.

Phil Barker
Newport on Tay, Scotland

Notes

1 Celtic is a famous Scottish football club from Glasgow. It has a historic association with the people of Ireland and Scots of Irish extraction, who mainly view themselves as members of the Catholic community.

2 My countryman, Bill Shankly, said, 'Some people think that football is a matter of life and death. I assure you it is much more serious than that'. His quip may reveal a great social truth. However, it reminds me of how many people would willingly genuflect before idols, rather than face their own reflection.

3 The Oxford English Dictionary (OED) defines 'ethics' as (variously) 'the moral principles by which a person is guided'. Although he had never heard of him, my father might well have been offering an everyday example of Jeremy Bentham's utilitarian dictum that: 'Ethics at large may be defined, the art of directing man's actions to the production of the greatest quantity of happiness' (OED).

4 Shephard B. '*After Daybreak: The Liberation of Belsen, 1945*', London: Pimlico, 2006.

5 Ethics: from the Greek *ethikos* (ἠθικόϛ), meaning – 'showing moral character'.

Acknowledgements

All moral enterprises are, ultimately, deeply personal affairs; no matter how many people might be involved in enacting them, or who might be affected as a result. I have been involved in the publication of two other books on mental health ethics, but the preparation of the manuscript for '*Mental Health Ethics: the human context*', proved deeply disturbing on a professional level, but oddly uplifting in a spiritual sense. This book changed me, and I am deeply grateful for having had the opportunity to play a part in its preparation.

Originally, I commissioned a chapter from an internationally renowned 'user–consumer advocate', who eventually had to drop out of the project. This led me to realise that I might have made a huge assumption that none of the other authors were in a position to represent the 'user–consumer' perspective. Some, if not all, authors might have experienced 'mental health' problems and might well have received professional help to address them. Indeed, many of the chapters offer deeply empathic accounts of the situation of 'patients' or 'clients', which suggests that perhaps some of this empathy originates from the author's own experience of difficulty and distress. It is appropriate, therefore, to express my gratitude to those authors, for allowing aspects of their own experience to reflect on their writing.

As an edited work my greatest privilege lay in reading, carefully, the contributions of the various authors: offering them some constructive, critical commentary. I hope that they found my words useful. Certainly, all were remarkably gracious in accepting my suggestions. In that sense, the authors are fine examples of true scholars.

It is appropriate, therefore, to acknowledge the gift of scholarship provided by all the contributors. It was my privilege to be the first to read their work, which they offered in the true spirit of collegiality. Everyone considered it their privilege to be invited to contribute to the book, but clearly the publishers and myself became the beneficiaries. To all the many authors, I extend my sincere thanks for their generosity of spirit, scholasticism and heartfelt considerations on mental health ethics.

I also acknowledge the sensitive yet efficient support provided by Grace McInnes and Khanam Virjee, from the publishers, Routledge, Taylor and Francis.

Finally, I would like to thank my wife, life-partner and colleague Poppy Buchanan-Barker, for her support over the past year. Together we learned, again, that life can be full of surprises. However, I learned, yet again, that no matter what surprises Life chooses to dish up, Poppy would still be there to lean on. No surprises there!

Acknowledgement

Grateful acknowledgement is made to Wiley-Blackwell for their permission to publish sections of a paper by John Cutcliffe and Paul Links in Chapter 22, which first appeared in the *International Journal of Mental Health Nursing*.

Editor's note

This book addresses mental health ethics from many different perspectives. This is only right and proper, given the uncertainty over any specific reading of the subject, and given the diverse – and often divergent – viewpoints of the various authors. As editor I chose the topics for all the chapters and provided a broad framework to which each of the authors worked. However, beyond that no effort was made to direct the authors or influence the core message of their chapter once submitted. This also is only right and fitting. If we are to develop our vision of the ethical landscape in mental health we must be open to challenges from others. We must also be prepared to live with uncertainty. There may be some ethical certainties, but encouraging people to agree on them often proves difficult.

As a result, I agree strongly with the ethical perspectives provided by some authors, but have concerns about those of others. I hope that my ethical unease helps to reflect the many ethical conflicts found in the field at large.

In many chapters certain words or phrases will be presented in 'scare quotes'. Most often these 'quotes' are intended to illustrate that: 'this is how this was described or defined by the author'. In effect, this is not *necessarily* what I would call it. On occasions, this might betray some disapproval of the term or phrase, but other times not. Hopefully, readers will be able to judge for themselves when any criticism is intended.

Section 1

Ethics and mental health

Section preface

Phil Barker

As we shall discover, most dictionaries define ethics as 'dealing with what is good or bad, right or wrong'. When applied to professions, ethics is concerned with 'moral duties or obligations' – what the professional *ought* to do in any given situation: the principles of conduct or standards of professional behaviour. Although professional ethics might appear special it is, in effect, merely a narrow description of the kind of 'moral conduct' considered 'right' or 'good' when applied to people in general.

The key lies in the word 'conduct', indicating how people *conduct* their affairs, both in relation to themselves, other people, the animal kingdom, if not also the planet that sustains us all. 'How *should* I act?' is the most ubiquitous ethical question, which might be asked in any situation. Although it is an unfashionable view, most human behaviour involves conduct. Aside from the small proportion of reflex behaviours, everything else that we 'do' involves choice or the possibility of choice.

Unfortunately, 'choice' has become something of a weasel word in the mental health field, where the idea is peddled that 'choice' is something that can be given or otherwise 'facilitated', when in reality it can only be restricted. Or at least, that is the case where people are free to conduct their lives, in whatever way they see fit.

This reminds us that the idea of 'psychiatric' or 'mental health' ethics is problematic, if not a contradiction in terms. In principle, ethics is only meaningful where people – or groups of people – are self-governing and have the opportunity to make choices free from any coercion. Rarely is this the case in the mental health field. The limits imposed on a person's exercise of freedom – however explicit – continue to haunt contemporary practice.

In this opening section, I seek to set the scene for the detailed examination of specific ethical dilemmas and related topics, which begin in Section 2.

In Chapter 1, I discuss some of the key ideas which have been developed over the centuries, and explore their relevance to the contemporary world of mental health. I propose that there are no *new* ethical dilemmas, far less any new theories to explain or resolve them. Almost everything that we believe today, concerning the moral challenges of everyday life and how we might respond to them, is a revised version of some older ideas about life and how it should be lived. Such philosophies have merely been revised to suit the language or the social context of some 'brave new world'.

In Chapter 2, I begin to examine the key ethical dilemma within the psychiatric or mental health field: that the fundamental assumptions concerning 'mental illness' and 'agency' – the person's capacity to act freely – risks rendering the idea of 'psychiatric/mental health ethics' meaningless. However, this is not a nihilistic view, merely a candid appraisal of the field at the present time. It is, of course, possible to aim for the development of such a genuine ethic. However, this will require major changes in the way professionals, and the services they represent, conduct themselves with the people embraced by such services.

In some senses our ideas about ethics have changed little over thousands of years. We continue to tussle with much the same problems as our ancestors and develop new theories that often differ little from those they seek to displace.

Finally, in Chapter 3 I discuss the extent to which moral dilemmas, regarding what *ought to be done*, vary across the different disciplines embraced by the field, and the many different situations, which professionals encounter. To what extent has our thinking about 'mental illness' really changed? To what extent are we merely recycling older, outmoded models of human problems: trying to avoid confronting the personal, social and political issues that we obscure with our increasingly technical concepts of 'psychiatric disorder'?

This chapter provides an introduction to the detailed examination of the professional context of ethical inquiry, which begins in Section 2.

1 Ethics

In search of the good life

Phil Barker

Of course, indifference can be tempting – more than that, seductive. It is so much easier to look away. It is so much easier to avoid such rude interruptions to our work, our dreams, our hopes. It is, after all, awkward, troublesome, to be involved in another person's pain and despair. Yet, for the person who is indifferent, his or her neighbors are of no consequence. And, therefore, their lives are meaningless. Their hidden or even visible anguish is of no interest. Indifference reduces the Other to an abstraction.[1]

(Elie Wiesel)

Everyday ethics

Damned to anguish

Ethics or moral philosophy may involve ordinary or everyday human dilemmas, but is in no way ordinary, far less easy to discuss. Ethics has been debated for thousands of years and different schools of ethical thought are associated with many different cultures as well as with individual philosophers. This diversity may fascinate the philosophy student but may prove frustrating for anyone seeking a unifying set of human values. The more one learns the more it seems that one set of views appears to negate all others. Indeed, there may well be no single *ethic* that can apply across all situations, societies or cultures. More importantly, there may be no single ethic that does not make life more difficult for you or me. Ethics can be a disturbing business.

All animals act in ways that have consequences for their immediate or long-term welfare, but only humans seem to anguish over 'dilemmas' or 'decisions', developing complex, often baffling, theories to explain their decision-making. Our capacity for language and communication creates this anguish. Without the ability to label, discuss and debate the decisions we make each day, life could well be simpler. Humans appear damned to think about themselves and life in general. As a result, making decisions becomes the most challenging aspect of being alive and being human.

Ethics involves enacting our private thoughts about ourselves, others and the world around us, and is almost as old as humankind. In that sense, it existed long before philosophical terms were coined and applied to such behaviour. The sheer complexity of much ethical terminology often obscures the ethical decision-making that goes on in everyday life. As a result, ethics is invariably viewed as a rarefied activity: a subject, like theology, studied outside of life itself, usually at university. This could not be further from the everyday ethical truth.

Today, ethics focuses on dilemmas that cause unrest in society. The *big* ethical questions continue to revolve around abortion, euthanasia, torture, warfare or the death penalty. With the emergence of concepts like 'assisted dying' or 'foetal stem cell research', some of these age-old dilemmas have grown even more complex. However, such 'big questions' are merely examples of issues with which people have wrestled down the ages. By no means are these the only ethical challenges we face in our lives. Every day people deliberate over whether or not to:

- put the cat out at night;
- give money to a beggar;
- return a wallet found in the street to its owner;
- pick up litter;
- correct a shop assistant who returns an excess of change;
- help someone who is being mugged;
- give information to the police concerning a crime;
- do a favour for someone;
- put an elderly relative into a care home;
- take public transport to work rather than use the family car.

Such deliberations involve our personal or shared *values* concerning, among other things:

- animal welfare
- charity
- honesty
- civic mindedness
- altruism
- public duty
- generosity
- loyalty
- eco-responsibility.

All such deliberations are forms of ethical decision-making, whether or not we label them in such terms.

Ethical thinking and moral doing

These examples illustrate how ethics governs most areas of everyday human life, where one person, or a group, does something *with*, *for* or *to* another person or group. Consequently, every area of social behaviour is governed by its own *code*: for example, 'business ethics', 'medical ethics', Christian ethics', Buddhist ethics', 'healthcare ethics' or 'sporting ethics'. These offer guidance regarding what might be seen to be 'right', 'proper' or otherwise 'necessary' within a specific sphere of human activity.

Most definitions of ethics describe:

- A *set of principles* that determine 'right conduct': what we *should do* in a certain situation.
- A *system* of moral values: *why* we *believe* a particular action is the right thing to do.

Although ethics is commonly viewed as something proscribed by philosophers, if not a specialist branch of philosophy itself, this can be a dangerous idea. We may develop the idea that ethics relates only to the 'big questions' mentioned. This may lead to the assumption that the challenging or awkward situations that make up our everyday lives raise no ethical issues. Alternatively, we may assume that if any such issues exist it is not our responsibility to address them. Many professionals assume that their professional code of conduct will resolve all the potential dilemmas they might encounter in their careers. As we discover in later chapters, this is a naive view and may leave the individual professional open to criticism. If professionals are not ethically vigilant in addressing the subtle conflicts encountered in practice, these may develop into serious threats to the welfare of those in the professional's care.

The assumption that ethics is not *my* personal responsibility often is linked to our social or cultural history. In societies, like the United Kingdom, where religion is or was influential, there is a tendency to assume that ethics is an extension of religious thought.[2] Different religions, and philosophers who embraced religious beliefs, may have contributed to the *development* of ethical theory, but their basis lies in age-old ideas about human nature. The Greek root of the word *ethics* (*ethikos*) means 'dealing with human nature', and relates to the overarching interest in the 'good life' first proposed by Aristotle,[3] which continues to entrance us to this day.[1] This begs the question: 'what is the *purpose of life?*' More specifically it invites us to ask 'what *ought* we to *do* to be a *good person?*'

When we come to consider ethical issues in mental health it would be reassuring to assume that these challenges and dilemmas might already have been addressed by 'medical ethics' or 'healthcare ethics'. However, the difficult history of psychiatry has generated its own distinctive ethical problems, which continue to haunt the contemporary mental health field (see Chapter 2). The question of what we *ought* to do in the name of ethical mental health care has no easy answer, or at least none that sits easily with contemporary legal, political and social attitudes towards the so-called 'mentally ill'.

Plus ca change . . .[5]

The term ethics can be used in different ways. We talk of someone embracing a 'working class *ethic* (singular)', implying the values associated with a particular social class. *Ethics* (plural) can also refer to the formal study of the choices people make in their lives: that is, 'moral philosophy'. In general, however, *ethics* refers to the rules or standards that govern the behaviour of an individual (*personal ethics*) or a group (e.g. *medical ethics*). Threaded through these differing definitions is a concern with *values* – either personal or collective.

Our social and cultural world is changing rapidly. Fifty years ago, 'homosexuality' was still a crime, and mentioned only in hushed tones, if at all. Today, 'homophobia' is, in some contexts, classed as a crime, and legislation exists in most countries to protect the rights of women and men who wish to confirm their same-sex relations through a civil ceremony. This might have bewildered my parents and grandparents, but so too would the widespread acceptance of divorce, cosmetic surgery, single-parenthood and drug-taking not to mention the contemporary obsession with 'celebrity'. Social mores have changed dramatically over the past half century leading politicians to lobby for a 'back to basics' approach or a revival of the 'family values' associated with the 'good old days'. (As we shall see, some moral philosophers express a similar kind of nostalgia.) Whether or not such 'basic' or 'family' values were widely accepted at any time in our history remains unclear. However, people from all walks of life continue to advocate and prosecute the kind of values they consider might make up the 'good life'. Few such people would call themselves 'moral philosophers', but their enduring concern for our understanding of 'right and proper conduct' shows that ethics remains the commonest form of 'everyday philosophy'.

Respecting the past – embracing the future

In trying to clarify what kind of values might help us address our myriad ethical dilemmas, there may be a virtue in acknowledging thinkers from the past. If nothing else, such reflection may help us avoid assuming that we have discovered something new, rather than merely having updated a much older way of thinking. As Fernandez-Armesto suggested:

> No one should feel ashamed of turning back to tradition. Memory of what previous generations have learned is the foundation of all possible progress. When traditions conflict, they need more care, not less: they should be keenly scrutinized, not casually discarded. Truth-finding techniques used throughout history are commended to us by the use once made of them. They remain useful, and the concepts of truth which have underlain them continue to deserve respect.[6]

To help us consider how to approach the particular ethical challenges that are encountered in the mental health field, it may be useful to summarise some of the key developments in the development of our understanding of ethics, or moral philosophy.[7]

A brief history of ethics

The Greek legacy

Alfred North Whitehead (1861–1947) famously said that the 'safest general characterisation of the European philosophical tradition is that it consists of a series of footnotes to Plato'.[8] Although bordering on exaggeration Whitehead was, perhaps, merely trying to locate the importance of Plato's thinking as a key influence on the Western tradition. This comment also reminds us that whereas science repeatedly supersedes the past, philosophy continues to draw on past influences and traditions. *Antony Flew* (1923–) clarified this link with the past by saying that: 'the whole *later development* of Western philosophy can be regarded as a series of extended footnotes to Plato (emphasis added)'.[9] Not only was Plato the first to have left an extensive body of work but, as Flew noted, it is almost impossible to define 'philosophy' without referring to his writings. Consequently, many of our contemporary ideas about society, the individual, rights and responsibilities, can be traced to the influence of Plato and other Greek philosophers from two and a half thousand years ago.

Socrates and self-discovery

The origin of ethics lies with *Socrates* (469–399 BC), who mentored *Plato* and, at least within the Western world, is recognised as the first philosopher to encourage both scholars and ordinary people to consider *how* they should live. Although little is known of his life,[10] as a young man he attended lectures on the science of the day, which concentrated on the physical nature of the universe. It became obvious to him that the resultant debates often involved circular arguments with few real conclusions. Moreover, he was concerned at the absence of any concern for the moral health of society, concluding that an understanding of the nature of human life was, by far, the most important form of knowledge. In his famous dictum, '*an unexamined life is not worth living*', he conveyed his belief that 'self-knowledge' was vital to any success in life. Like most Greeks he believed that people had a natural purpose (often called the *teleological* view[11]). He encouraged his fellow citizens to 'know thyself' – discovering the 'real selves' which lay within.

Although Socrates produced no philosophical writings his thought was documented by his pupil Plato, who described him as the 'gadfly', for the way he goaded the citizens of Athenian society; 'stinging' them into thinking for themselves. His belief that the wise man[12] was '*he who knows that he knows nothing*' became the basis of a sceptical form of inquiry and debate between people in which questions stimulated new lines of thought and more rational perspectives on a problem. Today, many forms of psychotherapy embrace this 'not knowing' approach – called 'the Socratic method' – as a way of helping people to explore new perspectives on their everyday human dilemmas. Unfortunately Socrates's support for 'not knowing' corresponded with a refusal to recognise the Greek gods. This was seen as an attempt to corrupt the youth of Athens and led to his trial at which he was condemned to death.[13]

Although Socrates may have begun the development of ethical inquiry, philosophers have since struggled with many of his core assumptions.

- How useful is discussion and debate for the acquisition of genuine knowledge?
- Is there any such thing as the 'true or inner self'?
- Is morality something that we discover or something we make up?
- Isn't morality concerned more with our relationships with one another and taking responsibility for how we act towards other people?

Plato and reason

Plato (428–348 BC) left Athens in disgust after the death of Socrates, returning a decade later to found his famous *Academy*, the model for all subsequent 'modern' universities. Plato had serious doubts about the validity of the democracy on which Athens was founded, where either mob rule or corrupt politicians held sway. In his key work '*The Republic*' Plato raised critical questions about the individual, the state and morality.[14]

Plato represented a key development in what we would now call 'rationalism'. Although he acknowledged the existence of empirical knowledge, gained through the senses, he believed that *reasoning* provided the means for developing a vastly superior understanding of the world. However, he also believed that only an elite class of philosophers could grapple with moral and political problems. Soon this would become the model for the powerful authority of the Christian church. The unwillingness of many 'ordinary' people to dispute moral problems, leaving this task to philosophers, theologians, politicians and other professional 'ethicists', is a contemporary example of the survival of Plato's model of the *Elites*.

Aristotle and common sense

Plato's student, *Aristotle* (384–322 BC), was more concerned with 'practical wisdom'[15] and proposed an ethical system that could be called 'self-realisationism'. Aristotle saw ethics very much as the concern of 'ordinary people', rather than Plato's philosopher-kings. In his *Nicomachean Ethics*[16] he discussed how if people could act in accordance with their true natures they would realise their full human potential, and would both *do* good and *be* content. Aristotle believed that human beings were 'programmed' with justice, fairness, courage and other virtues. However, people needed to choose a 'middle way' between the extremes of such virtues, where we might, for example, endanger ourselves or others, by being recklessly courageous or ridiculously fair. Critics have suggested that Aristotle's doctrine of the middle path is middle-aged, middle-class and middlebrow . . . the good man was in effect what came to be known in English as a 'gentleman' . . . one who is considerate of others, honest and decent, and possessed of integrity and sound principle.[17]

In most contemporary societies, Aristotle's ethical philosophy seems old-fashioned, especially where 'individualism' is prized over 'good citizenship' and morality is something that needs to be controlled, rather than viewed as a part of 'self-fulfilment'. However, his assumption that morality is something acquired, through diligent practice – like learning to play the piano – continues to prove attractive to some contemporary philosophers.[18]

Hellenism, hedonism and happiness

Although the Greek City States eventually collapsed and were replaced by military empires, Greek moral philosophy survived in different forms, especially in Hellenism, which comprised additions to Aristotle's ideas about happiness and fulfilment. Several different schools of *Hedonist* thought developed, all focused on how people might experience the greatest pleasure and the least pain. Today, the modern term 'hedonist' is associated with someone focused on self-gratification, regardless of the pain and expense to others. By contrast, many of the original hedonist thinkers were concerned with how pleasure and happiness might be maximised for the greatest number.

Aristippus (435–356 BCE) of Cyrene argued that happiness lay in *indifference* to ambition and possessions. The idea that fleeting desires should be indulged for fear that the opportunity might not be repeated, became known as Cyrenaic hedonism and found expression in the 'eat drink and be merry' outlook that prevails to this day. However, Aristippus was not exactly what we would call a 'hedonist' today. He believed that people had a responsibility to protect others from harm that might result from reckless pleasure-seeking. The good judgement and exercise of self-control necessary to temper powerful human desires was expressed through his motto: 'I *possess*, I am not possessed'.

Epicurus (341–270 BCE) rejected the extremism of the Cyrenaics, believing that some forms of pleasure-seeking could be detrimental, especially where indiscriminate indulgence might have negative consequences. By pursuing *moderation* in friendship and philosophical discussion, as much as in drinking and general merrymaking, the Epicureans were maintaining Aristotle's tradition. The greatest good, to Epicurus, was *prudence*, exercised through moderation and caution.[19] If pain and illness could be avoided then living was essentially good. Indeed, death was not something to be feared but rather *fear* was considered the source of most unhappiness. Roosevelt's famous saying, 'we have nothing to fear except fear itself', was an early twentieth century echo of the Epicurean philosophy.

Probably the most extreme, yet enduring, form of philosophy from the Hellenistic era was *Stoicism*.[20] Founded by *Zeno* (336–261 BCE) the Stoics had considerable influence on the Romans, especially *Cicero* and *Marcus Aurelius* in the first century AD and later medieval scholars. Although 'stoicism' is today equated with fatalism, in its original form this philosophy involved a powerful way of accepting life and all its trials. *Epictetus* (AD 55–135) is, arguably, the most well-known Stoic, epitomised by his famous sayings: '*difficult circumstances do not so much ennoble a man as reveal him*' and '*we are disturbed not by events, but by the view we take of them*'. This latter dictum became one of the philosophical mantras of the cognitive therapy movement.

For *Epictetus* the greatest good was contentment and serenity. Peace of mind was realised by mastering one's desires. *Epictetus* was born a slave but eventually freed by the Romans.

Perhaps this early life experience played a part in his view that we should not be a slave to the passions: if we cannot control our reactions to others and life in general, we shall never be completely free.

The Stoic philosophy focused on accepting the things that cannot be changed and doing something constructive in response to those that can be changed. This classic Stoical philosophy found a modern echo in the *Serenity Prayer*, attributed to the theologian *Karl Paul Reinhold Niebuhr* (1892–1971).[21]

The rise of Christianity

By the fourth century AD Christianity had become the official religion of the Roman Empire. Although the Church closed Plato's academy in Athens, at the same time by this time it had embraced much of Greek philosophy, which eventually found expression in many of the writings of the early Christian leaders, not least *St Augustine* (354–430) and later *St Thomas Aquinas* (1225–74) who were both influenced by Plato and Aristotle's ideas. However, up until the seventeenth century there was little further critical discussion of ethical principles since the question of 'how to live' had been settled by the Church and Christian teaching.

Humanism and the social contract

Socrates's original view was that people should 'think for themselves' rather than following blindly the dictates of authority. This became the foundation of *humanism*, which found its most powerful expression during the Renaissance, first in Italy in the fourteenth century and later throughout Europe. Like the Greeks questioning the role of the gods in human affairs, Renaissance humanism promoted scientific inquiry as the key means of understanding the world.

Niccolo Machiavelli's (1469–1527) infamous work *The Prince*[22] described the qualities rulers needed to gain and maintain power. Although interpreted by some as a satire, Machiavelli's book illustrated the ruthlessness that still appears to be central to the life of democratic politicians and unelected dictators alike. This led the English philosopher *Thomas Hobbes* (1588–1679) to propose that people were 'brutish' by nature, and needed to be tamed by society. In *Leviathan* Hobbes introduced the idea of the 'social contract', whereby people gave up some of their natural rights to maintain social order through governmental authority. This idea was developed further by *John Locke* (1632–1704) and *Jean-Jacques Rousseau* and later found its most powerful expression in Republicanism.[23]

Jean-Jacques Rousseau (1712–78) challenged Hobbes's bleak view of humanity, proposing that humans are born with a great potential for goodness, but needed appropriate education to draw this out. He saw civilisation as a corrupting force, promoting envy, greed and self-consciousness. His many critics – such as *Voltaire* – wrongly argued that he wanted people to return to 'walking on all fours', leading to the idea of the 'noble savage'.[24] Many subsequent writers contradicted both Hobbes and Rousseau, pointing out that many people develop courage, generosity and altruism, often from direct life experience. Indeed, this is not even peculiar to *Homo sapiens*. The obvious displays of affection, altruism and mutual defensiveness displayed by primates, are identical to the bonding and mutual supportiveness common to all human societies. The co-cooperativeness inherent in tribal and family systems clearly contradicts Hobbes's pessimistic view of people and the need for the 'social contract', but hardly supports Rousseau's romantic view. Indeed, morality may have evolved as part of the development of 'human nature' and continues to be maintained simply because of its usefulness to all kinds of human community.

Utilitarianism or consequentialism

In the eighteenth century *Jeremy Bentham* (1748–1832) and his disciple *John Stuart Mill* (1806–73) narrowed the ethical focus, once again, to address pain and pleasure. Their *utilitarian* philosophy was largely an extension of hedonist thinking and proposed that any act may be considered *right* if it tends to promote happiness and wrong if the reverse is the case. However, this referred to the happiness of everyone who might be associated with the act not just the performer. The utilitarian answer to the age-old question 'what ought a man to do?' was to act in such a way as to produce the best possible consequences for all concerned. As a result, their philosophy was often described as '*consequentialism*'. However, their theory was far more complex than it might first appear. The *circumstances*, both current and future, related to the act; the potential *effect on different parties* involved in the act; and how one determines the relative *value* of any consequence, are only a few of the potential issues involved in calculating what might be the 'greatest good'.

John Stuart Mill was concerned particularly with 'tyranny of the majority', not simply that posed by politicians. He believed that there was a need to protect people against:

> the tyranny of the prevailing opinion and feeling, against the tendency of society to impose, by other means than civil penalties, its own ideas and practices as rules of conduct on those who dissent from them; to fetter the development and, if possible, prevent the formation of any individuality not in harmony with its ways, and compel all characters to fashion themselves upon the model of its own.[25]

Mill believed that the only ground for using power against an individual was to prevent harm to others. His argument that, 'over himself, over his own body and mind, the individual is sovereign'[26] was to become the foundation of libertarianism. Under Bentham's original utilitarian system the rights of individuals and minorities might be threatened by favouring the majority view. Mill's essay *On Liberty* explored the need to provide the necessary political counterbalance required to foster a more pluralistic society.

Deontology – practical reason

Immanuel Kant (1724–1804) disagreed strongly with Utilitarianism, arguing that morality had little or nothing to do with the pursuit of 'happiness'. Instead, he developed a philosophical justification for the common sense view that morality was concerned with 'sticking to the rules'. Kant proposed that a moral act was one that stemmed from a sense of *duty*, rather than simply doing what we like. Commonly known as a *deontologist* (believer in rules or obligations) Kant adopted a highly *absolutist* position and argued that an act may be considered the right thing to do, *even* if it produces a bad consequence. Telling lies to save someone's life would be considered wrong, even if telling the truth resulted in harm to the person. His view that duty should be done for its own sake became known as the '*categorical imperative*'.

Kant developed his ideas through use of a 'universability test': 'what if everyone acted like this?' Therefore, if everyone *always* told the truth, the world would be a better place. If everyone told lies – even occasionally – then we would never know the truth. Kant proposed that: 'we should only act in accord with a given principle or set of principles if we can, at the same time, reasonably will that it should be binding on all others through space and time'.

Kant's philosophy has become the basis of much human rights legislation, although his critics have argued that he did not make it clear *why* we should do our duty.

Kant's ideas related only to rational beings, and so he exempted animals from any consideration. He believed that many people remained in a state of perpetual immaturity by refusing to have the courage to use their own understanding, whilst others exploited this situation by acting as their guardians.

> It is so convenient to be immature! If I have a book to have understanding in place of me, a spiritual adviser to have a conscience for me, a doctor to judge my diet for me and so on, I need not make any efforts at all. I need not think, so long as I can pay; others will soon enough take the tiresome job over for me.[27]

In contemporary society, where many of the 'tiresome jobs' associated with everyday living have been taken over by others, Kant's philosophy can seem idealistic. When we consider people with 'mental health problems', who might be viewed as not fully 'rational' (however this is defined), Kant's philosophy becomes even more challenging.

Radical scepticism

David Hume (1711–76) is classed as one of the giants of the Scottish Enlightenment. Nicknamed the 'great infidel' Hume's questioning stance to conventional belief brought him into conflict with the Church in Scotland, which interpreted his view as atheistic. Hume argued that there could never be such a thing as 'moral knowledge' promoting further the empiricist view that all genuine knowledge came through the senses. Hume challenged the view that logic might be used to 'prove' certain moral beliefs. Instead, he argued that morals derive from moral sentiments: the approval (esteem, praise) or disapproval (blame) expressed by onlookers. Hume argued that it is not the case that 'murder is wrong'. It is simply that I (and others) *disapprove* of murder. Reason is a slave to the passions. In that sense, moral beliefs are *psychological* rather than reasonable (or logical) as previous philosophers had argued.[28]

Modern-day critics have complained that Hume's philosophy leaves us with no rational means of condemning individual murders or events like the Holocaust, other than to say 'we disapprove'. However, although we cannot *prove* (empirically) that murder is wrong, this does not prevent us from sympathising or empathising with those harmed by murderous acts, or indeed any other form of 'inhumanity'. Such emotional connections lead to the development of legislation (and various social or community actions), which seeks to redress the consequences of murderous acts. In that sense Hume's 'passions' can be seen as the key factor in ethical behaviour.

Existentialism – no excuses

The traditional idea that human beings might have a *nature* was challenged by *existentialism*,[29] which proposed that we behave in particular ways because this is our *choice*, not because we are programmed by nature. Although not named until the 1940s, by the French philosopher *Gabriel Marcel* (1889–1973) existentialism became very much a twentieth century phenomenon. However, its formal roots lie in the works of *Soren Kierkegaard* (1813–55) and *Friedrich Nietzsche* (1844–1900), although countless others had addressed similar concerns for the centrality of 'existence' down the ages, including Buddha, St Augustine and Shakespeare. In a sophisticated extension of Stoic thinking, Kierkegaard said that everyone was responsible for giving meaning to their lives and should live life passionately and sincerely, however challenging the circumstances. Kierkegaard and Nietzsche saw life as meaningless, and hence the need to endow it with one's personal meaning. Later, writers like *Franz Kafka, Fyodor Dostoevsky* and *Albert Camus* further developed the theme of the human struggle with hopelessness and the absurdity of life itself.[30]

Existentialism is not a school of philosophy but a collective term applied retrospectively, often to writers who emphasised similar interests in finding 'self' and the meaning of life through *free will, choice* and *personal responsibility*. Beyond this common ground great differences exist among the key figures. Kierkegaard was devoutly religious, Nietzsche was anti-Christian, and Jean-Paul Sartre (1905–80) and Albert Camus (1913–60) were atheists and *Martin Heidegger* (1889–1976) infamously became a member of the Nazi party.[31]

In Sartre's highly influential view, if we deny the essential 'freedom' to make ourselves, thus giving our life its only meaning, we become *inauthentic* and guilty of '*bad faith*'. For Sartre, morality centred on the freedom of choice (*per se*), rather than on what, ultimately, was chosen or why. He recognised that all genuine actions ('authenticity') involved a struggle, which he called 'anguish' and which Kierkegaard had originally called *angst* (anxiety). Common existentialist propositions include the ideas that: people are at their best when *struggling* with their individual natures, fighting for life; all real decisions are *difficult* and may incur serious (perhaps unpleasant) consequences; personal *responsibility* and *self-discipline* are vital; all worldly desire is, ultimately, futile; and society and its various rules, limits and authorities, are irrelevant.

Existentialism enjoyed great popularity in the 1950s and 1960s, when the nature of the stark, anguished choices that had faced all those who fought against fascism, often at great cost to themselves, became clearer with the benefit of hindsight. However, the fundamentals of existentialist thought – personal responsibility, and the rejection of rules, systems, authority and especially 'gurus' – may prove troublesome for today's materialist culture, where human problems are frequently attributed to the influence of genetic, biological, social or political factors,[32] and people are encouraged to believe that they have 'rights' or 'entitlements' that others have an obligation to honour.[33]

Post-modernity and uncertainty

Post-war philosophy largely shifted its focus from the problem of knowledge to a concern with meaning. The original concern with 'human nature' found in ethical theories down the centuries generated new difficulties when differing, often competing, claims were made by psychologists, sociologists and anthropologists regarding what it *meant* to be 'human'. Despite the fact that *Sigmund Freud's* (1856–1939) theories about the influence of the 'subconscious' are often dismissed as wholly unscientific, clearly these ideas changed radically our understanding of people as moral agents. Rather than 'choosing', as the existentialists argued, Freud argued that people were *driven*, often by primitive psychic forces, which they neither were aware of nor understood.

The mass slaughter of the 'Great War', followed by the horrors of the Holocaust, suggested that Hobbes might have been right, and fostered a more cynical outlook on human nature. The Holocaust is widely accepted as the cut-off point between the old certainties of the past and the 'post-modern' era.[34,35] Robertson and Walter pointedly noted that:

The atrocities of the Nazi era and the atomic bombings of Japan cast a shadow over the morality of societies who had proclaimed themselves 'civilized'. Such claims had been historically justified in the light of the intellectual movement of the Enlightenment, where reason had triumphed over superstition, liberty over tyranny. In the wake of Auschwitz and Hiroshima, many were left to question how civilizations could be capable of such inhumanity.[36]

Although the term 'post-modern' was first used in late nineteenth century art criticism, it is commonly attributed to *Jean-Francois Lyotard* (1924–98), who challenged the traditional faith in 'grand narratives' – universal philosophical theories, such as the progress of history, scientific knowledge or absolute freedom. In multicultural societies, where information is streamed through a growing number of forms of mass-media, appreciation of widely differing perspectives (micro-narratives) becomes possible. Much of this had, however, been anticipated by *Marshall McLuhan* (1911–80) who had first predicted the creation of a 'global village'[37] which ultimately emerged through the Internet.

However, much 'post-modern' philosophy has been criticised for lacking clarity, being intentionally obscure[38] or in *Noam Chomsky's* (1928–) view: 'pretentious rhetoric that obscures fairly simple ideas through difficult writing'.[39,40] Those who think they can understand it find the key proposition of much post-modern philosophy – that there can be no overarching 'truths' – depressing or nihilistic. Or simply pointless – as the English philosopher *Bernard Williams* (1929–2003) noted: 'If you do not really believe in the existence of truth, what is the passion for truthfulness a passion for?'[41] He might also have observed that if there can be no truth then it would be impossible to lie, which might be very convenient, especially for those who, for whatever reason, wish to avoid taking responsibility for their actions.

Freud anticipated the 'post-modern' era – and the rise of fundamentalism – as a function of peoples' reliance on authority, whether religious or political. Edmundsun noted:

> One of the ways that some people attempt to resolve the crisis of authority is to believe in nothing at all – or to pretend to . . . this way of life, which sometimes goes under the name of postmodernism, denies the human hunger for belief entirely. As such, it starves the individual of what he desperately needs – authority in some form – and leaves him all the more open to being appropriated by this or that coercing system when the bad times come, as they will.[42]

Relativism and pragmatism

The central post-modern position that there are no overarching 'truths' – which so many have found depressing or nihilistic[13] – has often been compared to *relativism*:[14] what is called 'truth' is always relative to a particular frame of reference, such as a language or a culture. Relativism has been around at least since the ancient Greeks. *Protagoras* (490–420 BCE) claimed that: '*of all things the measure is Man, of the things that are, that they are, and of the things there are not, that they are not*'. However, even his contemporary Socrates noted the inherent paradox in such 'relativism': if no judgement could be 'objectively' true, then this would mean that relativism could not be 'true' either.[15]

In the modern era *Benedict de Spinoza* (1632–77) offered an illustration of relativism through his observation that music could be 'good' for someone who was melancholy, 'bad' (or evil) for someone who was mourning, and neither good nor bad to someone who was deaf.[16] However, relativism came to prominence in the twentieth century through Sartre's existentialist ethic: if the basis of any moral code lay in the individual's subjective moral core – 'following one's conscience' – then there could be as many moral codes as individuals to enact them.

Stated simply relativism seems obvious but not without serious implications. *Individuals* have different 'standards' regarding what they consider 'right and fitting' or 'evil and unacceptable' as do different *cultures* or *societies*; ranging from the minutiae of social etiquette to laws governing capital punishment. Anthropology also showed how most of the moral conventions discussed here so far applied only to European societies (or those, like the USA, which had developed from the 'Old World' model). Other, non-European (regrettably, often called 'primitive') societies had their own, very different, conventions and, by implication, morality. There could, therefore, be no overarching moral imperatives: it depended on the society or culture to which one belonged, or inhabited. In a similar, relativistic, vein *St Ambrose* was reputed to have said: '*When in Rome do as the Romans*'.

As people grew less reliant on the moral guidance offered by religion, Sartre's existentialism provided people with a rationale for individualism, albeit with its accompanying moral responsibilities. None of this was new. The revolt against the authority of the Catholic Church instigated by *Erasmus* and *Luther* in the sixteenth century employed Renaissance humanism to assert that religion should involve 'inward devotion' rather than the mere practice of rituals and ceremonies prescribed by authority figures. Individualism, wherever it was practised, for whatever reason, held the potential to disrupt convention and undermine authority. It is hardly surprising, therefore, that the Catholic Church continues to view relativism as morally threatening.[47]

At the end of the nineteenth century *Charles S. Peirce* (1839–1914) created the movement now known as *pragmatism*, the first and only school of philosophy to have developed in the USA[48] and significant contributions were made later by *William James* (1842–1910) and *John Dewey* (1859–1952). Pragmatism focused on the idea that all knowledge must be tested by its usefulness and rejected any form of absolutism and universality of thought. Within ethics pragmatism rejected the idea that there can be any universal ethical principle or universal value. Ethical principles could be no more than social constructs which have been found to be useful.

Pragmatism rejected most of the accepted views of traditional philosophy and, for that reason, often is bracketed with post-modernism. *Richard Rorty* (1931–2004) was the most eloquent advocate of pragmatism in the late twentieth century, defining it as the view that 'true' beliefs are those that work towards successful interaction with the world: those beliefs which help in the achievement of a culture's aims are those which can be justified. Rorty dismissed the whole truth-seeking history of philosophy. In a fairly straightforward illustration of his own pragmatic views he wrote:

> The trouble with aiming at truth is that you would not know when you had reached it, even if you had in fact reached it. But you *can* aim at ever more justification, the assuagement of ever more doubt. Analogously, you cannot aim at 'doing what is right', because you will never know whether you have hit the mark. Long after you are dead, better-informed and more sophisticated people may judge your action to have been a tragic mistake. . . . But you *can* aim at ever more sensitivity to pain, and ever greater satisfaction of ever more various needs.[49]

It has often been noted that the Italian fascist leader Mussolini attributed his moral philosophy to the influence of pragmatism,[50] with the implication that any individual or group might claim a pragmatic basis for even the vilest of 'cultural' practices.

A return to virtue ethics

The apparent lack of ethical boundaries in much twentieth century thought led many philosophers to call for ethics to refocus attention on an ethics which is 'agent-centred', concerned with moral character – 'what kind of *person* should I be?' – rather than 'act-centred' and concerned with the question 'what should I *do*? *Alasdair MacIntyre* (1929–) is one of the most well-known advocates of 'virtue ethics'. For MacIntyre, being a 'good' person is not about following rules but involves cultivating *habits* that assist in demonstrating good judgement – a contemporary reworking of Aristotelian ethics. MacIntyre accepts that there can be no return to the past, but he remains nostalgic for the Aristotelian 'virtues' model as the basis of communitarian values, which serves also as an important means of critiquing the individualistic focus of liberal modernity. In MacIntyre's view morality has become nothing more than the expression of individual whims. While moral language may still be used, it is not used to express moral claims as such but merely to promote particular preferences.[51] Indeed, MacIntyre anticipated the pernicious, socially destructive influence of political leaders, such as Margaret Thatcher, when he wrote:

> What matters at this stage is the construction of local forms of community within which civility and the intellectual and moral life can be sustained through the new dark ages which are already upon us. And if the tradition of the virtues was able to survive the horrors of the last dark ages, we are not entirely without grounds for hope. This time however the barbarians are not waiting beyond the frontiers; they have already been governing us for quite some time.[52]

MacIntyre acknowledged, however, that virtues were not timeless. Different ages and different kinds of society can generate a need for different virtues. However, other virtue ethicists have argued that most of the 'traditional' virtues – for example, courage, charity, temperance, fidelity, truthfulness, care and justice – retain their value and contribute not only to the survival of the group and community, but also hold direct benefits for the individual.[53]

Ethical theory

The history of ethics sketched out here is necessarily crude and selective. However, it suggests something of the range of conflicts, which have divided ethicists over the centuries. It may also suggest something of the extent to which philosophers agree on the key issues, even if they disagree about how these need to be addressed.

The contemporary field of ethics is commonly broken down into three areas of interest: *meta-ethics, normative ethics* and *applied ethics*.

Meta-ethics

The least clearly defined area of ethical theory, *meta-ethics* is concerned with the study of the meaning of moral language and the metaphysics of moral facts. *Meta-ethics* adopts a bird's-eye view of the whole ethical field. Are moral judgements 'objective' – belonging to some metaphysical or spiritual realm – or 'subjective' – created by humankind? Are the moral principles already described 'absolute' – fixed or universal – or more 'relative' in nature – determined by individuals or different cultures and traditions?

Another key focus in *meta-ethics* is the potentially psychological nature of ethical decision-making. What motivates people to be moral? What kind of psychological factors are involved, if any? Do people act primarily out of selfishness and a concern for their own welfare (*egoism*), or is moral behaviour fuelled by a concern for others (*altruism*)? Moreover, do people think carefully about their options and *then* make a *rational* decision? Or are their actions driven more by emotion: doing what 'feels' best for them, at that moment?

The reason-versus-emotion debate, highlighted by *David Hume* in the eighteenth century, fostered a critical consideration of the role of gender in ethical decision-making in the twentieth century. Does morality differ for men and women? All the philosophers cited in the preceding pages were men, very much in keeping with the history of philosophy itself. However, feminist philosophers drew attention to the very different ways that women and men make decisions in everyday life.[51] Women tend to be more spontaneous, making judgements based on an assessment of the prevailing circumstances,[55,56] whereas men tend to be more duty bound, largely unaffected by circumstances.

Normative ethics

The development of 'moral standards', which seek to regulate 'right' and 'wrong' behaviours, is the province of *normative ethics*, which aims to provide a general answer to the age-old question: 'how should I live?' or 'how ought I to act, morally speaking?' The key assumption in *normative ethics* is that there is only *one* ultimate criterion of moral conduct, whether a single *rule* or a set of *principles*. Three key areas of theories are commonly addressed: *virtue* theories, which were outlined earlier in the conclusion to the brief history of ethics; *duty* theories; and *consequentialist* theories. Before discussing these briefly I offer a summary of the 'Golden Rule', arguably the oldest example of a normative principle.

The Golden Rule: With examples to be found in ancient Egypt and Greece, as well as within the sacred texts of every major religion, the *Golden Rule* – '*do as you would be done by*'[57] – is the oldest example of a normative principle. Although its popularity in the Western world is unashamedly Christian, traceable to the Biblical invitation to 'love thy neighbour as thyself', humanists also recognise the value of practising the 'ethic of reciprocity'.

Countless everyday examples of the golden rule might be offered. I would not want someone to abuse me, steal my possessions, abandon me in my hour of need or allow me to starve. For the same reason I would not wish to see such actions visited upon others. However, as Bernard Shaw wittily observed, given that tastes vary so greatly between people, 'the golden rule is that there are no golden rules'. *Karl Popper* (1902–94) suggested that there was no need for such cynicism:

> Although we have no criterion of absolute rightness, we . . . can make progress in this realm. As in the realm of facts, we can make discoveries. That cruelty is always 'bad,' that it should always be avoided where possible: that the golden rule is a good standard which can perhaps even be improved, by *doing unto others, wherever possible, as they would want to be done by*; these are elementary and extremely important examples of discoveries in the realm of standards.[58]

The golden rule offers a *single principle* against which we might judge all actions. Popper argued that the use of a 'negative' version of the golden rule might even be more meaningful in everyday life: 'do NOT do unto others that which you would *not* want them to do unto you'.

What might be the ethical point of such a 'rule'? For Popper, it certainly did not mean that people's problems might be resolved, once and for all. He echoed the key principle of existentialism, noting that:

> (Once) men believed God to rule the world. This belief limited their responsibility. The new belief that they had to rule it themselves created for many a well nigh intolerable burden of responsibility.[59]

Whether they like it or not men and women are responsible for 'engineering' (in Popper's terms) the world they inhabit. The key question is: 'how will they acquit themselves of this responsibility?' With this in mind Popper wrote:

> It is our duty to help those who need our help, but it cannot be our duty to make others happy, since this does not depend on us, and it would mean all too often intruding on [their] privacy.[60]

Clearly, the golden rule does not provide 'answers' for every situation. Indeed, numerous critics of the golden rule have observed that, for example, a masochist who enjoys pain would inflict this on others, or a judge who cherishes liberty would set every prisoner free. However, the obvious criticism that we might not *know* what someone would want can be countered simply by *asking* them. Where this is not possible, for whatever reason, the golden rule invites us to be empathic if not also compassionate, providing a link with *virtue theory*.

Duty theories: Often described as deontological,[61] *duty theories* assert that all moral behaviour is based on some fundamental duty or obligation. It is our duty not to harm other people and we have an obligation to look after our children. These duties and obligations apply whether or not it is to our benefit.

The earliest examples[62] distinguished between *absolute* and *conditional* duties. Our duties (or obligations) to avoid harming others, treating them as equals and trying to promote their welfare, are all *absolute*. Alternatively, *conditional* duties relate to contractual agreements *between* people, such as 'keeping a promise'.

These ideas were developed into the principle of *rights* by *John Locke* (1632–1704) who argued that '*no one ought to harm another in his life, health, liberty or possessions*'. In 1776 *Thomas Jefferson* (1743–1826) reframed Locke's principle in drafting the American *Declaration of Independence*:

> We hold these truths to be self-evident, that all men are created equal, that they are endowed by their Creator with certain unalienable Rights, that among these are Life, Liberty and the pursuit of Happiness.[63]

These rights were *natural*, in the sense that they were not made or provided by governments; *universal*, in applying to people anywhere in the world; *equal*, in applying to everyone irrespective of gender, race, creed or ability; and most of all *inalienable* – they cannot be given over to someone else. In the American context the inalienable nature of such rights meant that slavery, considered by Aristotle to be a natural thing, could no longer be countenanced.[64]

Immanuel Kant is the most well-known deontologist, and refined earlier ideas about one's duty to oneself – such as making full use of one's talents; and duty to others – such as keeping promises. Kant believed in a single, overarching principle – the *categorical imperative* described earlier – which governs moral action, irrespective of our personal feelings. Although Kant described different versions of this *imperative* the requirement to treat people as an end in themselves, not as a means to some end, is most relevant to the field of health and social care. Kant anticipated the contemporary concern for 'dignity' when he defined this as an 'inner value'.

Kant developed the older distinction between duties and obligations by defining *perfect* and *imperfect* duties. The former are negative and absolute – we should not *murder* or *lie*; whereas the latter are positive and do not tell us to what *extent* we should fulfil them – we should treat people kindly and with respect *as far as possible*.

The Scots philosopher *William David Ross* (1877–1971) proposed seven duties that 'are part of the fundamental nature of the universe'.[65]

- *Beneficence*: help other people (increase pleasure, improve character).
- *Non-maleficence*: avoid harming other people.
- *Justice*: ensure people get what they deserve.
- *Self-improvement*: improve oneself.
- *Reparation*: recompense someone if you have acted wrongly towards them.
- *Gratitude*: benefit those people who have benefited us.
- *Promise-keeping*: keep both explicit and implicit promises, including the promise to tell the truth.

Ross acknowledged that these were *prima facie* duties, meaning that each principle is binding *unless* it conflicts with another moral principle. Where such a conflict arises we have to make a choice. The principles offer no guidance as to what course of action we should take in balancing the potential effects of one action against another.

Consequentialist theories: Whereas *duty* (or *deontological*) theories view 'rightness' or 'wrongness' as existing within the character of an action, *consequentialist* (or *utilitarian*) theories hold that the outcomes (consequences) of an action form the basis of any moral judgement, as represented by the common aphorism: '*the ends justify the means*'. Three different forms of consequentialism have been described, each with different implications.

1   *Ethical egoism* states that any action is morally right if its consequences are more favourable than unfavourable *only to the person* performing it.

For example, I tell a person (patient) and his family that a drug I know to have potentially harmful side effects is 'completely safe'. The person accepts the drug and both patient and family express their gratitude for my help, but in the fullness of time the person suffers damaging 'side effects'.

2   *Ethical altruism* states that any action is morally right if its consequences are more favourable than unfavourable *to everyone except the person performing the action*.

Alternatively, I tell a person and his family that a drug has the potential to be damaging if taken for any length of time. The family discusses my comments, and the person feels relieved and decides not to take the drug. However, I am criticised by my colleagues for undermining the team.

3   *Utilitarianism* states that any action is morally right *only* if the consequences of that action are more favourable than unfavourable *for all concerned*.

I am aware that the standard of care being offered by a nurse is putting certain patients at risk. I discuss this several times with the nurse to no effect. Finally, I report the matter to the team leader who takes the necessary action and the nurse duly improves her performance. I am praised by the team leader who notes that had I ignored this, both the team's reputation and the patients' health might have been damaged.

Each of these examples is extremely complicated, albeit for different reasons. If there is *absolutely* no concern for the possible negative effect of one's action on others, then *ethical egoism* becomes no more than a potentially dangerous form of 'self-interest'.[66] Alternatively, if our actions are determined always by their potential benefits to others, then we risk sacrificing ourselves, and *ethical altruism* risks becoming an ethic only for the 'sainted'. Finally, weighing up the possible 'costs' and 'benefits' of any action is rarely easy and, in the utilitarian example above, it is difficult to imagine how everyone might benefit. At the very least, the feelings of the nurse, whose conduct was considered to be deficient, will be injured, however temporarily. Perhaps for all of these reasons, *Gertrude Anscombe* (1919–2001), who is credited with coining the term 'consequentialism', observed that 'it is a necessary feature of *consequentialism* that it is a shallow philosophy'.

Utilitarianism is the most well-known and accepted form of *consequentialism*, developed originally by *Jeremy Bentham* and *John Stuart Mill*, in the eighteenth and nineteenth centuries, as described earlier in the historical overview. The 'utility' in *utilitarianism* is often equated with 'usefulness' and begs the question, 'Useful for what?' Most of the subsequent developments of utilitarianism, up to the present day, have focused on attempting to answer that question.

Bentham's original answer was to emphasise the usefulness of this theory in 'promoting pleasure and avoiding pain'. Although Bentham's ethic was originally defined as 'hedonic' (or hedonistic) utilitarianism, today the 'preference utilitarian' interprets the 'best consequences' in terms of 'preference satisfaction'. This means that 'good' is described as the satisfaction of each person's individual *preferences* or *desires*. The original question regarding 'usefulness' might be rephrased as: 'What *good* will come of this (action)?' However, since what is good depends solely on individual preferences, there can be nothing that is 'good' or 'bad' *per se*. Therefore, *preference utilitarianism* acknowledges that each person's experience of satisfaction will be unique.

There have been numerous criticisms of utilitarianism: appearing to make difficult choices seem easy; failing to acknowledge how special circumstances might influence a decision (especially where family or friends are involved); and holding a circular definition of what constitutes 'happiness' or 'the good'. However, such criticisms may fail to take account of the continued development and complexity of utilitarianism, especially within the field of 'practical ethics'.[67,68]

Moral principles and health care

As has already been noted, most of the everyday moral judgements involve an appeal to 'fairness' for all concerned or the 'welfare' of particular individuals. However, unwittingly, such appeals acknowledge many of the classic ethical principles discussed. The most popular distillation of such principles, developed specifically for the medical arena, was offered by Beauchamp and Childress,[69] who identified the need to respect *autonomy*, and to practice *non-maleficence, beneficence* and *justice*. As noted in the discussion of duty ethics above, Beauchamp and Childress's work popularised the philosophy of *WD Ross*[70] from the late 1920s.

- *Autonomy* derives from the Greek for 'self' and 'rule'. In health care this is taken to refer to the person's capacity for making independent decisions without being too overtly controlled or influenced by others.
- *Non-maleficence* derives from the Latin *primum non nocere*: 'first do no harm'. [Although commonly ascribed to Hippocrates, Herranz noted that this expression was first coined by the Parisian pathologist, *Auguste François Chomel* (1788–1858).[71]]
- *Beneficence* addresses the obligation to help others promote their legitimate interests and, more specifically, to advance their welfare.
- Finally, the principle of *justice* addresses the need to ensure that all such care and treatment is made available to all.

Beauchamp and Childress augmented these principles with four *rules*:

- *Veracity*: be truthful and honest at all times.
- *Privacy*: respect the person's right to keep secret details of his/her life circumstances, past and present.
- *Confidentiality*: ensure that all recorded details of the person's life and circumstances are managed to ensure confidentiality.
- *Fidelity*: strive to maintain the duty of care to the individual patient, however difficult the circumstances.

Like Ross's principles, all of Beauchamp and Childress's four principles also are *prima facie*. This approach offers no guidance for making such a choice, which often can be a source of dissatisfaction to those who hope that ethics might provide them with ordered rules or an easy answer to some dilemma.[72]

Some physicians consider that the 'Hippocratic ideals' on which Beauchamp and Childress's principles are based, no longer apply in medicine overall.[73] As most of the subsequent chapters in this book will illustrate, any attempt to pursue these principles and their accompanying rules in psychiatric (or 'mental health') practice generates the potential for considerable conflict. The traditional common sense notion that 'mad' people are bereft of reason, and therefore lack the capacity to make free and rational choices, remains at the heart of both psychiatric diagnosis (see Chapter 11) and contemporary mental health legislation (see Chapters 23–25). The implications for respecting *autonomy* need hardly be laboured further here. Similarly, much of the traditional focus of care and treatment focuses on safeguarding the public from 'mentally ill' persons, or protecting the 'patient' from him/herself, with the result that care and treatment is often coercive in nature. This carries considerable implications for the practice of *beneficence* and *non-maleficence*. Finally, the combined effect of the violation of the first three ethical principles begs major questions regarding the 'fairness' (*justice*) of psychiatric services: whose needs are being met – the person (patient), the family, the psychiatric/mental health professionals or the general public?

Applied ethics

Whereas meta-ethics and normative ethics are, unashamedly, theoretical in character, *applied ethics* – as the name implies – is concerned with the application of ethical reasoning to specific issues or areas of practical concern, addressing real-life situations. This relatively new discipline, which emerged in the 1970s, has many specialised fields, such as *bioethics, business ethics, sexual ethics* and *environmental ethics*. The alternative title – *practical ethics* – was popularised by *Peter Singer* (1946–) and includes consideration of areas as diverse as: the treatment of ethnic minorities, equality for women, the use of animals for food and research, the preservation of the natural environment, abortion, euthanasia and the obligation of the wealthy to help the poor.[74]

Meta-ethics dominated moral philosophy for the first half of the twentieth century, at least in the English-speaking world. However, the abstract focuses on the *language* of morality meant that ethics became ever more distant and technical, and actual moral problems were not addressed. This state of affairs was all the more surprising given that the period was marked, as Haldane noted, by: ' . . . two world wars, the rise of ideological totalitarianism, widespread attempts at genocide, and the development and use of weapons of mass destruction'.[75]

However, by the mid-1960s, especially in the USA, questions concerning civil rights, sexual ethics and the morality of warfare became prominent themes in public debates: 'What became clear, and was felt to be something of a scandal was that professional moral philosophy appeared to have nothing to say about these important moral issues'.[76]

As Beauchamp later noted, despite its recent origins, the topics that form the subject matter of applied (or practical) ethics have a perennial quality:

> Although moral philosophers have long discussed these problems, it is arguably the case that no major philosopher throughout the history of moral philosophy has developed a program or method of applied ethics . . . it is not obvious that applied ethics is the offspring of, or even dependent upon, general moral philosophy. Its early success in the 1970s owed more to arguments directed at pressing and emerging moral problems in society than to traditional theories of ethics. . . . The issues raised by civil rights, women's rights, animal rights, the consumer movement, the environmental movement and the rights of prisoners and the mentally ill often included ethical issues that stimulated the imagination of philosophers and non-philosophers alike.[77]

Despite Beauchamp's reference to 'the mentally ill' most of the major texts on applied ethics make no reference to 'mental health' or the traditional role of coercion in psychiatric practice.[78-81] This suggests that 'mental health problems' are either not conceived of as a social issue[82] or are viewed as less urgent than debates concerning the rights of people with disabilities[83] or immigration and pornography.[84] Or it might only indicate that philosophers have, so far, shown only a limited interest in this aspect of human experience.

Ethics and mental health

The moral status of medicine has been challenged on several fronts in recent times, perhaps most trenchantly by the Austrian philosopher *Ivan Illich* (1926–2002), who popularised the notion of *iatrogenic disease*[85] and criticised the medicalisation of many of the everyday problems of life, by Western medicine, especially in the areas of birth and death.[86] In a similar vein, Kennedy's classic text, *Unmasking Medicine*,[87] highlighted the spurious nature of the definition of disease, which underpinned most medical practice. This was especially evident in psychiatry, where Kennedy saw any diagnosis of 'mental illness' as bringing in its wake considerable social and political implications. Kennedy – a professor of law – echoed Illich's original critique by acknowledging that, despite its beneficent aims, and doctors' supporting claims to altruism, medicine could be, and often was, harmful.[88]

Over 30 years ago *Thomas S. Szasz* (1920–), the foremost philosopher of psychiatry,[89] re-affirmed the view that medicine was, fundamentally, a *moral undertaking*.[90] Only recently has it been accepted that this applies also to psychiatric medicine (and its latter day manifestation, 'mental health')[91] and extends also to areas such as counselling and psychotherapy.[92] It is over 200 years since psychiatry formed its uneasy alliance with medicine[93] and only recently has it acknowledged the social agenda inherent in the delivery of any 'mental health' service. However much medical and social concepts and procedures might be represented in its practice, mental health services continue to focus on age-old moral questions.[94]

> Although psychiatrists are unlikely to give direct advice about the right course of action, they will form an opinion of what is right and this will influence what they say and what questions they ask next; the patient will know if their doctor approves or not.
>
> '*How then should we live?*' is one of the fundamental questions, which we all have to consider and form our own values. Being aware of our values will help to prevent conflict with service users who may hold different values and assumptions about the world.[95]

However, psychiatry's inherent moral nature has long been apparent to historians. Indeed, despite its efforts to reinvent itself, through the regular arrival of new 'movements' and the promise of new 'therapeutic discoveries', psychiatry has long been viewed as morally suspect, if not downright criminal. The medical historian *Roy Porter* (1946–2002) wryly observed: 'psychiatry has been less than wholly successful in making sense of madness. This is no crime'. However, he added:

> What may have historically been a crime is the alacrity with which certain individual psychiatrists and in some ways the profession as a whole, backed by society's mandate, has taken upon itself the role of sorting out the mad, through the assertion that it possesses the answers. Have not the true fantasists been those psychiatrists who have claimed to hold the master-key to madness? In truth, such theories and therapies have all too often only proved a philosophical warhorse useful for riding roughshod over resistance and protests. The pontifications of psychiatry have all too often excommunicated the mad from human psychiatry, even when their own cries and complaints have been human, all too human.[96]

The novelist, Raymond Chandler, may have spoken for the silent majority when he said:

> I regard psychiatry as fifty percent bunk, thirty percent fraud, ten percent parrot talk, and the remaining ten percent just a fancy lingo for the common sense we have had for hundreds and perhaps thousands of years, if we ever had the guts to read it.[97]

Psychiatry's principal ethical failing has been, and perhaps continues to be, the widespread unwillingness to question its many ludicrous 'theories' and the heinous practices they so often supported.[98] Almost 20 years after Porter's despairing comments, The American journalist, Robert Whitaker echoed his sentiments:

> Stop telling those diagnosed with schizophrenia that they suffer from too much dopamine or serotonin activity and that the drugs put these brain chemicals back into

'balance'. That whole spiel is a form of medical fraud, and it is impossible to imagine any other group of patients – ill, say, with cancer or cardiovascular disease – being deceived in this way. . . . Hubris is everywhere, and in mad medicine, that has always been a prescription for disaster. In fact, if the past is any guide to the future, today we can be certain of only one thing. The day will come when people will look back at our current medicines for schizophrenia and the stories we tell to patients about their abnormal brain chemistry, and they will shake their heads in utter disbelief.[99]

In recent years some psychiatrists have come to acknowledge the moral and ethical problems resulting from the powers invested in, or assumed by, institutional psychiatry[100–102] and their observations have been echoed and developed by others, less constrained by the medical culture.[103–105]

The following chapters in this book seek to address a wide range of ethical and moral concerns, which in some way are related to, or affect practitioners; or are in some way relevant to the delivery of contemporary 'mental health' services. As these chapters will illustrate, there remains much to 'anguish' about. These chapters explore further the meaning of many of the traditional critiques of psychiatry, in the contemporary world of mental health. In doing so, the authors' ambition is to illustrate how the psychiatric and mental health field – as practised by a wide range of discipline, not only by psychiatrists – represents a special domain within 'applied ethics', which deserves a larger critical audience.

However, as Haldane has commented, such ambition is not without many, potential pitfalls.

> Although it is often supposed otherwise, even by those who should know better, moral philosophy is no easier to practise than any other area of the subject. . . . the suggestion of the Sophists and of some more contemporary applied ethicists – that there are skills the more or less mechanical employment of which will yield answers to moral questions – is both a disservice to philosophy and a corrupting influence on the consciences of those whom it claims to be assisting . . . there is a danger that when sophistry is exposed, people's reaction is not to seek better counsel but to conclude that there can be no sound reasoning about questions of value and conduct, supposing instead that these are just matters of personal preference.[106]

Perhaps, however, mental health ethics is far too important to be left to the professional philosopher, who to date has remained aloof if not entirely disinterested. Perhaps the ethical dilemmas involved can only be examined through the distorting lens of direct experience – whether by those involved in delivering a psychiatric or mental health 'service', or by those on the receiving end. As my late colleague *Steve Baldwin* (1962–2001)[107] and I wrote almost 20 years ago:

> Ethics are an everyday concept. Ethics are not, or should not, be some form of navel-gazing, or observation of the care setting from a remote vantage point. Raising questions about 'ethical issues' can, too often, be interpreted negatively as 'trouble-making'. In many situations the 'trouble' already exists, in the form of inadequate or inappropriate service. The emphasis of traditional ethical debates upon 'major' issues, such as abortion, euthanasia and sterilization, may have misled many workers into thinking that ethics are not the stuff of everyday life. For mental health workers ethics should underpin each and every action: no issue, however small, should be considered 'beneath' the ethical debate.[108]

Of course, as I suggested at the beginning of this chapter, it would be folly to believe that we would ever arrive at a 'new' understanding of these many, differing ethical challenges. As my colleague Ben Davidson and I noted:

> although we often think of our moral values as belonging distinctly to us, they are usually a distillation or complex product of the interaction of many age-old philosophies. As Hampshire[109] noted:

> It would be contrary to the evidence of history to think of conceptions of the good as developing in isolation, uninfluenced by rival conceptions. Moral ideas cross and re-cross imagined moral frontiers, sometimes finally obliterating them' . . . we are seeking to clarify our view of some constant of the human condition; a constant feature of human experience which might serve as the essential benchmark for all our ethical strife.[110]

Conclusion

Ethics deals with human nature, in particular the kind of conduct that represents the 'living of a good life'. Although ethics varies from one society or culture to the next there exists more common ground than differences. The academic study of ethics – as opposed to its everyday practice – has resulted in many, often significant, shifts in ethical thinking. However, with each review or challenge of the ethical orthodoxy, very similar ethical arguments re-emerge, suggesting that some 'constants' exist in the search for the ultimate definition of the 'good life'.

Despite repeated attempts to put ethics on a scientific footing, ethics does not, indeed cannot, represent *facts* – at least not in the accepted scientific sense. Ethics represents viewpoints or perspectives on the human condition. In effect, these are no more, or less, than *opinions*: not just those of esteemed philosophers, but of everyone who cares to consider the question, 'how should I live?'.

In that sense, ethics is simple and straightforward. However, when begged in the context of our everyday lives, and especially our relationships with others, any answer risks being neutered by a catalogue of 'ifs', 'buts' and 'maybes'. What is clear is that we cannot avoid asking such questions. Indifference may be tempting, if not seductive, but we know that this risks leading, eventually, to all manner of human horrors. To be ethical is to be human. If we shirk the challenge of ethics we risk sacrificing our right to be called human.

Notes

1 Wiesel E. *The Perils of Indifference*. White House Millennium Lecture, Washington, DC. Retrieved April 12, 1999, http://www.historyplace.com/speeches/wiesel.htm
2 Many ethics committees continue to hold a specific place for a minister of religion, and the field of bioethics, which first emerged in the early 1970s, was originally highly influenced by Christian ideas. See: Pellegrino ED. The origins of bioethics: Some personal reflections. *Kennedy Institute of Ethics Journal* 1999, *9 (1)* 73–88.
3 Thomson JAK. (Trans) *The Ethics of Aristotle*. Harmondsworth: Penguin Books, 1976.
4 Ferry L. *What is the Good Life?* Chicago, IL: University of Chicago Press, 2005.
5 Jean Baptise Alphonse Karry's famous epigram – '*plus ca change, plus c'est la meme chose*' (the more it changes the more it's the same thing) is commonly interpreted as 'the more things change, the more they remain the same'. This could be said of ethics, which has been the subject of many

changes of theoretical emphasis, but still appears to wrestle with the same topics. Chapter 2 discusses how, in the same way, psychiatry has revised its theories and philosophies down the years, but its key purpose has remained much the same.

6 Fernandez-Armesto F. *Truth: A History and a Guide for the Perplexed*. London: Black Swan, 1998, p. 223.

7 The 'history' offered here is necessarily crude and selective and is, unashamedly, Western, in origin. For a more considered discussion, see: MacIntyre A. *A Short History of Ethics: A History of Moral Philosophy from the Homeric Age to the Twentieth Century*. London: Routledge, 2002.

8 Whitehead AN. *Process and Reality*. New York, NY: The Free Press, 1979, p. 39.

9 Flew A. *An Introduction to Western Philosophy*. Indianapolis, IN: The Bobbs-Merrill Company, 1971, p. 41.

10 Kofman S. *Socrates: Fictions of a Philosopher*. Ithaca, NY: Cornell University Press, 1998.

11 From the Greek *telos* meaning 'end' or 'purpose'.

12 In keeping with traditional philosophical usage the term 'man' refers to humankind of both sexes.

13 Brickhouse TC. *Socrates on Trial*. Princeton, NJ: Princeton University Press, 1989.

14 Purshouse L. *Plato's Republic*. London: Continuum, 2007.

15 Aristotle. *Nicomachean Ethics* (2nd Edn) [Trans. T Irwin]. Indianapolis, IN: Hackett Publishing Co., 1985.

16 These were either edited by or dedicated to his son Nicomachus.

17 Grayling AC. *Ideas that Matter: A Personal Guide for the 21st Century*. London: Weidenfeld and Nicolson, 2009, p. 128.

18 MacIntyre A. *After Virtue: A Study in Moral Theory*. Notre Dame, IN: University of Notre Dame Press, 1984.

19 This idea retains its popularity in the contemporary political arena. See: Keegan W. *The Prudence of Mr Gordon Brown*. Chichester, West Sussex: John Wiley and Sons, 2003.

20 It took its name from the *Stoa poikile*, the painted hall in which their lectures were first given.

21 The original read: 'God give us grace, to accept with serenity the things that cannot be changed, courage to change the things that should be changed, and the wisdom to distinguish the one from the other'.

22 Machiavelli N. [Trans. G Bull] *The Prince*. London: Penguin Books, 2004.

23 Pettit P. *Republicanism: A Theory of Freedom and Government*. New York, NY: Oxford University Press, 1997.

24 Ellingson T. *The Myth of the Noble Savage*. Berkeley, CA: University of California Press, 2001.

25 Mill JS. *On Liberty* (1859) [Edited by Gertrude Himmelfarb]. London: Penguin Classics, 1985, p. 63.

26 Mill ibid. p. 69.

27 Kant I. *An Answer to the Question: What is Enlightenment?* London: Penguin Books, 2009, p. 1.

28 Millican P. (ed.). *Reading Hume on Human Understanding: Essays on the First Enquiry*. Oxford: Oxford University Press, 2002.

29 Solomon RC. (ed.). *Existentialism* (2nd Edn). New York, NY: Oxford University Press, 2004.

30 McBride WL. (ed.). *Existentialist Literature and Aesthetics*. New York, NY: Garland Publishing, 1997.

31 Faye E. *Heidegger: The Introduction of Nazism into Philosophy*. New Haven, CT: Yale University Press, 2009.

32 Nearly half of Canadians say that mental illness used as an excuse. Ottawa Citizen, August 18, 2008, http://www.canada.com/ottawacitizen/news/story.html?id=83527be3-ce9b-4534-92a0-2e508149bf7c

33 Fradella HF. *Mental Illness and Criminal Defenses of Excuse in Contemporary American Law*. Palo Alto, CA: Academica Press, 2007.

34 Mantel N. Ethics after Auschwitz: The Holocaust in history and representation. *Criticism* 2003, *45 (4)* 509–18.

35 Ziarek EP. Evil and testimony: Ethics after postmodernism. *Hypatia* 2003, *18 (2)* 197–204.

36 Robertson M and Walter G. Overview of psychiatric ethics VI: Newer approaches to the field. *Australasian Psychiatry* 2007, *15 (5)* 411–16.

37 Horrocks C. *Marshall McLuhan and Virtuality* (Postmodern Encounters). Cambridge: Icon Books, 2000.

38 Michel Foucault infamously described Jacques Derrida's writing as 'terrorist obscurantism': 'He writes so obscurely you can't tell what he's saying, that's the obscurantism part, and then when you criticize him, he can always say, "You didn't understand me; you're an idiot." That's the terrorism part'. [Quoted by John Searle in Postrel SR and Feser E. Reality principles: An interview with John R Searle. *Reason* Feb. 2000.]

39 http://www.chomsky.info/articles/1995----02.htm

40 In an infamous hoax, the physicist Alan Sokal expressed his rage towards 'postmodern philosophy' by submitting a paper, 'liberally salted with nonsense', to the journal *Social Text*. The paper, which argued that quantum gravity was no more than 'a social and linguistic construct' was published following peer-review. See: Sokal AD and Bricmont J. *Fashionable Nonsense: Postmodern Intellectuals' Abuse of Science*. New York: Picador, 1998.

41 Williams B. *Truth and Truthfulness*. Princeton, NJ: Princeton University Press, 2002.

42 Edmundsun M. *The Death of Sigmund Freud: Fascism, Psychoanalysis and the Rise of Fundamentalism*. London: Bloomsbury, 2007, p. 242.

43 Stangroom J and Benson O. *Why Truth Matters*. London: Continuum, 2007.

44 Levy N. *Moral Relativism: A Short Introduction*. Oxford: Oneworld Publications, 2002.

45 Fearn N. *Philosophy: The Latest Answers to the Oldest Questions*. London: Atlantic Books, 2005, pp. 132–3.

46 Spinoza B. [Trans. E Curley] *Ethics*. London: Penguin Classics, 2004.

47 Cardinal Joseph Ratzinger (later Pope Benedict XVI) suggested that society was moving towards 'a dictatorship of relativism which does not recognise anything as certain and which has as its highest goal one's own ego and one's own desires'. http://www.vatican.va/gpII/documents/homily-pro-eligendo-pontifice_20050418_en.html

48 To distinguish himself from William James and John Dewey Pierce re-named his philosophy *pragmaticism*.

49 Rorty R. *Philosophy and Social Hope*. Harmondsworth: Penguin, 1992, p. 82.

50 "pragmatism." *Encyclopædia Britannica. 2009. Encyclopædia Britannica Online*. December 3, 2009, http://www.britannica.com/EBchecked/topic/473717/pragmatism.

51 Gary K. Alasdair Macintyre: The epitaph of modernity. *Philosophy and Social Criticism* 1997, *23 (1)* 71–98.

52 MacIntyre A. *After Virtue: A Study in Moral Theory*. Notre Dame, IN: University of Notre Dame Press, 1981, p. 263.

53 Hursthouse R. *On Virtue Ethics*. Oxford: Oxford University Press, 2002.

54 Gilligan C. *In a Different Voice: Psychological Theory and Women's Development*. Cambridge, MA: Harvard University Press, 1982.

55 Noddings N. *Caring: A Feminine Approach to Ethics and Moral Education*. Berkeley, CA: University of California Press, 1984.

56 Held V. *The Ethics of Care: Personal, Political, and Global*. Oxford: Oxford University Press, 2006.

57 For a comprehensive discussion see: Wattles J. *The Golden Rule*. Oxford, Oxford University Press, 1996.

58 Popper K. *Addendum to The Open Society* (1945/1966) Vol 2: 386 (added emphasis).

59 Popper ibid. p. 24.

60 Popper ibid. p. 237.

61 From the Greek *deon* meaning 'duty'.

62 See for example: Schneewind JB. Pufendorf's place in the history of ethics. *Synthese* 1987, *72 (1)* 123–55.

63 Armitage D. *The Declaration of Independence: A Global History*. Cambridge, MA: Harvard University Press, 2007.

64 Finkleman P. *Slavery and the Founders: Race and Liberty in the Age of Jefferson* (2nd Edn). Armonk, NY: ME Sharpe, 2001.

65 Ross WD. *The Right and the Good*. Oxford: Clarendon Press, 1930, pp. 26–7.
66 Baier, for example, argued that this would be an unnecessarily simplistic view of ethical egoism. See: Baier K. Egoism. In P Singer (ed.). *A Companion to Ethics*. Oxford: Blackwell, 2001.
67 Shaw W. *Contemporary Ethics: Taking Account of Utilitarianism*. Oxford: Blackwell, 1999.
68 Singer P. *Practical Ethics* (2nd Edn). Cambridge, MA: Cambridge University Press, 1993.
69 Beauchamp TL and Childress JF. *Principles of Biomedical Ethics* (5th Edn). New York, NY: Oxford University Press, 2001.
70 Ross op. cit.
71 Herranz G. *The origin of "Primum non nocere"* Retrieved September 1, 2002, http://www.bmj.com/cgi/eletters/324/7351/1463
72 Gillon R. Medical ethics: Four principles plus attention to scope. *British Medical Journal* 1994, *309* 184.
73 Loefler I. Why the Hippocratic ideals are dead. *British Medical Journal* 2002, *324* 1463.
74 Singer op. cit. p. 1.
75 Haldane J. *Applied Ethics*. In N Bunnin and EP Tsui-James (eds.). *The Blackwell Companion to Philosophy*. Oxford: Blackwell, 1996, p. 724.
76 Haldane J. *Applied Ethics*. In N Bunnin and EP Tsui-James (eds.). *The Blackwell Companion to Philosophy*. Oxford: Blackwell, 1996, p. 724.
77 Frey RG and Wellman CH. (eds.). *A Companion to Applied Ethics*. Oxford: Blackwell, 2005, pp. 1–2.
78 Singer op. cit.
79 Singer P. *Applied Ethics*. Oxford: Oxford University Press, 1986.
80 LaFollette H. *Oxford Handbook of Practical Ethics*. Oxford: Oxford University Press, 2005.
81 Oderberg DS. *Applied Ethics: A Non-consequentialist Approach*. Oxford: Blackwell, 2000.
82 Fitzpatrick T. *Applied Ethics and Social Problems: Moral Questions of Birth, Society and Death*. Bristol: Policy Press, 2008.
83 LaFollette op. cit.
84 Cohen AI and Wellman CH. *Contemporary Debates in Applied Ethics*. Oxford: Blackwell, 2005.
85 Any condition caused by medical intervention.
86 Illich I. *Medical Nemesis*. London: Calder & Boyars, 1974.
87 Kennedy I. *The Unmasking of Medicine*. London: Allen and Unwin, 1981.
88 Bowman D. The Canon: Unmasking Medicine by Ian Kennedy. *Times Higher Education* 12 December, 2009, p. 49.
89 Hoeller K. (ed.). *Thomas Szasz: Philosopher of Psychiatry*. The Review of Existential Psychology & Psychiatry (Special Issue) 1997, Vols 1, 2 and 3.
90 Szasz TS. 'The Moral Physician' Chapter 1 in *The Theology of Medicine: The Political-philosophical Foundations of Medical Ethics*. New York, NY: Harper and Row, 1977.
91 Pearce S and Pickard H. The moral content of psychiatric treatment. *British Journal of Psychiatry* 2009, *195* 281–2. Retrieved 10 November, 2009, http://bjp.rcpsych.org/cgi/eletters/195/4/281#25655
92 Miller RB. *Facing Human Suffering: Psychology and Psychotherapy as Moral Engagement*. Washington, DC: American Psychological Association, 2004.
93 The definition of psychiatry as a branch of medicine can be traced to the work of Jean-Etienne Dominique Esquirol. See: Mora G. On the bicentenary of the birth of Esquirol (1772–1840), the first complete psychiatrist. *The American Journal of Psychiatry* 1972, *129 (5)* 562–7.
94 Pojman LP. *How Should We Live? An Introduction to Ethics*. Florence, KY: Wadsworth Publishing, 2004.
95 Gray AJ and Cox J. Psychiatry as a moral science. *E-letter to British Journal of Psychiatry* 28 October, 2009. Retrieved 12 December, 2009, http://bjp.rcpsych.org/cgi/eletters/195/4/281#25655
96 Porter R. *A Social History of Madness: Stories of the Insane*. London: Weidenfield and Nicolson, 1987, p. 233.
97 Hiney T and McShane F. (eds.). *The Raymond Chandler Papers: Selected Letters and Non-fiction*. New York: Atlantic Monthly Press, 2000, p. 174.
98 Szasz TS. *Coercion as Cure: A Critical History of Psychiatry*. New Brunswick, NJ: Transaction Publishers, 2007.

 99 Whitaker R. *Mad in America: Bad Science, Bad Medicine, and the Enduring Mistreatment of the Mentally Ill.* Cambridge, MA: Perseus Publishers, 2002.

100 Robitscher J. *The Powers of Psychiatry.* Boston, MA: Houghton Mifflin, 1980.

101 Bracken P and Thomas P. *Postpsychiatry: Mental Health in a Postmodern World.* Oxford: Oxford University Press, 2005.

102 Double D. The limits of psychiatry. *British Medical Journal* 2002, *324* 900–4.

103 Johnstone L. *Users and Abusers of Psychiatry: A Look at Psychiatric Practice* (2nd Edn). London: Brunner-Routledge, 2000.

104 Vatz RE and Schaler JA. Psychiatry's valid but dishonest reconsiderations. *USA Today* 2008, *136(2754)* 58–61.

105 Bentall RP. *Reconstructing Schizophrenia.* London: Routledge, 1990.

106 Haldane op. cit. p. 726.

107 Pickering H. Professor Steve Baldwin: Obituary. *Journal of Substance Use* 2001, *6 (2)* 134–5.

108 Barker P and Baldwin S. *Ethical Issues in Mental Health.* London: Chapman and Hall, 1991, p. 196.

109 Hampshire S. *Innocence and Experience.* London: Penguin, 1989, p. 156.

110 Barker P and Davidson B. *Psychiatric Nursing: Ethical Strife.* London: Arnold, 1998, p. 355.

2 The keystone of psychiatric ethics

Phil Barker

Every person lives in a world of social encounters, involving him in either face-to-face or mediated contacts with other participants. In each of these contacts he tends to act out what is sometimes called a *line* – that is, a pattern of verbal and non-verbal acts by which he expresses his view of the situation and through this his evaluation of the participants, especially himself. Regardless of whether the person intends to take a line, he will find that he has done so in effect. The other participants will assume that he has more or less wilfully *taken a stand*.

(Erving Goffman[1])

The shadow of psychiatric history

Common sense ethics

For the layperson ethics may appear straightforward and the many theories outlined in Chapter 1 might seem only to complicate matters. Ethics is about moral behaviour: 'right' and 'wrong'; 'good' or 'evil'. Sometimes this is concerned with the greatest 'good' in life: what really matters.[2] At other times it is concerned more with moral *obligations*: what people *ought* to do in particular circumstances – our *duties*. One might well ask: 'what is so difficult about any of this?' Making difficult decisions is the stuff of everyday life.

All people have beliefs and values, whether or not they describe them as ethical. Even the 'immoral/amoral' person is attached to some kind of moral code, however negative and self-serving this might appear to others. There is no real escape from ethics. We acquire the rudiments of our personal code from our families or culture, which we develop further by reflecting on critical events in our everyday lives: more of the ordinary stuff of our extraordinary existence.

As the opening quote from Erving Goffman suggests, *all* human encounters provide instances of moral behaviour. Whether or not this is *intentional*, far less based on philosophical reflection, our every action is likely to be judged by someone as an example of our having 'taken a stand': acting out our personal moral code.

The layperson might also be forgiven for thinking that any ethical problems that arise in the psychiatric or mental health field are also quite straightforward.

- When people become mentally *ill* they need some kind of 'treatment'.
- When mentally ill people don't want to take treatment, they need to be given this, just the same, *for their own good*.
- Mental health professionals are *responsible* for looking after mentally ill people, because they are unable to look after themselves.

People with a psychiatric diagnosis, their families and friends, and many mental health professionals also share these views. What could possibly be difficult about any of this? However, in the spirit of Socrates, all assumptions need to be examined carefully, if not exploded as myth. Assumptions about the province of psychiatry should be no exception.

The idea that 'mental illness is just like any other illness'[3] became a popular slogan, but it is no more than that. It may be comforting to assume that 'schizophrenia' is just like diabetes or 'borderline personality disorder' is similar to high blood pressure; and that both might respond well to medical treatment, offered by a General Practitioner (GP) or a hospital out-patient clinic. However, this would be wishful thinking. The complex personal, interpersonal and social problems that are given a psychiatric diagnosis bear no comparison with diabetes or hypertension. Aside from the differences in how such diagnoses are formulated, which will be shown later, most 'mental illnesses' carry a lot of historical baggage.[4]

Lay people, including some 'mentally ill' people, continue to maintain negative stereotypes concerning 'mad' patients[5] and even 'mad' psychiatrists.[6,7] These stereotypes are central to psychiatry's troubled legacy. Over the past 300 years, psychiatry[8] created, nurtured and frequently revised ideas about madness that became the basis of the stigmatising stereotypes[9] of 'mental illness,' which still persist.[10] If people with 'schizophrenia' are feared, or people with 'borderline personality disorder' are considered untrustworthy, then this is due largely to psychiatric mythology. Ironically, various government-sponsored programmes have been established to undo the effects of psychiatric stereotypes:[11] for example, that 'mentally ill' people are dangerous or stupid; indulgent or libidinous; or that 'mental illness' is incurable and runs in families. All such ideas were, originally, examples of psychiatric wisdom. Vestiges of these ideas are embedded within psychiatric diagnosis and some genetic theories.

Neither should we forget that 'mental illness' remains the only form of illness that can be 'treated' by force; against the person's expressed wishes, however well these might be expressed.[12] This exception provides the mental health field with an urgent need to consider carefully its ethical rules of engagement.

How people *think* about 'mental illness' and the 'mentally ill' – whether they be laypersons or mental health professionals – is tied, inextricably, to psychiatric history, which generated the language, concepts and psychobabble, that we use to talk about 'madness'. Psychiatric history also left an emotional legacy, which has influenced how we *feel* about 'mental illness' and the people it appears to affect. Whether we are in agreement with, or wholly opposed to its principles and practices, everyone stands in the shadow of this psychiatric history.

However paradoxical it might seem to the bewildered layperson, the mental health field is bedevilled by a singular set of ethical dilemmas, which distinguish it from mainstream *health care*; and from every other form of support embraced by the notion of *social care*.

Ethics concerns *human nature*, in particular the various rules, principles and codes that govern, influence or otherwise are related to human conduct.[13] 'Health care ethics'[14] and 'bioethics'[15] explore, if not actually explain, the myriad problems common to the health care field. However, many of the key texts – including the most popular books dedicated to 'practical ethics'[16,17] – rarely carry any serious consideration of psychiatry, psychology and mental health services in general. This suggests that health care ethicists and bio-ethicists either do not consider the ethical problems generated by psychiatry sufficiently serious to merit consideration, or that such problems are somehow considered beyond their purview.

The psychiatric field embraces a view of human nature, which distinguishes it from every other area of health or social care. This may account, at least in part, for psychiatry's virtual pariah status within mainstream ethics. The psychiatric *raison d'etre* – that some persons are 'mentally ill' and *need* 'treatment' by mental health professionals – is the source of all the ethical dilemmas in this field, many of which will be examined in later chapters.

Free to choose?

Given that the sub-title of this book is '*The Human Context*', the following short stories about persons[18] may help us begin to explore the psychiatric *world view*.

> *Billy*[19] is a 21-year-old dancer who develops a malignant tumour in his lower leg. His surgeon advises amputation of the leg above the knee. Despite the urging of his family and friends, Billy refuses to give his consent, saying 'I'll take my chances'.
>
> *Derek* also is 21 years old and for several years has wanted to join the army. His mother says that he has 'lost his mind to schizophrenia' and has been taking anti-psychotic medication for 3 years. Today he decides that he would 'rather die than carry on taking these drugs'. Against his family's wishes, and medical advice, he joins a group that offers to help wean him off medication.

Two young men, from the same country, and similar class and social backgrounds, who went to the same school, exit their teens in the glow of their 'promising futures'. Within a short time their lives are blighted by different kinds of tragedy, the nature of which insidiously begins to distinguish these young men who once had much in common.

The distinguishing feature is a single idea, albeit with a long, complicated and contested history – '*madness*'. In the oversimplified 'black-and-white' world of binary opposites people are *either*: 'rich or poor'; 'thin or fat'; 'clever or stupid'; '*sane* or *mad*'. If pressed, many people would locate themselves somewhere between these poles: sometimes like 'this' and at other times more like 'that'.

However, where 'mental illness' is concerned, many people find it necessary (if not easy), to define persons, unambiguously, as 'mad' or 'sane'. At what point someone moves from being 'sane' to 'mad' is, however, much less clear (see Chapter 11).

How such judgements are developed is undoubtedly ethical in nature. There is agreement among the families and professionals that something is 'wrong' with both Billy and Derek. The surgeon can declare, with some scientific certainty, that Billy's tumour is 'most definitely malignant'. This view is informed by a range of computer scans, cell biopsies, blood tests and so on. Indeed, the surgeon is not so much *making* a judgement, as summarising the stories, which the various objective tests have been telling, albeit in different languages. In a sense the doctor has not made the decision whether Billy is 'sick or well'. That decision has largely been made for him by his colleagues and their various tests and examinations. He merely confirms this decision by renaming their judgement with a clinical diagnosis.

By contrast, all the judgements regarding what is 'wrong' with Derek, and his possible 'need for treatment', were arrived at by a wholly different route. Various people *observed* him and *talked* to him – doctors, social workers, psychologists and nurses. From their observations and conversations a decision was made – individually or collectively – as to whether or not Derek was 'sick or well'. The final judgement – framed in the medical language of a diagnosis – may be regarded by family, friends, society at large, if not also Derek himself, as authoritative: based on years of experience. However, ultimately Derek's diagnosis was the *judgement* of one person or a group. No blood test, CT scans, electrocardiograms or any of the other 'objective measurements' recognised within health care played any part in deciding that he 'suffered from schizophrenia'.

These two stories raise a range of ethical questions. For example:

- Is it 'right' to allow Billy to 'take his chances', or let Derek stop taking his medication?
- Are Billy and Derek making 'emotional' decisions, which they will later regret?
- Are they both misguided or foolish?
- Are they being 'irrational' or 'impulsive'?
- Shouldn't someone try to 'change their minds': *make* them 'see sense'?

Later chapters discuss the legal powers that may be invoked to oblige people to accept 'treatment', whether or not they ask for this, or even refuse it (see Chapters 17, 23–25). Although the legislation varies slightly across countries, so-called 'mental health' laws embrace the same principle: a person's views may be overruled if they pose a threat to themselves or others.[20] The core assumption is that such persons are 'not of sound mind' (*non compos mentis*)[21] and therefore, incapable of managing their own affairs.

The situation can be more complex in the case of prisoners,[22] or people expressing a public wish to commit suicide.[23] However, in general there is no way that anyone can 'force' a person, like Billy, to accept or receive treatment. In that sense, the situation of those, like Derek, defined legally or diagnosed medically as 'mentally ill' has no parallel.

Complicating factors: women and culture

Consider two slightly different, but no less tragic stories.

> *Faridah* was 17 and planning to go to university to study psychology when her parents tried to arrange a marriage to her cousin. Much to her parents dismay she refused, left home and renounced the traditional religion of her family. Her father has disowned her and now she is working in a supermarket in a neighbouring town.
> *Lisa* is 24 and has lived with her partner, Miriam, for three years. They plan to confirm their relationship through a 'civil ceremony'. Lisa's mother does not agree with same-sex relations, far less 'gay marriages' and threatens never to speak to her again.

Although these stories are different from those of Derek and Billy, for many people they will elicit very similar questions:

- Do Faridah and Lisa 'know what they are doing'?
- Arranged marriages are part of Faridah's family tradition – why is she being so unreasonable?
- Lisa always knew that her mother did not approve of same-sex relations. Is she trying to upset her mother?
- Are Faridah and Lisa in need of some counselling, to talk through their problems with their families?
- Shouldn't someone try to make them both 'see sense' and change their minds?

In most parts of the world Billy would be free to reject medical advice even if he risked dying in the process. Derek, however, would likely end up being compelled to take medication – and might even be 'hospitalised' – through some legal measure, embedded within a

'Mental Health Act' (see Chapters 23–25). In some countries Faridah and Lisa would be free to lead their own lives, however they saw fit. In other countries, however, different kinds of interpersonal, social, religious and legal pressures might be invoked, in an attempt to influence (or control) them. As recently as the 1970s, both women might well have been diagnosed as 'mentally ill', purely on the basis of their defiance of parental authority or expression of sexuality.[21-26] Depending on how strongly their families advocated the need for 'treatment', both women might have been hospitalised against their wishes.[27]

A time traveller from the eighteenth century – before the emergence of modern psychiatry – might struggle to understand the stories about Billy and Derek. How could one person be free to risk dying by rejecting surgery while another could not stop taking some prescribed medication without risking a social or even a legal penalty? However, our time traveller might well share the views of Lisa and Faridah's families. Two hundred and fifty years ago the ritualised subjugation of women within families, especially by fathers, was commonplace; and sexual relations were only approved of within marriage, between a man and a woman. This serves to illustrate the extent to which some human dilemmas appear to endure across the centuries, while others clearly belong to certain periods in history, or are defined by specific cultural practice (see Chapter 21). However, even in contemporary, multicultural societies, the shadows of sexual repression and sexual prejudice still linger, threatening the liberty of women like Lisa and Faridah.

Agents and agencies – whose life is it anyway?

At one time or another all societies and cultures embraced the view that the person is the *agent* of his/her own life, or at least they applied this philosophy to some people, and denied it to others – like slaves. Today, the *Oscars Ceremony* and the *Nobel Prize*, Death Row and gaol sentences, would make no sense if it was not first assumed that people are responsible for their actions, and deserving of praise or punishment. In the twenty-first century, a person diagnosed with a 'mental health problem'[28] may have various *rights*: access to medical records; information about care and treatment; copies of care plans; support of a citizen advocate; financial support through 'disability benefits' and so on. However, in most societies, that person does *not* have to retain the right to take his/her own life, and risks being confined if mental health professionals become aware of such 'suicidal intent'[29] (see Chapter 22).

Most of the key religions – Judaism, Christianity and Islam – developed versions of the concept of *free will*, reinforcing the view that despite the overarching authority of God, ultimately, people were in charge of their own destiny; and could use this personal power to choose between right and wrong, 'salvation' or 'damnation'.[30] However, as an idea, 'free will' clearly pre-dates religion, whether ancient or modern. Religious doctrines have undoubtedly had a significant impact on the development of Western moral philosophy, and many of the key Western philosophers were religious believers. However, ethics and moral philosophy developed long before the establishment of any formal religious institutions. Given the twenty-first century assumption that 'mental illness' can be explained and treated 'scientifically', it is important to explore ethics from a secular perspective.[31]

Arguably, the most well-known ethical maxim is the *Golden Rule*: 'Treat others as you want to be treated'[32] (see Chapter 1). A close second would be John Stuart Mill's belief that all people should be free to decide how they live their lives, providing that their actions do not prejudice the freedoms of others.[33] Billy's situation might appear tragic. However, no matter how strongly his family and medical advisers might disagree with him, he can choose to live his own life, in the way he thinks fit – even if this might appear to involve signing his own death warrant.[34] Every day the news carries stories of people who have died 'by their own hand', however dramatic or drawn out the process may be. However, the 'celebrities' from the worlds of entertainment, the Arts or sport, who die from the effects of smoking, drinking, drug-taking or overeating, represent no more than the tip of an iceberg of people who die in similar circumstances. Public health campaigns related to smoking, exercise and diet became more aggressive at the start of the twenty-first century, but were stimulated more by the economics of health care, than any genuine concern for the welfare of individuals.[35]

Rarely, however, are those who die from 'self-inflicted' or 'lifestyle-related' problems described as *suicides*. The 200 or more people who leapt to their death when the Twin Towers in New York were collapsing are rarely, if ever, described as suicides, perhaps because naming their actions as such, is too hard to contemplate. Many commentators noted that these people had no choice. Such opinions may, unintentionally, demean the heroic gesture of those persons, trapped by fire and smoke, who leapt into space, taking their lives with them. The reluctance to compare these unfortunate people with those who 'take their lives' under quite different circumstances may illustrate the continued power of the taboo surrounding suicide (see Chapter 22).

Derek's decision to change the course of his life raises a vital issue, from which flows a host of other dilemmas. If psychiatric professionals decide that he is *not in his right mind* when he makes the decision to give up his medication regime, then he risks losing all control over his life. In the process, he loses all the freedoms Billy might take for granted. If he persists in rejecting the counsel of his family and the advice of his doctors, then force – in different guises – may be used against him, in the guise of 'compulsory treatment' – *for his own good*.

The rational argument for equal rights for women has been proposed, for over 200 years, originally by women (*Mary Wollstonecraft*[36]) and later by men (*John Stuart Mill*[37]). Despite the influences of the second wave of 'feminist' consciousness in the 1960s, and the radical lesbian voices of the 1970s, gender equality and complete freedom of sexual expression remain aspirations, rather than givens. However, 50 years ago we would not even be discussing Faridah and Lisa's stories, when the subjection of almost all women and the suppression of sexual freedoms were more commonplace. More importantly, in most parts of the Western world, the practice of 'pathologising' such women as 'mentally ill' has largely been abandoned.

The person problem

The mind, the person and the brain

Various philosophers have noted, in different ways, that there are only two 'things' in the world: *things* that have substance, weight and so on and *relationships*, which clearly have none of these. This assertion is central to the psychiatric/mental health world, where relationships lie at the heart of virtually everything done in the name of caring, helping and treating – indeed, the whole catalogue of psychiatric–psychotherapeutic 'interventions'. This view also underlies Szasz's original critique of the concept of 'mental illness'. Physical 'things', like the body, become ill or diseased. The mind, which is not a 'thing' cannot, by definition become 'ill'. The idea of 'mental illness' can be nothing more than a metaphor.[38]

The mind is a concept, like time, which clearly *signifies* something important to the living of our lives, but which is not a 'thing' in itself, separate from us. We talk about *time*, which 'passes' or 'drags' and which appears all too real: without time we would not age and wrinkle. But where is it? Although we can measure its 'passing' by watching a clock, we cannot pick it up, hold it or weigh it. However, I still appear to age, even when I am not watching the clock and would still grow old even if every timepiece were removed from the world. So, whatever time *is*, it is not dependent on the existence of clocks and watches. Time does not exist, or at least not in the same sense that my watch exists. The 'mind' belongs in the same category as time or numbers: concepts we have invented to signify some of the relationships we appear to have with the world of our experience, which ultimately may lie beyond our capacity to understand them.

There is not space, here, to address these issues in anything other than a very superficial manner. However, their implications need to be noted since they *signal* the key, enduring philosophical problem of the psychiatric/mental health field: what is the *relationship* of the mind to the brain, if any? In the shadow of this question lie concerns with the 'self' and the 'person', concepts that have, traditionally, been sheltered by the umbrella, catch-all concept of 'mind'.

Although the idea that 'mental illness' is a disease of the brain is hardly new, it was revived greatly by the proclamation in the USA of the *Decade of the Brain* (1990–9).[39] As a direct result, efforts have accelerated over the past 20 years to attempt to explain 'mental illness' by reference to discrete aspects of brain function. As the neuroscientist Alastair Compston noted, such an endeavour carries in its wake a wide range of ethical and legal dilemmas.

> If behaviour in the individual is just robotic brain function, are we simply the slaves of ion flux across cell membranes and chemical activity at synapses; or is there free-will? Is it appropriate for society to seek retribution and compensation when individual behaviour is aberrant, and the product of a deranged brain or mind?[10]

The enigma of the self

Harry Stack Sullivan (1892–1949) was the first to propose a formal theory of interpersonal relationships,[11] proposing that what was called 'mental illness' involved a person's *problems in living*.[12] Sullivan anticipated Szasz by locating 'mental illness' within human relationships. These problems, in Sullivan's view, could be viewed as the person having problems in relating to (or living with) him or herself (*intra*personal), or in relating to (living with) other persons (*inter*personal). Sullivan also coined the term 'self-system', which refers to the complex store of information a person has about him or herself, other persons, and relationships with others, the person's position and various roles in society, rights, values, rules governing relationship to others and the world in general. Not least, in the context of our discussion here, Sullivan proposed that the 'self-system'[13] also is the repository of the person's moral principles. In Sullivan's theory, the individual is involved in an ongoing struggle to maintain consistency within the self-system. When this breaks down – on any of the levels already noted – the individual experiences anxiety, which then leads to all manner of attempts to restore balance within the threatened self-system. Often, these attempts at restoring balance are seen, by others as strange, odd, abnormal or dysfunctional, and so become labelled as manifestations (or symptoms) of 'mental illness'.

Sullivan's theory is pertinent to our discussion of ethics for two reasons. He proposed – in the spirit of the existentialists – that *who* we are is what we *do*.[11] People exist in their relationships – with self and others. Second, he illustrated the ways that persons *learned* to be themselves, thus emphasising the developmental nature of *personhood*.

However, for those not versed in, or uncomfortable with, psychoanalytic theory, Sullivan appears to shed little light on what exactly is the 'self'. Today, we are preciously close to accepting that the 'self' is somehow embedded *in* the brain,[15] or is no more than the *workings* of the brain. The Nobel Prize-winning neuroscientist *Francis Crick* (1916–2004) was typical of reductionist thinkers of the modern era when he proposed that: '"you", your joys and your sorrows, your memories and your ambitions, your sense of personal identity and free will, are in fact no more than the behaviour of vast assembly of nerve cells and their associated molecules'.[16]

Whereas Sullivan proposed that persons were to be found in their relationships (ephemeral things), in Crick's view they were 'no more than' the workings of their brains (physical things). Contrary to Crick's claim that his hypothesis was 'astonishing', Szasz noted that his 'scientific' approach had produced nothing new:

> If Crick thinks this is a new idea, it is because he is ignorant of the history of the mind and especially of the history of madness. Hippocrates (fourth century BC) had already asserted that the mind is a function of the brain, a facile equation that never lost its appeal.[17]

Every 'new' idea, theory or model of the mind that is proposed appears to bear striking similarities to much older notions of the *psyche*, the *soul* or the *self*. Even contemporary neuropsychiatric attempts, like Crick's, to locate the mind *in* the brain sound like echoes of Descartes's claim that the seat of the soul lay in the pineal gland; a proposition that today we consider ludicrous. In time, contemporary neuroscientific claims to explain the 'mind' will likely appear equally ludicrous.

Psychiatry, psychology and especially psychotherapy have devoted considerable effort to examining, exploring and defining the notion of the 'self', which has long been viewed as integral to the problems variously called 'mental illness'.[48] However, in Harre's view:

> one's sense of self is not an ego's intuition of itself. To have a sense of self is to have a sense of one's location as a person, in each of several arrays of other beings, relevant to personhood. It is to have a sense of one's point of view, at any moment a location in space from which one perceives and acts upon the world, including that part that lies within one's own skin. But the phrase a 'sense of self' is also used for the sense one has of oneself as possessing a unique set of attributes which, though they change nevertheless remain as a whole distinctive of just the one person. 'The self', in this sense, is not an entity either. It is the collected attributes of a person.[19]

For Harre, the 'self' is a *useful fiction*, but no more than that. We make our 'selves' up as we talk – about our world of experience, about others who inhabit it and most of all about our 'selves'. The 'self' is, literally, a personal *construction* – something made up by the *person*.

Harre's view on *personhood* appears to be a twentieth century revision of John Locke's original definition from 300 years ago: 'what "person" stands for . . . is a thinking intelligent being, that has reason and reflection, and can consider itself as itself, the same thinking thing, in different times and places'.[50]

However straightforward this might appear, there remains much disagreement. As the ethicist, Mary Anne Warren has noted:

> While there is little agreement about exactly what 'person' means, most philosophical analyses of the concept of person suggest that persons are beings that are not only sentient but also possessed of more sophisticated mental capacities, such as those that are often subsumed under the concepts of rationality and self-awareness.[51]

However casually we talk about 'persons' and the myriad 'personal' aspects of our every-day lives, this expression may conceal much uncertainty concerning 'who' and 'what' we are.

Persons and other animals

In her influential essay, *On the Moral and Legal Status of Abortion*, Warren listed five traits that she considered relevant to the notion of personhood[52]:

- *consciousness* and the capacity to feel pain;
- developed *reasoning* ability;
- self-motivated *activity*;
- the capacity to *communicate* – in creative ways; and
- the presence of *self-concepts* (self-awareness).

In Warren's view anything that meets all of these criteria is certainly a person.[53] Yet, she argued, a thing could fail to meet *some* of these criteria and still be regarded as a person. Crucially, she argued that any 'thing' that fails to meet *all* of these criteria is definitely *not* a person. Versions of Warren's views are central to most, if not all, 'pro-abortion' arguments. The early stage foetus clearly satisfies *none* of Warren's personhood criteria, and the late stage foetus satisfies no more criteria than many non-human animals to which the 'right to life' is not accorded.[54] If it is acceptable to kill, and eat, animals that have *some* of the characteristics of personhood, what could be wrong with killing a foetus that has none of these characteristics?

The idea that we should have special rules regarding the care of humans has been called *speciesism*, especially by those upholding 'animal rights' in general and opposition to the use of animals in medical research, in particular.[55]

Peter Singer (1946–), the philosopher most associated with 'animal rights' and speciesism[56] extended the debate over abortion of the foetus to include new-born infants and seriously disabled children. Given that personhood required rationality, autonomy and self-consciousness, Singer argued that:

> Infants lack these characteristics. Killing them, therefore, cannot be equated with killing normal human beings, or any other self-conscious beings. This conclusion is not limited to infants who, because of irreversible intellectual disabilities, will never be rational, self-conscious beings . . . . No infant – disabled or not – has a strong claim to life as beings capable of seeing themselves as distinct entities, existing over time.[57]

Singer's distinctive utilitarian philosophy points out the irrational nature of our 'species blindness' over vivisection. It is considered acceptable to experiment on highly sentient animals, like monkeys, but the idea of abortion, far less the idea of experimenting on severely disabled children, is considered by many to be nothing short of horrific.[58] Not surprisingly, Singer's views have been challenged by various disability groups, who see a strong resemblance between his ideas and those of the eugenics movement of the early twentieth century and the Nazi genocide. Indeed, it was argued that American eugenicists inspired and supported the Nazi racial 'purification laws, but failed to appreciate how this led, inevitably, to the Holocaust.[59]

Many people with a diagnosis of 'mental illness' are either considered to be disabled or consider themselves to be so. It would be folly, also, to forget that the 'elimination' of *both* physically and 'mentally' disabled (insane) people was a key focus of Nazi eugenics. Surprisingly, however, Singer has never commented specifically on the situation of people with 'mental illness', far less the ethics of psychiatry.

The main relevance of Singer's ethics for the psychiatric/mental health field lies in the definition of personhood, especially the emphasis on rationality, which has long been central to mental health legislation. The American Law and philosophy professor, Michael S. Moore, offered a typical example when he argued that:

> Since mental illness negates our assumption of rationality, we do not hold the mentally ill responsible. It is not so much that we excuse them from a prima facie case of responsibility; rather, by being unable to regard them as fully rational beings, we cannot affirm the essential condition to viewing them as moral agents to begin with. In this the mentally ill join (to a decreasing degree) infants, wild beasts, plants, and stones – none of which are responsible because of the absence of any assumption of rationality.[60]

In today's politically correct climate Moore's views can appear offensive. However, the idea that 'mentally ill' people cannot be held responsible for their actions is more popular than ever, although few realise that, by offering such a dispensation, they are relegating such people from the human race. In that sense, nothing much has changed.

Given Singer's considerable writings on life and death issues,[61] Szasz took him to task over his 'silence' on the civil rights violation endemic to psychiatry, and especially the various suicide prevention programmes spawned by psychiatric thinking.[62] Concerning Singer's approval of the idea of 'physician-assisted suicide' Szasz wrote:

> In the past, church and state regulated suicide. Today, medicine and the state regulate it. Singer wants to expand the power of the therapeutic state: 'If acts of euthanasia could only be carried out by a member of the medical profession, with the concurrence of a second doctor, it is not likely that the propensity to kill would spread unchecked throughout the community'. Once again, I refrain from comment.[63]

Where a person decides, to use David Hume's famous phrase, that 'life is no longer worth living', *and* this judgement might involve some 'terminal illness', Singer approves of 'physician assisted suicide'. However, Szasz noted: '. . . individuals who try to kill themselves but fail – that is, who attempt to commit "physician-unassisted suicide" – are punished by psychiatric imprisonment and torture'.[64]

Szasz continued:

> Death control or ending one's life because that is what one wants is a personal matter. If we treat suicide as a medical matter, dispensing suicide by prescription, we do not give control over ending one's life to the person who wants to kill himself; we give it to the state and its medical agents . . . 'Liberty', declared Acton, 'is the prevention of control by others.' Either the state controls the means for suicide and thus deprives persons of a fundamental right to self-determination, or we control it and *assume responsibility for the manner of our own death.* Giving physician-agents of the state the power to prevent suicide by psychiatric coercion *and* the power to provide 'suicide' by medical prescription does not enhance patient autonomy, as Singer claims. It enhances the prestige and power of the state and its bureaucratic agents.[65]

As noted earlier, contemporary mental health services are obliged to guarantee 'patients' a range of 'rights'. However, the right to control over one's life is not among them. Some contemporary social scientists, especially those who endorse a 'post-modern' perspective, will see this concern with individual *rights*, if not the whole idea of the individual person, as rather old-fashioned; the legacy of Enlightenment values and thinking. With a nod towards the 'post-modern' critique, one such social scientist noted:

> The Enlightenment exemplified a distinctive 'age of reason' during the eighteenth century . . . . Progressive ideas about the freedom of the individual and rationalism vied with religion and superstition to explain the natural world . . . .. Society was construed as being in a state of perpetual advancement towards a better future, and the individual was *adorned* not only with rights, but also with the responsibility for his or her own actions and destiny.[66]

Such a view can, however, be seen as narrow, if not distorted:

> The Enlightenment did not originate in the 18th century: it owed much to Antiquity, to the Middle Ages, to the Renaissance and to the seismic shifts of the 16th, 17th and 18th centuries. It was therefore largely concerned with . . . the taking on board of views that had been in conflict, with a rediscovery and reinterpretation of Classical Antiquity, with the reception of what was ancient and modern and with abstractions (such as ideas of what constituted freedom and equality).[67]

With their concerns for the individual, rights and rationalism, both Singer and Szasz are clearly 'Enlightenment' thinkers. Does this mean that their philosophical arguments are no longer valid? Undoubtedly not! It is impossible to discuss, far less propose new perspectives on human nature without invoking the past. It has become popular to dismiss, if not actually disparage, the philosophical and scientific legacy of the Enlightenment. However, such 'post-modern' perspectives appear to function only within the hallowed halls of academe, and have little to offer the everyday reality as people know it. As the psychiatrist, *Joanna Moncrieff* has observed:

> Relativist and post-modern analyses are ultimately unsatisfactory because, by suggesting that all forms of knowledge are ultimately ungrounded, there is no basis for deciding between different theories of the nature of madness and how to manage it.[68]

It is self-evident that a person's actions are influenced, to varying degrees, by biology and social environment. No person can exist without a body; and no person's acts can be executed in a vacuum. The 'post-modern' criticisms of the concept of the 'individual' appear, at the very least, to trivialise any consideration of human behaviour. At worst, they risk dehumanising all our worldly acts.

- If *I*, as an 'individual', am not responsible for *my* actions, then who (or what) is?
- If I cannot *own* my actions, what does this mean for *me*, as a discrete human being?

Persons, citizens and the shadow of eugenics

That human beings could 'torture' an experimental animal but have qualms about turning off life support, for a severely disabled child (or adult) appears to bewilder philosophers like

Peter Singer who views such attitudes as *irrational*. However, Singer appears to assume that humans exercise 'rationality' in all their relations with one another. Clearly this is not the case. As Singer's philosophical ancestor David Hume made clear, 'reason is, and ought only to be the slave of the passions': we are driven by emotion.

When someone forgives a family member – or even a stranger – who has harmed them, this often appears wholly irrational to the dispassionate onlooker. One has to work hard, philosophically speaking, to expose any 'rational' basis for acts of forgiveness, generosity, altruism and heroism. People engage in such acts, often spontaneously, not because they will bring in their wake some kind of good fortune. Often, people appear to 'lose out' from such acts, or at least reap no obvious benefit. Such acts appear to be driven by the person's perception of some kind of connection between themselves and the object of their actions, *not* because they have sat back, reflected philosophically, and finally decided that this is the *rational* thing to do. This interpersonal dynamic can, and frequently is, extended to animals, which humans frequently admit to the human zone, thereby making them honorary citizens.

Farmers may be comfortable with ferrying sheep or pigs in great number, in cramped conditions, to their slaughter, but would never transport their dogs in a similar manner, far less kill them in abattoirs. As the contemporary English philosopher, *AC Grayling* has noted[69] this exemplifies the honorary citizenship of dogs, a species which has, for thousands of years, been viewed as part of the 'human family', although clearly not by everyone. When the family dog, hamster or parrot dies, only a rare few would consider eating it. But the same people have no difficulty in cooking and eating steak, bacon or chicken. This may well be 'irrational', but is merely a further illustration of the complex web of relationships woven as part of our social lives, which can include cross-species relationships.

It is obvious that many people with severely physically or intellectually disabled family members or friends – including those in a coma or persistent vegetative state – have no difficulty in accepting such individuals as *persons*, despite their failure to fulfil the philosopher's criteria for personhood. Even when such individuals make no obvious contribution to society, their existence continues to be valued by family, friends and other compassionate outsiders.

Ironically, when Singer's mother developed Alzheimer's she reached a point where she no longer recognised Singer, his sister or her grandchildren, and effectively had lost the ability to reason. In such a state, she too failed to meet Singer's definition of a person. According to his ethical theory, she ought to have been killed or left to die, at least in principle. From Singer's utilitarian perspective it would be wasteful to devote time, money and effort on her care, which could have been better spent on improving the lives of other people.

So much for utilitarian theory. In the everyday world of reality Singer and his sister hired a team of home healthcare aides to look after their mother, ultimately spending tens of thousands of dollars in the process. When pressed on this decision Singer said, 'I think this has made me see how the issues of someone with these kinds of problems are really very difficult . . ... Perhaps it is more difficult than I thought before, because it is different when it's your mother'.[70]

Despite his insistent urging to put our feelings to one side – to be 'rational – clearly Singer didn't follow his own advice when it came to his mother. It is slightly ironic that the 'father' of the idea of 'practical ethics' should appear so impractical when asked to address an ethical dilemma concerning his mother. However, having had time to reflect Singer responded later to this criticisms by saying that it was more a case that he had 'disobeyed' his own rules and therefore had 'acted unethically'. This seems preciously close to adopting the position of: 'don't do as I *do*, but do as I *say*'. It seems worth questioning the value of any ethical theory that only 'works' in the abstract, rather than in actual, perhaps highly 'personal' situations.

Of course, not everyone will appreciate how value can be attached to individuals who appear to have so little to contribute in return, whether they are disabled children or people with dementia. In1915, the novelist *Virginia Woolf* (1882–1941) described a walk in her diary:

> On the towpath we met & had to pass a long line of imbeciles. The first was a very tall young man, just queer enough to look twice at, but no more; the second shuffled and looked aside; & then one realised that every one in that long line was a miserable inef-fective shuffling creature, with no forehead, or no chin, & an imbecile grin, or a wild suspicious stare. It was perfectly horrible. They should certainly be killed.[71]

A few years earlier, in 1910, *Winston Churchill* (1874–1965) was a Cabinet Minister when he wrote a letter to *Herbert Asquith* (1881–1947), the Prime Minister, noting that:

> the unnatural and increasingly rapid growth of the feeble-minded and insane classes, coupled as it is with a steady restriction among all the thrifty, energetic and superior stocks, constitutes a national and race danger which it is impossible to exaggerate.[72]

Churchill's 'solution' was that 'the source from which all the streams of madness is fed should be cut off and sealed'[73] – through mass sterilisation. For some contemporary com-mentators, the views of Churchill and Woolf have not so much gone away as been reframed by contemporary science.[74,75]

Churchill's recommended policy of mass sterilisation was never enacted but a version of this did become the first stage in the Nazis' infamous extermination policy '*lebensunwertes Leben*': life unworthy of life.

> Of the five identifiable steps by which the Nazis carried out the principle of 'life unworthy of life,' coercive sterilization was the first. There followed the killing of 'impaired' children in hospitals; and then the killing of 'impaired' adults, mostly col-lected from mental hospitals, in centers especially equipped with carbon monoxide gas. This project was extended (in the same killing centers) to 'impaired' inmates of con-centration and extermination camps and, finally, to mass killings in the extermination camps themselves.[76]

The Nazi guards and their supporters who herded the '*lebensunwertes Leben*' into cattle trucks as part of the 'Final Solution', were acting 'rationally'. Their actions fitted their 'racial purity' ideology like a glove. In terms of ethics the Holocaust provides the most extreme example of 'empathy failure': the inability, or unwillingness, of one person to appreciate the intrinsic human nature of other persons, however different they might appear.

The Nazis merely took to the extreme the philosophy of 'selective breeding' first proposed by *Francis Galton* (1822–1911)[77] in the late nineteenth century, drawing on the evolutionary studies of his half-cousin, *Charles Darwin* (1809–82). Up until the 1940s this was a popular idea and many people – famous for their artistic or intellectual qualities – expressed a similar lack of empathy through their support of *eugenics*.[78]

The drive to enhance, improve or otherwise 'cleanse' populations is hardly new. As the American geneticist, *Elof Axel Carlson* noted, the 300-year old 'belief that some people are socially unfit by virtue of defective biology . . . echoes an earlier theory of degeneracy dating back to biblical antiquity, when people were deemed unfit because of some transgression against God or God's law'.[79]

In our gene-fascinated age, Carlson's 'bad idea' – and its many 'well-intentioned' supporters – is unlikely to go away.

The altar of good intentions

Neither should we forget that the history of psychiatry is chock full of examples of ludicrous, reductionist models of human being, which were used to control and contain people, when relating to their pain and distress proved too challenging. In this history are embedded the names of countless distinguished individuals who also claimed to be acting in the 'best interests' of the mad, insane or 'mentally ill'. However, many of these 'pioneers' shared the views of the eugenicists and Nazi executioners in failing to recognise *as persons* the people in their care.

Chapter 3 considers some of the lessons that might be learnt from psychiatric history, many of which superbly illustrate the proverb, 'the road to hell is paved with good intentions'. By way of introduction, I conclude this chapter with the sobering example of *Viktor Frankl* (1905–97) who was a psychiatrist whose spiritual epiphany in the Nazi concentration camps became the basis of all his subsequent work.[80,81]

Frankl became a legendary figure through his autobiographical writings and his exposition of logotherapy: his own brand of existential psychotherapy,[82] which focused on helping people to discover, or reveal, the meaning[83] of their experiences, especially suffering. Frankl remains, for many, a near-sainted example of someone whose personal experience transformed his vision of what psychiatry could or should be.

However, towards the end of his life Frankl appeared to fall victim to the same hubris that possessed his Nazi captors. Towards the end of his life Frankl proudly wrote:

> I have signed authorisations for lobotomies without having cause to regret it. In a few cases, I have even carried out transorbital lobotomy. However, I promise you that the human dignity of our patients is not violated in this way . . . . What matters is not the technique or therapeutic approach as such, be it drug treatment or shock treatment, but the spirit in which it is being carried out.[84]

By 1969, when Frankl made these comments, it had become all too clear that 'transorbital lobotomy' had been the crudest form of soul-murder possible, and had been perpetrated on a staggering scale in the USA, by a relatively small number of psychiatrists. Sadly, Frankl was among them.[85–87] His example reminds us that we might do well to be suspicious of anyone who claims to know what is 'best for us', especially when they appear to have fallen in love with their own reflection.

Ironically, much earlier in 1946 Frankl had famously written that:

> an incurable psychotic individual may lose his usefulness but yet retain the dignity of a human being. *This is my psychiatric credo*. Without it I should not think it worthwhile to be a psychiatrist. For whose sake? Just for the sake of a damaged brain machine which cannot be repaired? If the patient were not definitely more, euthanasia would be justified.[88]

Despite his best intentions, Frankl's subsequent actions offered another example of how great moral authorities do not always practice what they preach.[89,90]

Conclusion

In this chapter I have outlined the key ethical problem in psychiatry: the use of coercion, both subtle and overt, to control, contain or otherwise 'treat' a person deemed to be 'mentally ill'. This aspect of psychiatric/mental health practice distinguishes it from all other forms of medical and social care, where any illicit contact between professional and patient risks being classed as 'assault and battery'.

Various justifications are made routinely for the use of coercion. However, in every case this entails – indeed requires – a diminishment of the status of the 'patient' as a *person*. This affects the way in which all others view the person/patient and opens the way to a wide range of ways of relating to the person, which would prove impossible under any other circumstances. This is, without doubt, the most unpalatable ethical truth in the mental health field.

The commonest defence is that force is used only *as a last resort*, in an effort to *act in the best interests* of the 'patient'. To draw an analogy between the use of psychiatric force and *rape* may prove unsettling for some and offensive to others. Such an analogy, however disturbing, helps put the nature of the coercive 'relationship' in context.

In the twenty-first century Western world a burgeoning catalogue of legislation seeks either to prevent 'sexual harassment' or to mete out punishment to transgressors. Such 'harassment' can range from ways of talking to, or about, another person, to unwanted physical contact. The excuse that 'no harm was intended' or that the intention was 'affectionate or loving', rarely cuts much ice.

The reason is simple. The person is assumed to be the 'owner' not simply of the *body* but also of *feelings*, which can be 'injured' by unwelcome or uninvited attention. Although some sexist exceptions persist, bolstered by the notion of 'cultural differences', in most societies unwelcome or uninvited sexual overtures are classed as criminal acts. Despite the philosophical confusion over the definition of a 'person', most people accept that all adults are *agents*; the captain of the metaphorical ship of their lives. Any attack, however slight, poses an existential and potentially physical threat to the person and all that she or he stands for.

The attribution of a diagnosis of 'mental illness' implies that the individual is *irrational* or *unreasonable* and lacks the capacities necessary to *self-govern*: to be an agent or *person*. In such circumstances, it is argued, force may be used as a *humane* intervention: thus saving the person from himself or herself.

Expressing his doubts about such 'humanitarian' theory, which he believed was 'a dangerous illusion and disguises the possibility of cruelty and injustice without end', the Christian scholar *CS Lewis* (1898–1963) wrote:

> Of all the tyrannies a tyranny sincerely exercised for the good of its victims may be the most oppressive. It may be better to live under robber barons than under omnipotent moral busybodies . . . those who torment us for our own good will torment us without end for they do so with the approval of their own conscience. They may be more likely to go to Heaven yet at the same time likelier to make a Hell of earth. Their very kindness stings with intolerable insult. To be 'cured' against one's will and cured of states which we may not regard as disease is to be put on a level with those who have not yet reached the age of reason or those who never will; to be classed with infants, imbeciles, and domestic animals.[91]

Lewis's protest translates easily to the mental health field, where interest in clarifying the nature of the 'states' which such 'humanitarian' interventions seek to 'cure', has all but vanished. Instead, terms like 'mental illness', 'psychiatric disorder', 'mental health prob-lems', 'mental health difficulties and even 'mental health illness' are used interchangeably, rendering each of them largely meaningless.

To avoid being viewed as an interfering 'busybody' far less a 'robber baron', all mental health professionals must be ethically vigilant. It is their moral responsibility to articulate clearly the basis of their ethical reasoning which, as Bloch and his colleagues rightly observed, changes from one situation and 'patient' to the next. The implicit psychiatric assumption that the 'patient' is not 'in his right mind' and therefore cannot be held 'respon-sible' provides the key justification for almost every aspect of psychiatric/mental health practice. This assumption, therefore, also holds the key to unlocking most, if not all, of the ethical dilemmas in the field, where the general guidance provided in various 'codes of pro-fessional practice' will likely prove inadequate, as Bloch and his colleagues suggested.[92] If professionals are dissatisfied with such guidance or the prevailing ethics of their colleagues or society in general, it could be argued that it becomes their moral duty to make a challenge to the orthodoxy. To fail to do so risks being seen as offering support, however implicit, to unethical practice.[93]

As noted in Chapter 1 ethics are *opinions*, not facts. However carefully developed and reinforced by supporting evidence, no ethical perspective can be proven or disproven like a scientific formula. This explains the frequent changes in the course of ethics down the ages, as competing arguments have sought to override the received wisdom of the day. In the human context of mental health practice, every mental health professional, if not also 'users' or 'consumers' of such services, are potential architects for the design or redevelopment of an ethical code fit for the contemporary world. This work might be enabled further by con-tributions from the professional philosopher, but the key responsibility for shaping ethical practice lies with practitioners themselves.

Notes

1 Goffman E. 'On face-work: An analysis of ritual elements in social interaction'. In Goffman E. (Ed.). *Interaction Ritual: Essays on Face-to-Face Behaviour*. New York, NY: Pantheon, 1982: p. 5 (emphasis added).

2 This is commonly referred to as 'the good life'. In the *Nicomachean Ethics*, Aristotle compared 'living the good life', with an archer attempting to aim an arrow. The archer needs a target to aim at to determine whether or not his aim is 'true'. Similarly, people are more likely to live a good life if they know what makes a human life good. (Aristotle *Nicomachean Ethics*. Translated by Terence Irwin. Indianapolis IN: Hackett Publishing Co., 1985.)

3 The 'Practical Psychiatrist' website offers a typical example: 'The thing is, mental illness is just like any other illness. It has a biological basis just like diabetes or high blood pressure'. The Practical Psychiatrist: A commonsense guide to psychiatry (Cited 2009 December 22th) Available from: http://psystone.com/

4 Sartorius N, and Schulze H. *Reducing the Stigma of Mental Illness: A Report from a Global Programme of the World Psychiatric Association*. Cambridge, MA: Cambridge University Press, 2005.

5 Freidl M, Lang T, and Scherer M. How psychiatric patients perceive the public's stereotype of mental illness. *Social Psychiatry and Psychiatric Epidemiology* 2003: 38(5), 269–75.

6 Morgan G. Why people are often reluctant to see a psychiatrist. *Psychiatric Bulletin* 2006: 30, 346–7.

7 Walter G. The stereotype of the mad psychiatrist. *Australian and New Zealand Journal of Psychiatry* 1989: 23(4), 547–54.

8 The term here refers to *all* the professional disciplines involved in the development of psychiatric theory and the delivery of psychiatric practice.

9 Goffman E. *Stigma: Notes on the Management of Spoiled Identity*. Englewood Cliffs, NJ: Prentice Hall, 1963.

10 Byrne P. Stigma of mental illness and ways of diminishing it. *Advances in Psychiatric Treatment* 2000: 6, 65–72.

11 An example from England is available at: http://www.time-to-change.org.uk/ (Cited 2009 December 22) and from Scotland at: http://www.seemescotland.org.uk/ (Cited 2009 December 22).

12 http://www.mindfreedom.org/

13 McLeish K. *Key Ideas in Human Thought*. London: Bloomsbury, 1993.

14 Deveterre RJ. *Practical Decision Making in Health Care Ethics: Cases and Concepts*. Washington, DC: Georgetown University Press, 2000.

15 Kuhse H and Singer P. (Eds). *A Companion to Bioethics*. Oxford: Wiley-Blackwell, 2001.

16 Singer P. *Practical Ethics* (2nd ed.). Cambridge, MA: Cambridge University Press, 1999.

17 LaFollette H. (Ed.). *The Oxford Handbook of Practical Ethics*. Oxford: Oxford University Press, 2003.

18 Apart from 'making it personal', the term *person* seems the most elegant and parsimonious way of referring to, or addressing, an 'individual human being'.

19 All names used here are pseudonyms.

20 The 'threat to self and others' is a fairly recent criterion. Historically, people could be, and often were, hospitalised and 'treated' coercively, whether or not they were manifestly 'dangerous'. See: Shorter E. *A History of Psychiatry: From the Age of the Asylum to the Era of Prozac*. San Francisco, CA: Jossey Bass, 1998; Porter R. *Madness: A Brief History*. Oxford: Oxford University Press, 2003; Szasz TS. *Coercion as Cure: A Critical History of Psychiatry*. New Brunswick, NJ: Transaction Publishers, 2007.

21 Post-classical Latin *non compos mentis* – not master of one's mind (from thirteenth century in British sources, usually in *non fuit compos mentis suae* 'he (or she) was not of sound mind', and variants. Oxford English Dictionary: http://www.oed.com (Accessed 2009 December 26th).

22 The *World Medical Association Declaration on Hunger Strikers* states: 'It is ethical to allow a determined hunger striker to die in dignity rather than submit that person to repeated interventions against his or her will'. http://en.wikipedia.org/wiki/Hunger_strike#Legal_situation (Accessed 2009 December 20th). However, not all national medical associations are bound by such guidance, and may choose to pursue alternative strategies.

23 The original 'criminal' nature of suicide is maintained by the phrase: to 'commit suicide'. Usually, it is mainly crimes that are committed. In the United Kingdom suicide was only decriminalised in 1961 and in the Republic of Ireland in 1993.

24 Chesler P. *Women and Madness*. New York, NY: Four Walls Eight Windows, 1997.

25 Showalter E. *The Female Malady: Women, Madness and English Culture, 1830–1980*. London: Virago Press, 1987.

26 Appignanesi L. *Mad, Bad and Sad: A History of Women and the Mind Doctors from 1800*. London: Virago Press, 2009.

27 Homosexuality was a 'psychiatric disorder' (i.e. 'mental illness') until the mid-1970s. See: Bayer R. *Homosexuality and the Politics of Psychiatric Diagnosis* New York, NY: Basic Books, 1981. Wives who opposed their husbands or daughters who opposed their fathers (especially over matters of a sexual nature) were commonly diagnosed as 'hysterical', 'neurotic' or even 'schizophrenic'. See: Showalter op. cit.

28 In principle, this popular euphemism for 'mental illness' covers everything from the most minor anxiety to suicidal despair.

29 Attempted suicide was only decriminalised in the United Kingdom in 1961 and in Ireland in 1993. However, attempted suicide remains a criminal offence in some countries.

30 Basinger D. *The Case for Freewill Theism: A Philosophical Assessment*. Downers Grove, IL: InterVarsity Press, 1996.

31 On a personal level, I find much of the contemporary critiques of religion – especially from the Dawkins and Hitchens camp – to be petty, adolescent and sanctimonious. (Dawkins R. *The God Delusion*. London: Bantam Press, 2006; Hitchens C. *God is not Great*. London: Atlantic Books, 2007).

As a libertarian I believe that people are free to believe in, support and fund any religion they choose – in the same way that they are free to choose their political, sporting and cultural affiliations. The contemporary discourse around 'mental health' is, however, underpinned by a set of 'scientific' assumptions. Therefore, it is important to challenge these assertions/assumptions in a wholly secular manner.

32 See: Gensler H. *Formal Ethics*. London: Routledge, 1996.

33 Mill JS. *On Liberty*. New York, NY: Cosimo Classics, 2005.

34 In the famous song from the musical '*Hair*' (1968) Nina Simone sang '*What have I got, nobody can take away . . . I've got freedom, I've got life*'. In a related vein, David Hume famously said: 'No man ever threw away life, while it was worth keeping'. See: Hume D. *On Suicide*. London: Penguin Books, 2005.

35 A significant lobby exists for the imposition of 'fat taxes' on 'junk foods', similar to those imposed on alcohol, gambling and smoking. See: Waist banned: Does a tax on junk food make sense? *The Economist*, July 30th, 2009.

36 Wollstonecraft M. *A Vindication of the Rights of Women*. London: Penguin 1992 (orig. 1792).

37 Alexander E. (Ed.). Mill JS. *The Subjection of Women*. New Brunswick, NJ: Transaction Publishers, 2001 (orig. 1869).

38 Szasz TS. *The Myth of Mental Illness: Foundations of a Theory of Personal Conduct* (Revised Edition). New York, NY: Harper Perennial, 1984.

39 Proclaimed by President George Bush Snr. http://www.loc.gov/loc/brain/proclaim.html (Accessed 2009 December 29th).

40 Compston A. Editorial. *Brain* 2005: 128, 1741–2.

41 Sullivan HS. *The Interpersonal Theory of Psychiatry*. New York, NY: WW Norton and Co., 1953.

42 Evan FB. *Harry Stack Sullivan: Interpersonal Theory and Psychotherapy*. London: Routledge, 1996.

43 All our contemporary notions of 'self-esteem', 'self-concept' and so on are traceable to Sullivan's work in the pre-Second World War period.

44 Albeit an idea that is as old as Socrates.

45 Descartes famously located the seat of the soul in the pineal gland.

46 Crick F. *The Astonishing Hypothesis: The Scientific Search for the Soul*. New York, NY: Charles Scribner's Sons, 1994: p. 3.

47 Szasz TS. *The Meaning of Mind: Language, Morality and Neuroscience*. Westport, CT: Praeger, 1996: p. 84.

48 Laing famously tried to redefine psychosis in general and schizophrenia in particular, as a problem involving the 'divided self'. See: Laing RD. *The Divided Self: An Existential Study of Sanity and Madness*. London: Penguin, 1990.

49 Harre R. *The Singular Self: An Introduction to the Psychology of Personhood*. London: Sage, 1998: p. 4.

50 Locke J. *An Essay Concerning Human Understanding*. Oxford: Oxford University Press, 1690: xxvii:9, 302.

51 Warren MA. *Moral Status: Obligations to Persons and Other Living Things*. Oxford: Oxford University Press, 1997: p. 18.

52 Warren MA. On the moral and legal status of abortion. *Monist* 1973: 57, 43–61.

53 Warren developed these criteria as part of a 'thought experiment' where aliens tried to determine whether 'things' encountered on Earth were humans or not.

54 Some non-human animals are considered almost 'equivalent' to humans. This was shown when the English journalist AA Gill caused a furore when he wrote about shooting a baboon 'to see what it would be like to kill someone'. http://www.guardian.co.uk/world/2009/oct/26/aa-gill-shot-baboon (Accessed 2009 December 27th).

55 Ryder RD. *Victims of Science: The Use of Animals in Research*. London: Davis-Poynter, 1975.

56 Singer P. *Animal Liberation: A New Ethics for Our Treatment of Animals*. New York, NY: Harper Perennial Modern Classics, 2009.

57 Singer P. *Practical Ethics* (2nd ed.). Cambridge, MA: Cambridge University Press, 1993: p. 182.

58 Singer has, to my understanding, never *recommended* experimentation on disabled children, but has included various 'thought experiments' that embrace comparisons between such children and higher-order primates.

59 Kühl S. *The Nazi Connection*. New York, NY: Oxford University Press, 2002: p. 192.

60 Moore MS. Some myths about 'mental illness'. *Archives of General Psychiatry* 1975: 32, 1483–97.

61 Singer P. Changing ethics in life and death decision making. *Society* 2001: 38(5), 9–15.

62 Szasz TS. The 'Medical Ethics' of Peter Singer. *Society* 2001: 38(5), 20–5.

63 Szsaz ibid. p. 25.

64 Szasz ibid. p. 24.

65 Szasz ibid. p. 25.

66 Morrall P. *Madness and Murder*. London: Whurr, 2000: p. 2 (emphasis added).

67 Curl JS. Review: In defence of the Enlightenment. *Times Higher Education Supplement* 2009 December 31st. http://www.timeshighereducation.co.uk/story.asp?storyCode=409761&sectioncode=26 (Accessed 2010 January 7th).

68 Moncrieff J. *The Myth of the Chemical Cure: A Critique of Psychiatric Drug Treatment*. London: Palgrave-Macmillan, 2009: p. 238.

69 Grayling AC. *The Meaning of Things*. London: Phoenix, 2002: p. 85.

70 Specter M. 'Profiles: The Dangerous Philosopher'. *New Yorker* 1999 September 6th, p. 55.

71 Bell AO. (Ed.). *The Diary of Virginia Woolf*. London: Hogarth Press, 1977: Vol. I, p. 13.

72 http://www.winstonchurchill.org/support/the-churchill-centre/publications/finest-hour-online/594-churchill-and-eugenics (Accessed 2009 December 30th).

73 Ibid.

74 Dominic Lawson: We're hiding from the truth: Eugenics lives on. http://www.independent.co.uk/opinion/commentators/dominic-lawson/dominic-lawson-were-hiding-from-the-truth-eugenics-lives-on-834608.html (Accessed 2009 December 30th).

75 Shakespeare T. Back to the Future? New Genetics and Disabled People. *Critical Social Policy* 1995: 46, 22–35.

76 Lifton RJ. *The Nazi Doctors: Medical Killing and the Psychology of Genocide*. New York, NY: Basic Books, 1986: p. 21.

77 Bynum WF. The childless father of eugenics. *Science* 2002: 296, 472.

78 In addition to Woolf and Churchill this group included: TS Eliot, John Maynard Keynes, Linus Pauling, Theodore Roosevelt, Bertrand Russell, George Bernard Shaw, Marie Stopes, HG Wells, Woodrow Wilson and Emile Zola.

79 Carlson EA. *The Unfit: A History of a Bad Idea*. Cold Spring Harbor, NY: Cold Spring Harbor Laboratory Press, 2001.

80 Frankl V. *Man's Search for Meaning*. London: Rider, 2004.

81 However, Pytell has noted that Frankl's time in Auschwitz has been questioned, along with other aspects of his pre-war life. See: Pytell T. Transcending the angel beast: Viktor Frankl and humanistic psychology. *Psychoanalytic Psychology* 2006: 23(3), 490–503.

82 Frankl V. *The Doctor and The Soul: From Psychotherapy to Logotherapy*. New York, NY: Vintage Books, 1986.

83 *Logos* (Gr) 'meaning'.

84 Frankl V. 'Nothing but' – On reductionism and nihilism. *Encounter (London)* 1969: 33, 51–6.

85 Some have tried to excuse the work of Walter Freeman, who popularised the 'ice pick' technique, used on thousands of 'patients': El-Hai J. *The Lobotomist: Medical Maverick Genius and His Tragic Quest to Rid the World of Mental Illness*. New York, NY: Wiley, 2007.

86 For a critical history of lobotomy, see: Szasz TS. Ch. 6 Lobotomy in *Coercion as Cure: A Critical History of Psychiatry*. New Brunswick, NJ: Transaction Publishers, 2007.

87 For a useful account of lobotomy from a psychiatric survivor's perspective, see: Miller J. Psychiatry as a tool of repression. *Science for the People* March/April 1983: 14–34. Available at: http://psychiatrized.org/LeonardRoyFrank/MiscArticlesOnPsychiatry/psychiateyasa toolofrepression.pdf (Accessed 2010 January 6th).

88 Frankl *Man's Search for Meaning*. op. cit. p. 135 (emphasis added).

89 Pytell T. op. cit.

90 May R. Letter to the Editor. *Journal of Humanistic Psychology* 1979: 19(4), 85.

91 Lewis CS. 'The Humanitarian Theory of Punishment'. In Lewis CS. (Ed.). *God in the Dock*. Grand Rapids, MI: Wm B Eerdmans Publishing, 1970: pp. 287–300.
92 Bloch S. (Ref) see Chapter 3.
93 The legal defence that the plaintiff was effectively 'only following orders' was used first by the Nazi accused at Nuremberg in 1945 and has become known as the *Nuremberg Defence*. The problems of using such a defence in professional practice are explored further in Chapter 3.

3   Who cares any more anyway?

Phil Barker

The comfort of codes and customs

Who decides what is right?

The public might be forgiven for believing that all 'mental health professionals' are ethically minded and that their practice is bounded by powerful ethical codes, informed by the latest developments in medical ethics. Indeed, this might also be an accurate representation of the professional's self-image. When ethical problems emerge, it is assumed that professionals will have worked out how to deal with them. As noted in Chapter 2, what could possibly be so difficult?

In their popular textbook on psychiatric ethics, Bloch, Chodoff and Green took a different view, acknowledging that psychiatric life rarely was that straightforward:

> It is always tempting, but equally hazardous, to assist the psychiatrist by offering guide-lines for ethical conduct. Immutable ethical rules are simply not available. Rather, ethi-cal decision-making depends on the individual in association with professional peers and their well-considered reflections to act in morally appropriate ways. Guidelines may be set but are, unlike laws, unenforceable. Moreover, a code of ethics or conduct can only be expressed in general terms. Psychiatrists remain responsible for making ethical decisions in specific cases.[1]

This seems no more than common sense. General rules – or codes – however useful in general, often are lacking when it comes to the particular. Individuals differ from one to another as do the situations in which they find themselves. Decisions concerning 'what to do' must, obviously, be *person-specific* and *situation-dependent*.

Ethical theories might offer some general guidance, but in Bloch, Chodoff and Green's view, they have limited practical usefulness:

> While these theories may be entirely coherent and thoroughly well-argued, the question still arises as to how they apply to concrete day-to-day situations. We could argue that for psychiatrists who face challenging and complex circumstances, every situation is unique and precludes the application of general principles or guidelines of conduct.[2]

In a couple of sentences, the legacy of thousands of years of philosophising about ethics is dismissed, along with the more contemporary theorising that has emerged from the world of 'practical ethics'.[3] How practitioners, whether psychiatrists or other disciplines, begin to address the complexity of person-specific *and* situation-dependent ethical dilemmas, is unclear.

However, having advocated the virtual abandonment of all theoretical principles or institutional guidance, Bloch, Chodoff and Green acknowledge that their idea of a wholly personalised form of ethical decision-making could become a considerable ethical chore:

> Adherence to this 'situational' or case-by-case approach has the virtue of appreciating the special features involved but its considerable disadvantage is its exhausting quality, calling as it does on the psychiatrist to reach an ethical position *vis-à-vis* every one of his patients, their families and colleagues. Such an onslaught of incessant decision-making would soon lead to a paralysis of clinical action.[4]

It is tempting to assume, like Bloch, Chodoff and Green, that we can develop an original view of any given situation, wholly autonomously. This could hardly be further from the truth. We may be responsible for enacting our individual beliefs, but those beliefs are usually 'hand-me-downs' – borrowed from influential family members, teachers within formal education, our community and, not least, our culture. Even if we set out to be ethical dissidents, rejecting such acquired beliefs, they still act as vital irritants for the generation of what we might believe to be our 'personal philosophy'. If all contemporary academic philosophy is no more than 'footnotes to Plato' (see Chapter 1) then the idea that anyone might develop an 'original' ethical view of any contemporary situation, borders on the grandiose.

Who cares anyway?

I have spent a lot of time discussing the various challenges thrown up by life; the awkward decisions we are required to make; and the general feeling of dissatisfaction that invariably comes in their wake. I discovered that some people happily admit to having little understanding of ethics; others believe that they understand ethics completely; and the rest confess little or no interest: 'What has any of this to do with me?' As Bertrand Russell allegedly said: 'Many people would rather die than think: In fact they do so'.[5] The aggregate view seems to be that ethics is 'not a problem', as that annoying pleasantry would have it.

This mix of modesty, arrogance and ignorance illustrates why the ethical debate has been sustained for thousands of years, across all societies and cultures, ancient and modern. People may *know* that certain actions are inherently 'right' and others are inherently 'wrong'. Explaining *why* they believe this proves impossible for some, is all too obvious for others, and the rest – perhaps the majority – simply could not care less.

Whistle-blowing and conscience

Few professionals would openly advocate the virtues of ignorance. By definition 'professionals' are expected to know *what* constitutes acceptable, professional practice, even if they cannot explain *why* this is so. A Code of Conduct may not exactly be the equivalent of an ethical Oracle, but it does provide professionals with a set of 'dos and don'ts', which might help those who are too lazy to think through the issues for themselves. That said, blind observance of such a code may provide professionals with a feeling of security, but whether or not such codes have much in common with 'ethics' is open to debate. There may well be a very wide gulf between 'acting ethically' and 'following an ethical code'.

In 1982 a group of 15 psychiatric nurses at Wexham Park Hospital in England were suspended, and their Senior Nursing Officer subsequently was sacked, after they refused to restrain and forcibly inject a detained woman patient with a tranquillising drug.[6] In the nurses' view the woman *neither* needed the drug *nor* was detained properly. When her case was reviewed by a mental health tribunal two months later, the woman was declared 'sane' and it was noted that she had *not*, indeed, been properly sectioned. She was immediately released from hospital. It was noted that: 'one of the reasons the psychiatrist gave for requiring the woman to be forcibly injected with a heavy tranquilliser was that she might leave her husband and not return to the marital home'.[7] The case became a 'cause celebre' in psychiatric circles, mainly because the senior nursing officer who was sacked, *Paul Walsh*, was depicted as having a 'challenging attitude' towards the authority of psychiatrists; although subsequent events clearly vindicated his actions in supporting his nursing colleagues in refusing to restrain and forcibly inject the woman patient. As far as I am aware, Walsh and his colleagues were never congratulated for upholding an appreciation of liberty that is, at least historically, a classic English virtue.[8]

In 1990 another nurse, *Graham Pink*, wrote first to his senior manager, then to the minister for health, and eventually to the Prime Minister, in an effort to raise his concerns about the inadequate care being provided to elderly people. When he gained no response, he wrote a 'whistle-blowing' article for the *Guardian* newspaper. Some months later he was sacked by his health authority for 'breaching confidentiality'.[9] Ironically, Pink became a celebrated figure for his ethical stance. Almost 20 years later he was voted one of the most influential nurses in the world.[10]

In 2008 a community psychiatric nurse and chair of the *Unison* union, *Karen Reissmann*, was sacked in a similar fashion to Graham Pink, for criticising the policies of her service.[11]

In 2005 another nurse, *Margaret Haywood*, had secretly filmed the appalling standards of care of older people for a BBC *Panorama* programme. She was reported to the Nursing and Midwifery Council (NMC), subsequently struck off, and was no longer able to work as a nurse.[12] Ironically, the programme stimulated such widespread concern, among nurses and the general public, that Haywood was hailed as another heroic whistle-blower, but the NMC was unrepentant.[13] If the law is not an ass, legislators of all shades often are ruled by an asinine mentality. *Plus ca change. . . !*

Not only nurses are vulnerable, should they decide to follow their own conscience, rather than simply toe the party line. The psychiatrist, *Duncan Double* (see Chapter 4), was suspended in 2001 for six months from his National Health Service (NHS) job in Norwich, England. This followed concerns raised by general practitioners over Double's way of working with suicidal patients. Double's employers told him his practice was 'unsafe': that he needed retraining in 'organic psychiatry' and that he must undergo clinical supervision for one year. Double was told that if he did not agree he would be disciplined.[14]

Even the layperson might wonder what relevance 'organic psychiatry' would have for the care of 'suicidal persons'. In effect, Dr Double's employers were telling him to be more like a 'proper doctor', despite the obvious fact that psychiatry is not anything like a 'proper' medical discipline. As many authors will illustrate in other chapters, psychiatry is about 'problems in living' and suicide is, without doubt, one example of how people elect to deal with such problems. How 'organic psychiatry' – the study of brain pathology – could help Dr Double offer a better service to suicidal persons is beyond me; and probably beyond most suicidologists.

Attempts to control the professional life of psychiatrists are fairly unusual. Other disciplines – such as nurses – appear to be much more heavily controlled: by 'professional codes', whether explicit or implicit. Or it may be that the enforcement of such codes is more draconian in the case of nurses; more in keeping with a military discipline, than one founded on caring and compassion. Certainly, little care or compassion was shown towards the nursing 'whistle-blowers' mentioned above. At other times, some of the punitive treatment of nurses viewed as having breached their professional code appears downright silly.

In 2009 a nurse was threatened with suspension for wearing a crucifix, and thus breaching the hospital's 'dress code'.[15] Yet another nurse was suspended and threatened with possible dismissal after she asked an elderly woman if she wished her to pray for her recovery.[16] All the examples offered here would be laughable but for the threat they posed to the individual professional and her or his livelihood.

The sleep of reason[17]

The trade in lunacy: early beginnings

It is impossible to discuss mental health ethics without an appreciation of the history of psychiatry, which overshadows the contemporary field, serving as the source of most of our contemporary ethical problems. A common misconception – among lay public and professionals alike – is that the 'mentally ill' – like 'the poor' – have always been with us, and that 'services', of some description, have always existed for such people. History tells a very different story.[18]

History is peopled with characters noted for their distinctive, unusual or otherwise eccentric behaviour. Indeed, without such distinctions heroes and villains alike would be ignored by the historian. These features were accepted, at the time, as defining characteristics: how such an individual might be recognised. Although not the first, Freud popularised the idea that there might be something 'wrong' with some historical characters, by retrospectively 'analysing' them and their personal foibles. He started this dubious form of 'psycho-biography' with an 'analysis' of Leonardo da Vinci.[19] Using contemporary descriptions, coupled with some autobiographical material, Freud 'diagnosed' Leonardo's 'homosexual pathology'. Of course, now that homosexuality is no longer viewed as an aberration, far less an 'illness', Freud's study seems quaint and narrow minded.[20] Similar 'psycho-biographies' have been developed for various historical characters, all with the aim of retrospectively 'diagnosing', among other things, their 'depression', 'manic depression' or 'psychopathy'.[21] Such a gross misuse of history betrays a lack of understanding of the way social phenomena – like the birth and development of psychiatry and psychology – are embedded within particular societies, cultures and epochs. Particular forms of behaviour have been viewed as queer or frightening down the ages. However, with the birth of psychiatry, the perception of many of these patterns of behaviour changed dramatically, as they were cast as evidence of 'psychopathology'.

No serious discussion of mental health ethics can begin without acknowledging that psychiatry did not *discover* 'mental illness', but *invented* it. Although much has changed over the past 300 years, *all* contemporary ideas concerning 'mental health' derive from that original invention; translating or reframing the original psychiatric prejudice for a new generation.

The birth of the age of madness

Shakespeare's characters have become popular targets for such retrospective psycho-biographies.[22] Ironically, the Elizabethan era was more tolerant of eccentricity than our own, supposedly more 'modern', times. Although distinctive, Shakespeare's fictional characters – in keeping with the real people who served as his models – were widely accepted for 'who' and 'what' they were. Although all sorts of social distinctions and barriers may have existed, the idea of separating off people on the basis of their behaviour alone had not yet been countenanced.

Many authors trace the origins of contemporary psychiatry to Bedlam, or the Bethlem Hospital in London, which began to cater for a few people 'deprived of reason' in the fourteenth century. The present Bethlem and Maudsley Hospital likes to talk about its contribution to 'mental healthcare in London, a story which stretches back at least 760 years.'[23] This is somewhat disingenuous. For at least the first 300 years, the Priory of St Mary of Bethlehem, housed only a few people, in atrocious conditions. Only, after the establishment of the Bethlem at Moorfields, at the end of the seventeenth century, could the 'history' of modern-day psychiatric services be said to have begun.

As Porter acknowledged:

> Through the Middle Ages and well beyond, crazy people had rarely had any special, formal provision made for them. Refuges specifically for lunatics were almost unknown. . . . Mostly, however, lunatics were looked after (or neglected) within the family, kept under the watch of the village community, or were simply allowed to wander (the English 'Tom o' Bedlam').[24]

The most elegant history of the 'birth of the Age of Madness', as we now understand it, was offered by Szasz, who saw this clearly as a post-Shakespearean development; related to the demise of the feudal order, the rise of commerce, secularism and the growth of the state, at the beginning of the eighteenth century.[25] Ironically, the first to be so detained was a small group of wealthy people, kept in their own homes or housed in the private homes of 'asylum keepers' – usually clergymen or apothecaries. In either case the need for 'care' was determined by their families, not requested by the individuals themselves. Often described as the earliest examples of 'psychiatric patients', these individuals were considered a problem by their families and, for a significant charge, asylum keepers were contracted to resolve the 'problem': taking the person out of the family, if not society as a whole. The beneficiaries were both the asylum keepers, who were well-paid for their service, and the families, many of whom inherited the person's wealth by default. Although small in number this group marked the beginnings of the 'trade in lunacy'.[26]

However, as society changed, becoming more complex, the focus soon fell upon:

> *Lonely individuals* – persons without land or occupation, without home, family or means of subsistence – (who) became *visible*. Called beggars, vagrants or vagabonds, their presence *disturbed* the majority of the people living more fortunate lives. The result was the segregation of this inchoate group of individuals with only one feature in common: poverty-homelessness. What was the justification for depriving them of liberty? Homelessness. Called 'vagabondage', the condition/conduct was criminalized, and the offenders were confined in poorhouses and jails. Soon self-appointed benefactors arose who felt that this de facto imprisonment without trial was inappropriate for modernizing societies: with authority and power being transferred from doctors of theology (i.e. clergymen) to doctors of medicine, the reformers 'recognized' that these masses of unwanted individuals were being cared for by physicians, specifically 'mad-doctors'. This social rethinking led to the great institutionalization movement of the nineteenth century, that is, the construction of large public insane asylums and the confinement in them of all kinds of persons who disturbed the social order. Because the incarceration rested on medical-legal justification, physicians sought to identify the diseases that caused people to become insane, and jurists sought to refine the legal principles and practical procedures to rationalize and 'improve' commitment procedures.[27]

The early 'mad-doctors' saw an opportunity to capitalise on the growing 'trade in lunacy', by translating the 'moral problem' of madness into a *medical* one. As the influence of the

Enlightenment grew, with its emphasis on reason and science, the new 'mad-doctors' developed medical (as opposed to theological) models of madness. Thus began the so-called 'scientific' study and treatment of 'mental illness' that continues to the present day. Although the diagnostic catalogue of 'disorders' continues to grow (see Chapter 11), and new theories and models of causation and 'therapy' displace the old, the human reality of 'madness' continues to be obscured by the metaphor of 'mental illness'.

Plus ca change . . . [28]

The care of the 'mad/insane/mentally ill' has changed little in three centuries. Today, wealthy individuals or their families may still buy services at home or in 'private clinics'. However, the majority, especially the poor or disadvantaged, are 'served' by institutional services, whether private or public – either in hospitals or in the community. The popular view is that all such services are focused on 'treating' the 'illnesses' of people who become 'psychiatric patients', a reflection of the common misconception that 'mental illness' is just like any other illness.[29] In reality, most such 'patients' are 'managed' by a team whose key aim is to minimise 'risks', avoid public scandal and limit the possibility of litigation for malpractice. In principle, many Western societies – like the United Kingdom – comfort themselves that the old days of coercion are over and most 'patients' are 'treated' on a voluntary basis. This optimistic view is founded on a limited understanding of mental health legislation. Anyone who rejects offers of psychiatric help – for whatever reason – may find themselves compelled to accept treatment under a provision of the 'mental health act'. Indeed, many Western countries have extended the range of 'compulsory treatment orders' from the hospital to the community (see Chapters 23–25).

For over 30 years it has been assumed that a process of 'deinstitutionalisation' was completing its course, with a full transition to 'community care' as its ultimate objective. Priebe and Turner challenged this common view,[30] arguing instead that a process of 'reinstitutionalisation' was being established. This is shown through:

- *increases* in the amount of forensic provision, especially within the private sector;
- *increases* in compulsory treatment across most European countries, including the United Kingdom;
- *increases* in the use of 'supported housing' as a replacement for old-style 'asylum' facilities;
- *increases* in the use of 'outreach' services to establish institutions 'not defined by bricks and mortar'; and
- using 'early intervention' methods to create a new group of psychiatric patients from within a group who, otherwise, might have avoided psychiatric services.

Moreover, despite a drop in the number of voluntary admissions and NHS psychiatric beds in England, there has been an increase of 20 per cent in the use of powers of detention for 'mental disorders' in the period 1996–2006.[31] If people will not act in their own 'best interests', society – or its agents – will try to make them 'see reason'. The parallels with George Orwell's nightmare vision in *1984* are all too evident.

Attitudinally, little has changed either. 'Patients' continue to be defined by the extent to which they are viewed as a problem by their immediate family or by the wider society. Those who actively solicit help in dealing with their problems are, increasingly, defined as having *only* 'common mental disorders' (e.g. anxiety or depression). Such 'minor mental health problems' (the 'worried well') are distinguished from '*serious* mental illness'.[32]

Szasz has suggested that the most appropriate functional description of mental hospitals or other institutional systems of 'mental health care' would be 'orphanages for adults':

> Formerly, a child who had no parents or relatives willing to care for him was sent to an orphanage. He was treated in this way not because he suffered from a condition called 'orphanhood' but because he could not care for himself and no one was willing to care for him. Today's adult orphanage – the domicile we euphemistically call a 'mental hospital' or 'mental health center' – serves an analogous function. Moreover, the mental patient is housed in a mental hospital not only because he cannot or does not care for himself ('properly') but because mental health experts and government agents tell people that the 'victim' suffers from a condition called 'mental illness' that requires 'medical treatment'. Virtually everyone believes this explanation-rationalization-justification.[33]

Although many might baulk at this title – especially the politically correct mental health lobby – later chapters will demonstrate that the key attitudinal problem in mental health continues to be *paternalism*: people are still treated *as if* they were unable to act for themselves – that is, as if they were children.

Foucault's error and the myth of antipsychiatry

Despite the substantial evidence supporting the development of the 'trade in lunacy' and its evolution into contemporary psychiatry, this history was *dislocated* by the influential, but wholly erroneous thesis offered by Foucault[34] who represented the imprisonment of the Parisian rabble under Louis XIII, as a form of warfare between the 'haves and have-nots'. As Szasz has noted[35] the *Hôpitaux Général* had neither doctors nor nurses, nor medical treatments of any kind. Indeed, such 'hospitals' made no pretence at being 'medical', far less 'therapeutic' establishments. However, Foucault's tendentious 'history' found much support among those with socialist, collectivist or other leftist pretensions.

The key attraction of Foucault's thesis lay in its potential to *politicise* psychiatry. Left-leaning psychiatrists in the 1960s applauded Foucault's *Madness and Civilisation*, recognising its emphasis on class as a potential prop for their attempts to realign mainstream psychiatry. The so-called British 'antipsychiatrists' – Ronnie Laing and David Cooper – are often incorrectly aligned with Thomas Szasz and Michel Foucault to form the core of this 'movement'. Ironically, Foucault made it clear that he shared 'no community' either with them, or with Franco Basaglia, the Italian advocate of 'Democratic Psychiatry'. Foucault was, without doubt, *anti*pathetic to many things, not least capitalism, democracy, liberalism and libertarianism, but he denied any support for 'antipsychiatry'. As Szasz details at length, Foucault maintained his support for the traditional principles of psychiatry, refusing to reject the concept of 'mental illness' or the abolition of coercive psychiatric practices.[36] Ultimately, he pledged his support for the Iranian (Islamist) revolution, which he saw as less oppressive and dishonest than his own Western society. Given that he was openly gay, and eventually died of AIDS, while Iran still classed homosexuality as a capital offence, Foucault's pledge of support was curious to say the least.[37]

If any 'alternative' to mainstream psychiatry ever existed, it undoubtedly lay in the work of Basaglia and his push for radical, allegedly Marxist, reform of the Italian psychiatric system. However, despite his alleged radicalism, Basaglia had no interest in dismantling psychiatry, but sought only to reshape it in his own image.[38] Basaglia never dispensed with the notion of 'mental illness'. Using a classic Marxist argument he merely shifted the causal explanation to society. Basaglia was replicating the kind of 'false liberation' first delivered by Philippe Pinel in France 200 years earlier. He used his influence on the Italian legal system to transfer the power of control over psychiatric patients from the hospital to the community, where he (Basaglia) would become the ultimate authority figure.

Today, some traces of Basaglia's Marxist influence are to be found in 'Democratic Psychiatry': a loose 'movement' emphasising 'social' alternatives to mainstream psychiatry, self-help and political activism.[39] Sadly, however much they emphasise socialist ideals, they offer little challenge to the main psychiatric power base – the use of coercion enshrined in mental health legislation (see Chapters 23–25).

Drugs – 'moral treatment in pill form'

Despite the troubled history of 'mental illness' and its 'treatment', in the twenty-first century most people accept that 'mental illness' is 'treatable' and that drugs represent the treatment of choice. This may be true for politicians, legislators, most mental health professionals and many families of the 'mentally ill', but is rarely true for those required to take such drugs.

Psychiatric drugs (see Chapter 15) are the only 'mind-altering' substances that people do *not* take by choice. Increasing numbers of people risk prosecution by their efforts to acquire heroin, cocaine, marijuana and other mind-altering drugs. Those for whom such drugs are not just a youthful 'experiment', often end up taking them on a long-term basis, in considerable quantities, as 'recreational drugs'. However, no one goes looking for illicit supplies of 'antipsychotics' or 'antidepressants'. The reasons are obvious. Drugs like heroin, lysergic acid diethylamide (LSD) and cocaine help people relax, give boosts of energy, or 'entertain' them, with short-term 'mind-bending' effects. By contrast, psychiatric drugs have notoriously disturbing effects: slurred speech, loss of sensation, impotence and lethargy in the short term; and trembling, shaking, rigidity, seizures and shuffling, all evidence of brain damage, in the longer term. We should not forget that, for many people, long-term use of such drugs results in chronic health problems, like diabetes, and early death. The repeated references to 'side effects' of psychiatric drugs are disingenuous. Where the constituents of such drugs did not, originally, possess brain-damaging potential, they were developed in such a way that this became their key function. The developers of the early neuroleptic drugs compared them to a 'chemical lobotomy', and were impressed by the 'emotional indifference' shown by patients given the drug.[40]

The age of traumas, syndromes, disorders and addictions

The medical view of humanity has a distinct moral bias. People are only fully accepted *if* they are healthy. If people become 'sick' they must demonstrate their ambition to *recover*, for example, by accepting treatment; or risk being penalised in some way. As the costs of health care escalate, calls for people to 'take responsibility' for their health – especially through exercise, diet, stopping smoking and curbing the use of alcohol and drugs – become an everyday occurrence.[11]

The recovery 'movement'[12] began as an offshoot of the psychiatric 'survivor' and 'self-help' movements, and was heavily committed to 'taking responsibility'. Slowly, however, 'recovery' has been taken over (or 'colonised') by government health officials, who seek to develop recovery 'outcome indicators' for services, and recovery 'targets' for professional staff. Moreover, some governments have narrowed the original definitions of recovery to 'returning to work', 'coming off benefits' or otherwise being seen to make a useful contribution to society.[13] Language is merely a tool for communication. The colonisation of 'recovery' is another example of how bureaucrats can transform a 'radical' term to suit their political ends.

Psychiatry has never been concerned with some autonomous, independent 'enemy', which slowly insinuates its way into our lives – like prostate cancer. Instead, it has always been concerned with people's behaviour – or rather the aspects of their behaviour that proves threatening to others, or disturbing to the people themselves. Unlike genuine diseases – which emerge, develop and thrive independent of human influence – 'mental illness' cannot exist outside of a social context. The philosopher asks: 'if a tree falls in the forest, and no one is there to hear it, does it make a sound?' (attributed to George Berkely (1685–1753)). We might well ask: 'can someone go "crazy" on a desert island, if no one is there to notice this?'.

The events called 'mental illnesses' are indisputably interpersonal or social in character. People may die of a 'silent disease', which only shows up on autopsy. People do not die of 'silent' forms of mental illness, only discovered by a post-mortem. If physical illness is ultimately identified by tissue culture or other forms of laboratory analysis, 'mental illness' is known through interpersonal relationships. If you 'disturb' me, *I* suspect that *you* might be 'disturbed'; or vice versa. The psychiatrist can only confirm or reject my hunch through another interpersonal relationship: by talking to you. Almost anything that *you* do that 'disturbs' *me* (or vice versa) might, ultimately, be classified as a form of 'mental illness' (see Chapter 11).

This is hardly a novel observation. In the year I entered the psychiatric field, Thomas Szasz observed that:

> After the turn of the century, and especially following each of the two world wars, the pace of (this) psychiatric conquest increased rapidly. The result is that, today, particularly in the affluent West, all of the difficulties and problems of living are considered psychiatric diseases, and everyone (but the diagnosticians) is considered mentally ill. Indeed, it is no exaggeration to say that life itself is now viewed as an illness that begins with conception and ends with death, requiring at every step along the way, the skilful assistance of physicians and, especially, mental health professionals.[14]

Developing Szasz's theme, the sociologist, Frank Furedi, suggested that a 'therapy culture' had emerged,[15] reflecting a burgeoning interest in people making *public confessions*. At first, this was confined to celebrities, keen to excuse their dissolute behaviour by attributing it to some 'illness'. Over time pressure has been put on almost everyone to admit their weaknesses, express his/her grief, anger or frustrations, or otherwise search for 'explanations' of relationship or family breakdown, through 'therapy'. Such a narcissistic culture cannot survive without 'disorders' to serve as the focus of 'therapy'. As Szasz first suggested, the therapy culture is a gigantic job-creation programme for all 'mental health professionals'.

Furedi agreed:

> Recent decades have seen the discovery of an unprecedented number of new types of illnesses. This is the age of traumas, syndromes, disorders and addictions. The diagnosis of post traumatic stress disorder (PTSD), depression, addiction, chronic fatigue syndrome, attention deficit hyperactivity disorder (ADHD), and multiple personality disorder (MPD), are being applied to a wide section of the population. In the early 1970s, MPD was a rare diagnosis – less than a dozen cases in the previous years; by the 1990s, thousands of people were diagnosed as multiples. Alcoholism was initially

represented as the disease of the addicted individual. Since the 1980s, the children of alcoholics, their partners and carers, are diagnosed as codependent . . .. Once primarily associated with women, depression is now represented as an infirmity that also afflicts children, students and men. Until recently, the diagnosis of ADHD was confined to children. It has now been reinvented as a condition that also afflicts adults. This elaboration of the impact of mental disorders is matched by the growth in the number of routine experiences that are said to cause psychological damage.[46]

This begs the question: who is *not* 'disturbed' or 'disordered' in some way? Furedi recounts the story of the Aberfan disaster in Wales in 1966, when 116 schoolchildren and 28 adults were engulfed by a coal-tip slide. A year after the disaster, a family and child psychologist noted that all the surviving children, who had resumed their education within a fortnight, seemed 'normal and adjusted'. Indeed, the general consensus was that the villagers had managed to deal with their distress admirably, with very little outside help.

Thirty-five years later, Furedi noted that researchers were now criticising the local psychiatrist at the time of the disaster, for *not encouraging* people to 'realise they needed help': 'Since the 1990s the history of Aberfan is being rewritten in line with today's therapeutic ethos. . . . A collection of recently conducted interviews of Aberfan survivors suggest that, retrospectively, people have discovered past traumas'.[47]

Doubtless, any clever interviewer could 'help' the last few survivors of the Great War, the London 'blitz', or others who have displayed some 'Dunkirk spirit', 'uncover' some deeply embedded and unresolved 'trauma'. An alternative view might be that such 'uncovering' is, rather, a process of *reconstruction*: transforming an image of oneself as a resilient and resourceful person into one possessed by frailty and vulnerability. Of course, people will only go to the trouble of making such 'transformations' if it is in their 'best interests'. The glut of 'confessional' books, tapes and film scripts suggests that society has a huge appetite for stories of pain and suffering, rewarding the 'sufferers' with a fleeting celebrity. No crystal ball is needed to forecast that such 'appetites' and the accompanying 'fame' are likely to be transitory; and will be replaced by some new fashion in human grotesquery.

People who have overcome, or 'filed away' some grotesquely challenging events, undermine the whole therapy industry. They exemplify the possibility that people who have experienced all manner of problems in living, can 'get on with' their lives, perhaps with the support of friends or family or even people who have been in the same boat.[48] This should not surprise us. The people captured on film or camera, in the wake of some personal or communal disaster, often evoke strong feelings of pity, but these images invariably strike us as heroic. Since time immemorial, people in all parts of the world have displayed their capacity to survive the trials and tribulations imposed by life. The dogged resistance of 'psychiatric survivors', with their faith in 'mutual support', merely serves as another illustration of such human resourcefulness and resilience.

People may show great resilience in the face of major physical illness, but inevitably this will be short lived. Few people 'recover' from cancer or heart disease without medical treatment. By contrast, all the indications are that much psychiatric, psychotherapeutic or counselling 'treatment' makes little real difference. Indeed, the WHO global study[49] of schizophrenia – considered to be the most malignant form of 'mental illness' – found that people in 'underdeveloped' countries often recovered from a first episode of 'schizophrenia' without receiving any drug treatment, whereas in affluent countries like the United Kingdom or the USA, people risked beginning a lifelong 'career' as an incurable 'schizophrenic'. These findings match Mosher's view that: 'It appears justified to expect recovery for most persons with early-episode psychosis, if the proper conditions exist around them'.[50] Jablensky and Sartorius, who led the WHO global study, commented:

> The sobering experience of high rates of chronic disability and dependency associated with schizophrenia in high-income countries, despite access to costly biomedical treatment, suggests that something essential to recovery is missing in the social fabric.[51]

None of this is surprising. Almost all the available studies of people hospitalised with a psychotic diagnosis in the pre-neuroleptic era (pre-1960s) show that around two-thirds made good social recoveries.[52] Indeed, outcomes for people with this diagnosis are worse now than before the introduction of neuroleptic drugs.[53]

The moral of all such stories, whether drawn from research or personal accounts,[54] is that people can and do recover from what are perceived to be 'serious mental illnesses', either with the social support of others, or through some 'talking cure'.[55] However, we should not forget that although the various talking cures are described as 'therapies', they involve nothing more than two (or more) people talking. The apparent usefulness of social support or conversation for helping people 'get over' serious problems clearly indicates that such problems cannot be considered to be 'illnesses'. So far, there is no indication that simply talking about cancer, unstable diabetes or cardiopulmonary disease results in an amelioration of such conditions.

Conclusion

Madness may have been part of human life for thousands of years, but our interpretations of it have changed greatly: a victim of fads and fashions if not also political ambition. If history tells us anything about the plight of the so-called 'mentally ill', it is that there is never a shortage of people keen to exert power over them: whether by developing some treatment to control their 'symptoms', or to enslave them in endless rounds of 'therapy'.

Whereas madness once referred only to a small number of people, its contemporary descendant – 'mental health problems' – could be applied to most of society's members. The term 'mental health' has been used so generally as to become generally useless.

The mental health field is highly politicised, not least because of the links with big business – like the pharmaceutical industry – but also because the burgeoning empire of medical, nursing, social care staff and therapists depends, for its very existence, on a regular supply of 'patients', 'clients' or 'service users'. There are plenty of reasons to believe that people could be much more self-sufficient in dealing, autonomously, with the problems they encounter in their lives. However, where people are not actively coerced into receiving care and treatment, which perhaps they do not want, they are encouraged to think they need such help, and risk becoming dependent on professional or technical solutions, rather than drawing on their natural sources of support.

Most of the major shifts in thinking about 'mental illness' and 'mental health' have occurred in the last 50 years. Today, almost every conceivable problem, which people encounter in their lives, or create through some reckless act, risks being labelled a 'mental health problem'. As will be shown in later chapters, people no longer: experience difficulties in growing up or growing old; grapple with the apparent meaninglessness of life; and use other people as a means for fulfilling their own, selfish, needs. Instead, perennial human problems are translated from moral dilemmas into manifestations of some form of 'mental illness', 'psychiatric disorder' or 'psychological dysfunction'. Most Western societies readily accept this psychiatric revision of the human story and establish Think Tanks to plan how to service these 'new' disorders, and government departments to monitor the performance of professionals in delivering such services.

The examples of the 'whistle-blowers' mentioned earlier show how difficult it is to 'care' for and about our fellow women and men. Those willing to 'stand up and be counted' over some ethical issue risk being punished or penalised, often by their own professional colleagues. Instead, ridiculous codes of 'political correctness' police ever more sterile forms of care and treatment, much of which may be irrelevant to the actual everyday concerns of the people who are the 'patients'.

As Thomas Szasz noted recently, none of this should surprise us:

> It is a truism that the interests of the individual, his family, and the state often conflict. Medicalizing interpersonal conflicts – that is, disagreements among family members, the members of society, and between citizens and the state – threatens to destroy respect not only for persons as responsible moral agents, but also for the state as an arbiter and dispenser of justice. Let us never forget that the state is an organ of coercion with a monopoly on force – for good or ill. The more the state empowers doctors, the more physicians will strengthen the state (by authenticating political preferences as health values), and the more the resulting union of medicine and the state will enfeeble the individual (by depriving him of the right to reject interventions classified as therapeutic). If that is the kind of society we want, that is the kind we shall get – and deserve.[56]

At one level, ethics can be read as the observance of some moral code, perhaps laid down for us by our professional 'masters'. Many will be content to observe such a code, as an expression of their professionalism. Others will see such codes as no more than a starting point: crude summaries of complex issues, which need to be engaged with, dynamically, so that we might understand better what action is required of us. Those who decide to explore their ethical dilemmas are likely to end up begging all manner of questions, and risk becoming seen as 'whistle-blowers' and 'trouble-shooters' if not simply 'trouble-makers'. They might well ponder the 'rights' and 'wrongs' of psychiatric diagnosis, especially the patent fakery involved in framing problems in living as some kind of 'illness' or 'disorder'. They might worry about the dangers posed by the 'therapy culture'; and the risk that by interpreting people's problems as a cue for 'expert intervention', we risk demeaning people by failing to appreciate their capacity to cope with most human disasters. By begging such questions, they will take the ethical debate out of the narrow confines of the 'professional–patient' relationship, and relocate it within society, where it belongs. The answers that may begin to emerge might help shape the kind of society we want – rather than the one we deserve, because of our passivity.

Notes

1 Bloch S, Chodoff P and Green S. *Psychiatric Ethics* (3rd Edn). Oxford: Oxford University Press, 1999, p. 3.
2 Bloch, Chodoff and Green ibid. p. 2.
3 Singer P. *Practical Ethics* (2nd Edn). Cambridge, MA: Cambridge University Press, 1993.
4 Bloch, Chodoff and Green op. cit. p. 2.
5 Attributed: source unknown.
6 See: Barker P. Judgement on the road to advocacy. *Nursing Times* 2001, *97 (12)*, 35.

7   From the Hansard report of the parliamentary debate, October 18th 1982: http://hansard.millbank-systems.com/commons/1982/oct/18/conscience-clause-for-forcible-restraint#S6CV0029P0_19821018_HOC_439 (Accessed 2010 January 11th).

8   Mill JS. *On Liberty* (1859) [Edited by Gertrude Himmelfarb]. London: Penguin Classics, 1985.

9   'Yours sincerely F G Pink' Society Guardian, 11th April 1990: http://www.guardian.co.uk/society/1990/apr/11/guardiansocietysupplement (Accessed 2010 January 11th).

10 'Nursing Champions: The NT Diamond 20' December 2008: http://www.nursingtimes.net/nursing-champions-the-nt-diamond-20/1943974.article (Accessed 2010 January 11th).

11 Shifrin T. 'Go whistle' Society Guardian, 12th March 2008: http://www.guardian.co.uk/society/2008/mar/12/nhs.health

12 http://www.nursingtimes.net/whats-new-in-nursing/management/bbc-defends-undercover-nurse-as-nmc-probes-confidentiality-breach/5000519.article (Accessed 2010 January 11th).

13 http://www.nursingtimes.net/nmc-defends-decision-to-strike-off-undercover-nurse-margaret-haywood/5000608.article (Accessed 2010 January 11th).

14 Double D. 'Critical Psychiatry: Challenging the biomedical dominance of psychiatry'. In Double D (Ed.) *Critical Psychiatry: The Limits of Madness*. Basingstoke, Hampshire: Palgrave Macmillan, 2006, pp. 14–15.

15 http://news.bbc.co.uk/1/hi/england/devon/8265321.stm

16 This seemed doubly ironic, given nursing's historical relationship with different religious groups. http://news.bbc.co.uk/1/hi/england/somerset/7863699.stm (Accessed 2010 January 2nd).

17 In his etching '*El sueno de la razon produce monstruos*' (The sleep of reason brings forth monsters) Goya illustrated, allegorically, what happens when reason is suppressed: All manner of folly and ignorance let fly.

18 The history offered here is necessarily brief and selective. See: Porter R. *A Brief History of Madness*. Oxford: Oxford University Press, 2003; Scull A. *Most Solitary of Afflictions: Madness and Society in Britain 1700–1900*. London: Yale University Press, 2005; Wallace ER and Gach J. *History of Psychiatry and Medical Psychology*. New York, NY: Springer, 2008.

19 Freud S. (Edited by J Strachey) *Leonardo da Vinci and a Memory of His Childhood*. New York, NY: WW Norton and Company, 1990.

20 Freud retained a strong prejudice against 'homosexuals' to the end of his life.

21 See: Storr A. *The Dynamics of Creation*. New York, NY: Ballantine Books, 1993; Thiher A. *Revels in Madness: Insanity in Medicine and Literature*. Ann Arbor, MI: University of Michigan Press, 2003.

22 Cummings Study Guides refer to: 'Shakespeare's knowledge of both physical and mental illness', despite the fact that the term – 'mental illness' – was not to be coined for another 200 years. http://www.cummingsstudyguides.net/xMedicine.html

23 http://www.slam.nhs.uk/about/history.aspx

24 Porter R. *A Social History of Madness London: Stories of the Insane*. London: Weidenfield and Nicolson, 1987.

25 Szasz TS. *Coercion as Cure: A Critical History of Psychiatry*. New Brunswick, NJ: Transaction Publishers, 2007

26 Parry-Jones WL. *The Trade in Lunacy: A Study of Private Madhouses in England in the Eighteenth and Nineteenth Centuries*. London: Routledge and Kegan Paul, 1972.

27 Szasz TS. *Antipsychiatry: Quackery Squared*. Syracuse, NY: Syracuse University Press, 2009, p. 150.

28 English – 'The more things change the more they remain the same'.

29 For a typical example of such reasoning, see: http://psystone.com 'The thing is, mental illness is just like any other illness. It has a biologic basis just like diabetes or high blood pressure'.

30 Priebe S and Turner T. Editorial: Reinstitutionalisation in mental health care: This largely unnotices process requires debate and evaluation. *British Medical Journal* 2003, *326*, 175–6.

31 Keown P, Mercer G and Scott J. Retrospective analysis of hospital episode statistics, involuntary admission under the Mental Health Act 1983, and number of psychiatric beds in England 1996–2006. *British Medical Journal* 2008, *337*, a1837.

32 It once was conventional to distinguish between 'neuroses' and 'psychoses' on this basis. People who were *disturbed* by their experiences were neurotic; those who *disturbed* other people were psychotic.

33 Szasz op. cit. p. 151.

34 Foucault M. *Madness and Civilization: A History of Insanity in the Age of Reason* [Translated by R Howard]. New York, NY: Pantheon, 1963.

35 Szasz op. cit. p. 29.

36 Szasz op. cit.

37 Szasz op. cit. pp. 129–32.

38 Scheper-Hughes N and Lovell AM. (Eds). *Psychiatry Inside Out: Selected writings of Franco Basaglia*. New York, NY: Columbia University Press, 1987.

39 http://www.asylumonline.net/

40 Rosenbloom M. Chlorpromazine and the psychopharmacologic revolution. *The Journal of the American Medical Association* 2002, *287*, 1860–1.

41 http://www.superliving.co.uk/health/take-responsibility-for-your-own-health.html (Accessed 23rd March 2010).

42 Many who describe themselves as 'psychiatric survivors' or 'service users' – especially in the United Kingdom – deny that any *formal* recovery movement ever existed. Here, I use the term in a loose sense, to acknowledge the range of groups and individuals who espoused broadly 'recovery-focused' ideals. See: Pembroke L 'Recovery is a Trojan Horse' http://www.psychminded.co.uk/news/news2009/sept09/mental-health-recovery001.htm

43 Barker P and Buchanan-Barker P. Death by assimilation. *Asylum* 2003, *13 (3)*, 10–13.

44 Szasz TS. *Ideology and Insanity*. Harmondsworth, UK: Penguin, 1974, p. 4.

45 Furedi F. *Therapy Culture: Cultivating Vulnerability in and Uncertain Age*. London: Routledge, 2004.

46 Furedi ibid. 111–12.

47 Furedi ibid.

48 Chamberlin J. *On Our Own*. London: Mind, 1988.

49 Jablensky A, Sartorius N, Ernberg G, *et al*. Schizophrenia: Manifestations, incidence and course in different cultures. A World Health Organization ten-country study. *Psychological Medicine. Monograph Supplement* 1992, *20*, 1–97.

50 Mosher L. Non-hospital intervention with first episode psychosis. In J Read, LR Mosher and RP Bentall (Eds) *Models of Madness: Psychological, Social and Biological Approaches to Schizophrenia*. London: Routledge, 2004, p. 35.

51 Jablensky A and Sartorius N. What did the WHO studies really find? *Schizophrenia Bulletin* 2008, *34 (2)*, 253–5.

52 Mosher op. cit. p. 350.

53 Hegarty J. One hundred years of schizophrenia: A meta-analysis of the outcome literature. *American Journal of Psychiatry* 1994, *151*, 1409–16.

54 The documentary film 'Take these broken wings: Recovery from schizophrenia without medication', describes the recovery of several people, including Joanne Greenberg, author of 'I never promised you a rose garden'. Available from: http://www.pccs-books.co.uk/product.php?xProd=481&xSec=4

55 Barker P. *Talking Cures: A Guide to the Psychotherapies for Health Care Professionals*. London: NT Books, 1999.

56 Szasz TS. *The Myth of Mental Illness: Foundations of a Theory of Personal Conduct*. 50th Anniversary Edition. New York, NY: Harper Perennial, 2010, p. 283.

Section 1 – Ethical dilemmas

Phil Barker

People have always looked after the sick and infirm of their community, but formal attempts to care for 'mentally ill' people is a fairly recent development. The reasons *why* asylums, psychiatric hospital and clinics were established had more to do with politics and social control than compassion. Indeed, all the ethical dilemmas within psychiatry, psychology and psychotherapy involve conflicts between a belief in the virtues of *care* and *compassion* on the one hand, and the perceived need for *control* and *coercion* on the other.

Among the ethical dilemmas raised in Section 1 are the following:

How should I live?

Socrates's original question reminds us that, despite the influences of legislation, professional codes and cultural conventions, ethics is a personal affair. How do we reconcile all the possible conflicts between what others think or say we should do, and the voice of our own conscience?

Am I my brother's / sister's keeper?

Much ethical thinking in the Western world is influenced by Christian ideas, and so Cain's question is highly apposite. The idea that we *should* look after our 'brothers' and 'sisters' because they are unable to look after themselves is deeply embedded in psychiatric thinking. How do we know that they cannot be more self-sufficient? Who gives us the right to take responsibility away from another person; to live their lives on their behalf?

Is ethics just about 'being a nice person'?

Since being ethical implies doing 'good' one might easily assume that this translates into being 'nice', 'gentle' and 'kind'. All these may be appropriate. Often our need to do the 'right' thing will bring us into conflict with others. Being ethical may involve more 'trouble-making' than bringing comfort to others. Might the challenge of being ethical take you out of your 'comfort zone'?

How far should I go?

Most whistle-blowers, like those mentioned in Chapter 3, are applauded by sections of the general public, but ostracised by their own colleagues. In time, the virtue of their ethical stance may be recognised, but by then considerable damage may have been done to their reputation and livelihood. How far would you go to defend what you thought was right and just?

Is ethics not simply 'common sense'?

The language of philosophers can often be tortuous and ethical theories often seem to over-complicate fairly simple ideas. To those with strong moral convictions, ideas of 'right' and 'wrong' appear straightforward. To those who can see 'both sides of the argument', the issues are more complicated. Undoubtedly, moral conduct depends on us making sense of a challenging situation. However, if that sense was 'common' we would not, repeatedly, encounter the same old problems. What will you do when your 'common sense' is not shared by others?

Section 2

The professional context

Section preface

Phil Barker

Contemporary mental health care is usually a team effort. Depending on the setting, team membership may be diverse or restricted but, increasingly, different professionals bring a range of skills and knowledge to bear on the service; some acting only as a support to other team members, as in the delivery of team supervision.

Individual or group psychotherapy or counselling, offered in a clinic or consulting room, may involve only one therapist or counsellor. However, in almost all other mental health services – from an 'acute' ward based in a general hospital through to community follow-up in a person's own home – a range of different professionals are likely to be involved. People may spend more time receiving care, support or treatment, from one dedicated professional (a 'key worker' or therapist), but the nature of the service offered and its underlying philosophy usually belong to the whole team.

As noted in Section 1, 50 years ago people entering a psychiatric hospital would likely have encountered only psychiatrists, nurses, porters and cleaners. Today they meet a wide range of professionals, and in many settings this will include 'user-advocates' or 'peer support workers': people with direct experience of psychiatric care, who offer a very different kind of support, based largely on their own experience of psychiatry.

Although responsibility for a person's care and treatment may belong to the team, some responsibilities will be shared between members; some weighing more heavily on some team members than others. Experience, qualifications, expertise and status within the organisation are also likely to affect the extent to which one professional is expected to shoulder responsibilities. As a result, job titles, professional affiliations, degree of seniority and workload all are likely to affect team members' views of their work, including the ethical dilemmas that arise from trying to fulfil their professional obligations.

Section 2 profiles seven disciplines who represent, in my view, the key *professional* contributions to contemporary mental health care. As the various chapters will reveal, much common ground exists between these professionals; but each recognises some special issues, which are linked in some way, to his/her particular discipline.

Psychiatrists have been viewed as 'father figures' for over a century, a reflection of Sigmund Freud's psychoanalytic stamp of authority. That Freud was not a psychiatrist is irrelevant. Most lay people associate almost every aspect of psychiatric practice with his influence. Whether or not they crave this power and authority, psychiatrists will be accorded the highest rank among all mental health professionals. People, who become patients, will expect them to wave some magic wand, dispense wise truths, or otherwise 'fix' them. For those psychiatrists with more modest or egalitarian ambitions, this can be a difficult cross to bear.

Mental health nurses – once known as 'mental' or 'psychiatric' nurses, have long been seen as the psychiatrist's *aide de camp*. Perhaps they are still trying to escape from the iconic glare of

Nurse Ratched, in '*One flew over the cuckoo's nest*'. Perhaps they believe that by refocusing on 'mental health' rather than 'madness' or 'psychiatric disorder', they will be viewed more positively. Arguably, nurses face the greatest ethical challenge, since they are expected to be an almost constant presence in the clinical arena; and are expected to be able to deal with every critical event which might arise. Nurses are all too easily cast as angels or Earth-mothers, whether they are women or men.

The problems of living, which are cast as 'mental illnesses', always arise in a person's everyday life: in his/her family; among his/her friends and colleagues; within his/her parent culture or natural community. **Social workers** are, traditionally, the group that is expected to understand and engage with the wider social world of the person in care. Much of their work is practical and pragmatic, but is embedded in an ever-evolving set of theories about social work practice.

Psychologists are often mistaken for psychiatrists, and vice versa. This can also be traced back to Freud's influence. The lay public may be unable to tell the difference but the professional distance between psychologists and psychiatrists can be considerable. Many psychologists are uncomfortable with the medicalisation of problems of living; and try to refocus on more pragmatic and practical ways of helping people deal with the distress they encounter in their lives. Often associated with the provision of cognitive behavioural therapy, hopefully psychologists have much more to offer: especially in helping both the team, and the person, make sense of 'psychological distress'.

Although all mental health professionals offer support that might be described as therapeutic, **psychotherapists** and **counsellors** offer a dedicated therapy service, although the distinction between these two disciplines remains unclear. For the purposes of this book, both will be cast as the '**therapist**'. Working in close emotional proximity to people who are highly distressed and vulnerable, carries its own particular challenges. The analyst's couch may be consigned to history, but the atmosphere of the consulting room still haunts contemporary therapy practice.

The **occupational therapist** is expected to help people maintain their connection to everyday living: the real world they have left outside the psychiatric walls. Like the social worker, much of their work is practical and pragmatic, but has a more specific focus on aspects of everyday living that are critical if people are to regain their independence, confidence and a sense of self-sufficiency.

Although psychiatry and psychology were, originally, focused on some kind of 'soul' work, the *psyche* has largely been overshadowed by more mundane concerns. Not surprisingly, however, many people still feel that they have been overtaken by some spiritual crisis. If their 'mental illness' is not, fundamentally, spiritual in nature, then the experience of breakdown carries distinct spiritual overtones. The role of the **chaplain** in a multi-faith, multicultural society is not easily defined, but probably involves an honest encounter with the distressed person. Or at least, such encounters may be more honest and open than is possible for other disciplines, weighed down as they are by theories and models concerning 'what to do'.

Ideally, I should have commissioned a chapter on the ethical dilemmas facing the **team** as a collective unit. Perhaps the honest, reflections of the individuals here, will *suggest* some of the implications for cordiality and conflict that might emerge within the team, as a living unit.

4 The psychiatrist

Duncan Double

What are we talking about?

The mental illness of King George III (1738–1820) is commonly said to have helped to focus public and political attention on the problems of the mentally ill.[1] The hypothesis that this illness was due to porphyria may well be a myth.[2] The king was under great strain following the loss of the American colonies, particularly as he had insisted that the American war be extended to prevent further protests over British taxes. Following serious bouts of illness, he became permanently deranged in 1810 and his son then acted as regent.

Although famous physicians failed to treat the king successfully during his first illness in 1788–9, Francis Willis became celebrated for curing and mastering the king's madness. The king was not excused Willis's standard treatments of the time, such as restraint in a straight-jacket and blistering of the skin. His intervention met with opposition from other physicians. They minimised his reputation by pointing out that he had been ordained as a priest before practising medicine, and that he apparently gained financially from taking upper-class luna-tics into his private asylum even before obtaining his medical degrees (see Chapter 3).

Noteworthy complaints from other physicians included that Willis allowed the king to read *King Lear* and to shave himself with an ordinary razor.[3] However, such gentler methods and greater liberty seemed to have gained the king's confidence. A traditional anecdote is that, when asked what he would have done if the king had become violent with the razor, Willis replied that he would have controlled him with his gaze. The regime at his asylum involved manual work in the stables and fields of the estate, with the patient labourers dressed in coats, waistcoats, breeches, stockings and powdered wigs.

Mental health services have developed since Willis's time, particularly through the replace-ment of asylum provision by community care. However, the ethical environment of his psy-chiatric practice may not be that dissimilar from the present day. Psychiatry manages madness on behalf of society, and it therefore has a tendency to exaggerate its authority for control, as illustrated by Willis's belief in the dominant power of his gaze. How to manage risk, such as the question of who is responsible if an incapable patient harms himself because he has access to a shaving razor, is a particularly modern, central concern. Justifications are still made for custodial practice, including the need for sedation and seclusion, even if the straightjacket is no longer in regular use in developed services.

However much it may at times wish that it could, psychiatry cannot escape its social role. Its authority for compulsory detention and treatment is legitimated in the *Mental Health Act*. Its power is also kept in check by provisions within the Act, such as appeal against detention, which are designed to protect patients' rights (see Chapters 23–27). There has always been a tension between restraint and freedom in psychiatric practice. There may be good intentions but practice easily slips into paternalism, as reflected by putting patients into unnatural dress at Willis's asylum.

In this chapter I want to explore some of these ethical issues for psychiatrists raised by this anecdote; not in a comprehensive way, but to highlight the extent to which treating people as objects may have ethical implications for psychiatric practice. I acknowledge the subtleties and complexities of behaving ethically in practice, rather than assume that it is always easy to do what is right for patients. Nonetheless, it is not my intention to avoid the need to make judgements about professional behaviour.

From asylum to community care

To set the role of psychiatry in context it is important to understand its history (see Chapter 3). Modern psychiatry has its origins in the state provision of the asylums. In the United Kingdom, the first was opened in Nottingham in 1812. The *Lunacy and County Asylums Act* 1845 made it mandatory for each borough and county to provide adequate asylum accommodation at public expense for its pauper lunatic population. Despite the emphasis on asylum provision, there always was some turnover of patients in the asylum and boarding-out of chronic cases and trial discharge played a role.[4]

Doctors have always had a key part in the asylums and in psychiatric care in general. Even at the Retreat in York, opened by the Quaker and layman, William Tuke, in 1796, the original superintendent was a retired medical practitioner, although he died after 2 months. The Retreat was famed for its humane treatment of patients, using 'reason and kindness' to create a management regime which minimised the use of restraint. However, it was not set up to challenge the medical profession, whose role has always been key. The original superintendent was replaced by an apothecary, and there was a visiting physician who attended the Institution several times a week from when it opened[5] (see also Chapter 3).

The Asylum Journal of Mental Science was first published in 1855 by authority of The Association of Medical Officers of Asylums and Hospitals for the Insane, which had been formed in 1841. The Royal College of Psychiatrists now publishes this journal as the *British Journal of Psychiatry*.

Voluntary admission was only possible after the *Mental Treatment Act* 1930. Even then, application needed to be made in writing to the person in charge of the hospital. The *Mental Health Act* 1959 set the foundations for modern psychiatric treatment and made informal admission the usual method of admission.

Although asylums initially may have been built with good intentions, they quickly became overcrowded institutions. The motivation for the rundown of the traditional asylum, or 'dehospitalisation', was ethical – what has been called the 'dismay and disgust with the old asylum system'.[6] I prefer the term 'dehospitalisation' to 'deinstitutionalisation', as patients are often still cared for in smaller, semi-institutional settings, and in that sense are not completely deinstitutionalised.

Scandals about poor care in psychiatric hospitals were a powerful motivator for community care.[7] The peak of the mental health population in the United Kingdom and USA was the mid-1950s and later in other Western countries.[8] A *World Health Organisation* report[9] in 1953 recognised that hospitals needed to become more of a therapeutic community. After this time, the doors of the old asylums started to be unlocked.

What most concerned the critics of the asylums were the effects of cutting people off from the wider society, making them apathetic, submissive and lacking in initiative and interest. Custodial care may compound people's mental health problems. As the numbers of people reduced, the traditional asylum became increasingly irrelevant to the bulk of mental health problems. This does not mean that the same institutionalising pressures do not affect modern community practice and I will take up this issue further when I discuss the ethical problems inherent in professional relationships and other aspects of community services.

What are the ethical problems of psychiatry?

Mental health professionals face the challenge of dealing with people who may be in a vulnerable and desperate state. The potential intimacy of relationship, which is easily exploited, can mean that professionals may gratify their own needs, such as sexual and financial needs, rather than really be motivated by helping others (see Chapter 8).

For example, in a nationwide survey of American psychiatrists, 7.1 per cent of male and 3.1 per cent of female respondents admitted to sexual contact with their own patients.[10] These high figures show that sexual prohibition in mental health therapy and care, although an absolute moral and ethical standard, is clearly an issue that needs to be considered in the training of doctors. At the beginning of their training, 25 per cent of medical students were found to be prepared to contemplate that intimacies with patients may be acceptable if genuineness of feeling existed between the two parties.[11]

Furthermore, financial ties, in particular, between the pharmaceutical industry and academic psychiatry, provide personal as well as institutional income, creating a conflict of interest that pervades mental health practice. The drug companies pay 'key opinion leaders', whose jobs include writing journal articles and speaking at medical education meetings. For example, Joseph Biederman, Professor of Psychiatry at Harvard Medical School and chief of Pediatric Psychopharmacology at Harvard's Massachusetts General Hospital, has influenced psychiatric practice to the extent that children as young as 2 years old are now being diagnosed with bipolar disorder and treated with a cocktail of drugs, many of which are prescribed 'off licence'. Through Congressional investigations by Senator Charles Grassley, it has been disclosed that Biederman received $1.6 million in consulting and speaking fees between 2000 and 2007.[12]

While sexual contact and financial exploitation may be the most extreme forms of boundary violation, much other professional behaviour may take advantage of the dependency of the patient on the doctor and the inherent power differential. It may not be surprising that an anti-rational approach is taken to dealing with the problem of illness. The wish is for a simple, quick, cheap, painless and complete cure. However, in these circumstances, the ethical responsibility of doctors is not to make grandiose claims and not to play up to ideas that they are magically omnipotent.[13]

The mainstream claim, that mental disorders can be entirely explained in neurobiological terms, has been justified by the argument that an emphasis on impersonal brain mechanisms eliminates feelings of guilt or shame in those with psychiatric disorders, as well as avoiding the tendency to blame individuals, such as parents, for causing the problems.[14] However, by focusing on the brain rather than the person, biological psychiatry may reduce any sense of personhood and agency. There are, therefore, ethical implications of believing that everything we do is at the will of the brain. Reducing mentally ill people to the need to rectify a neurochemical imbalance in the brain misdirects attention away from the difficult task of understanding the reasons for their problems. This is particularly the case with psychosis, which is difficult to understand and empathise with in a rational way.

In Paradise Square in Sheffield, there is a plaque commemorating the translation of Philippe Pinel's seminal work *A treatise on insanity* by Dr D.D. Davis in 1806.[15] The original was published in French a few years earlier. Pinel was clear that mental illness was a psychological problem and that psychiatry focused on 'lesions of the functions of understanding'.

I mention the case of Pinel to emphasise that there has always been a psychosocial approach in psychiatry, right from its modern foundations.

Pinel's approach was called '*traitement moral*', which was translated as moral treatment, meaning psychological, in the sense of 'through the emotions', not moralising, treatment. He viewed case histories of asylum inmates with understanding and respectful kindness, although he was still determined to break any resistance of patients.[16]

There has always been a tension between custodial and therapeutic practice in psychiatry. Jean Baptiste Pussin, the director of the Bicêtre, a public hospice for men near Paris, where Pinel worked as 'physician of the infirmaries', first replaced iron shackles with straightjackets in 1797.[17] Pinel followed Pussin's example 3 years later at the Salpêtrière, the public hospice for women, where he then served as physician-in-chief. Pussin used repressive measures but claimed he controlled patients without mistreatment. The idea of Pinel as the liberator of the insane has become fixed in two well-known paintings, entitled 'Pinel orders the chains removed from the insane at Bicêtre' by Charles Muller, dated 1849, and 'Pinel frees the madwomen at the Salpêtrière' by Tony Robert-Fleury, painted as late as 1878.

Pinel was sceptical about the aetiological importance of brain changes in mental illness. His psychosocial perspective was the basis for his humanitarian intent. The theoretical model of mental illness held by professionals can have implications for their ethical practice. However, this does not mean that I do not recognise that psychiatrists with different theoretical orientations cannot treat patients ethically and with kindness. For example, Vincenzio Chiaguri (1759–1826), although having a somaticist understanding of mental illness that differed from Pinel, expected patients to be treated with respect. He outlawed chains as a means of restraint, even before Pinel, in 1793, at Santa Dorotea, the hospital he directed before moving to the Bonifazio in Florence.[18]

Can psychiatrists ever escape their history?

When King George III relapsed in 1801, Willis's sons treated him. The following epigram became well-known:

> The king receives three doctors daily –
> Willis, Heberden, and Baillie:
> Three distinguished clever men –
> Baillie, Willis, Heberden:
> Doubtful which more sure to kill is
> Baillie, Heberden, or Willis.

There can be disastrous consequences of investing faith in the omnipotence of doctors. Therapeutic zeal has led to the justification of all sorts of groundless, and sometimes damaging, if not lethal, medical interventions. Doctors should not exploit patients, but abuse may well be endemic in psychiatric practice. Psychiatry may not easily be able to escape this unethical history. This predicament may be related to its tendency to emphasise physical treatment (see Chapters 14, 15 and 21).

Medical emphasis on physical treatment

Medical authority has had an influential, if not dominant, role in mental health practice. As mentioned above, there has always been a range of views within the profession. Although the majority view has been to focus on somatic treatment, the psychosocial emphasis on the mind has also always been present, as we saw with the example of Philippe Pinel. Nonetheless, the somatic perspective has led to the development of various physical treatments over the years.

For example, hydrotherapy was used to treat disturbed patients by using baths of different temperatures, and packs, which meant wrapping patients in sheets and blankets. The theory was that a well-equipped hydrotherapy outfit could reduce the use of mechanical and chemical restraint.

Dorothea Buck-Zerchin,[19] who was sterilised without consent in 1936 at a Hospital for Nervous and Mood Diseases in Germany, described the treatment she received there. This included:

> buckets of cold water poured over our heads, with lengthy baths in a tub covered with a canvas that bore a stiff high collar in which my neck was fixed for 23 hours . . .. Rest was given with wet packs . . .. A wet pack meant to be bound into cold, wet sheets so tightly that one could no longer move at all. From our body temperature, the sheets would become first warm and then hot. I would cry out in rage at this senseless restraint in these hot sheets.

Buck-Zerchin does not describe her state of mind at the time. Presumably her treatment was intended to help control her disturbance. The 'sharp end' of psychiatry still includes control and restraint, seclusion and forced injections. Maybe it is better to see these interventions as a failure of treatment, rather than as treatment itself (see Chapter 13).

Another example of physical treatment is insulin coma therapy, which was seen as a means of bringing psychiatry closer to mainstream medicine. Patients were put into a hypoglycaemic coma through administration of dangerously large doses of insulin in a special insulin unit. They were then lifted back to consciousness with a sugar solution. The treatment was used for two decades until the 1950s when clinical trials questioned its effectiveness.[20]

Electroconvulsive therapy (ECT) is the only somatic therapy still in general use. It involves giving patients an epileptic fit through administering electric shock to the head. It is now used with a short-acting anaesthetic and muscle relaxant, but not when first introduced. Initially it was used for schizophrenia, but now for psychotic depression (see Chapter 14).

Surgical intervention may not be the most obvious treatment for mental disorder. Looking at its development in a little more detail may help us to understand what the enthusiasm for physical treatments in psychiatry is all about. We may think that some physical treatments sound excessive, but the motivation has been to intervene in what is seen as a desperate situation.

Lobotomy – or operating to partially separate the frontal lobes from the rest of the brain – was thought to take the 'sting' out of mental disorder, by removing disabling fear.[21] Walter Freeman (1895–1972), an American psychiatrist, developed the transorbital or 'ice pick' lobotomy, by performing the operation by accessing the frontal lobes through the eye socket. As far as he was concerned, this was a minor operation and he toured the country performing several operations in a day, even in public.[22] Aggressive treatments are justified by the apparent results, and the damage they cause is overlooked (see Chapter 2).

Less well known is the phase of surgery on other parts of the body that preceded that on the brain itself. Henry Cotton (1876–1933), an eminent and notorious American psychiatrist, believed that the cause of mental illness was the systemic effects of largely hidden chronic infections.[23] Septic foci, therefore, must be searched for and eradicated. Particular attention was paid to removing the teeth and tonsils.

Even if many people were sceptical about the causal connection, Cotton argued that detoxification was none the less beneficial, and that patients were relieved when they found that their mental condition was the result of poisoning by infection. Cotton's theory of focal infection may have met its demise because of the drastic, and not infrequently fatal, operation of colectomy: removal of the colon.

We may think we are now protected from the dangers and blindness of wish-fulfilling expectations in the era of the randomised controlled trial. However, simplistic and biologically reductionist accounts of mental disorder, which underpinned the work of Cotton, still sustain modern pharmacotherapy. For example, it is commonly said that psychotropic medication corrects chemical imbalances in the brain. This theory is as much without proof and requires as much faith and self-deception as that of Cotton (see Chapter 15).

Perhaps we can learn from our sense of outrage about the damage caused by the overenthusiastic physical treatments of the past. I think the lesson is that even a psychosocial understanding of mental illness, if it is to be influential, needs to have a strong ethical foundation.

What is the point of psychiatric medicine?

Psychiatry diagnoses and treats mentally ill people. I want to look briefly at the specific ethical implications of both diagnosis and treatment, in particular the use of medication.

In everyday practice, moving on too soon to making a diagnosis can foreclose understanding of a person's problems. 'The answer' has not necessarily been found by giving a single-word label for a person's difficulties. Most psychiatrists assume that there are discrete entities that correspond to the different psychiatric diagnoses. In reality, there may be no absolute differentiation between normality and mental illness. Furthermore, there is considerable overlap between different diagnoses.

It is important not to reify a psychiatric diagnosis by regarding it as an entity of some kind. Diagnosis can easily become the first step in the objectification of a person, with obvious ethical implications. Speculating about the biological basis of mental illness, and the supposed biochemical imbalance or other brain abnormality behind it, is a myth (see Chapter 11). The biomedical diagnostic process is self-protective and may avoid dealing with the difficulties of understanding the meaning of a person's problems. At least potentially, the ethical implication is that it reduces persons to their brains.

Doctors do not just prescribe medication in their treatment of patients. Of course, their relationship with patients and how they interact with others involved with patients also have an influence. However, medication is the particular aspect of mental health treatment most associated with doctors, although supplementary prescribing has now been extended to UK nurses and pharmacists[24] (see Chapter 15).

Medication is often prescribed in life crises. When people are desperate they will accept almost anything that is proposed to help them. Medication reinforces defensive mechanisms against overwhelming anxiety. Expectations alone that medication will produce improvement may themselves produce apparent benefit. In other words, placebo effects can be powerful.

Ethical implications of the use of medication arise because of bias in clinical trials, leading to data being interpreted in a more positive way than it should be. The degree to which psychotropic medications are merely placebos with side effects is rarely considered.[25]

However, the extent to which this is true has ethical implications, because of the, at least potential, exploitation of patients.

The problem of relying on placebo is that it may prevent patients from dealing with their problems and create a dependency and vulnerability to discontinuation reactions. Because people believe in the drug, taking it becomes a habit. Any change threatens an equilibrium related to a complex set of meanings that their medications have acquired. People often stay on medication, maybe several at once, even though their actual benefit is questionable. It can be more of a problem than it is worth to stop medication.

As I have said, medication is not the only treatment used by psychiatrists. At the other end of the spectrum of psychophysical treatment, there are also ethical implications of the use of psychological therapy. Psychoanalysis, for example, at times, has been deterministic in its scientific understanding of human nature, with the potential to objectify people as much as medication treatment. The ethical implications of focusing on the person need to be considered for all psychiatric treatments.

What are the ethical challenges inherent in professional relationships?

Psychiatrists work in teams and form just one of the professions providing mental health services. Organisational factors also have ethical implications for their practice.

In particular, as I outlined above, the political context now focuses on community care, rather than hospital provision. The rundown of the traditional psychiatric hospitals tapped into an anxiety about loss of control of the mentally ill in the community. In particular, a central concern of UK mental health policy has become public safety due to homicides by psychiatric patients. There is an independent inquiry into every such case[26] (see Chapter 29). The effect of these inquiries has been to introduce an ever more rigid and bureaucratic interpretation of the *Care Programme Approach* and risk assessment, despite the difficulties of showing that any deficiencies in this regard are in fact related to outcome.[27]

More generally, our modern identity is expressed in the 'Risk Society'.[28] We find it difficult just to accept that things we do not want to happen have happened. As expectations of what can be achieved have risen, our increasingly technological society switches blame onto services provided by society that it thinks should have prevented the misfortune.

The ethical implications of these institutional pressures are that professional behaviour may not necessarily be in the interests of patients, because it becomes more important for professionals to defend themselves against criticism. There is a problem about being too risk averse. Psychiatry learnt this lesson when it opened the doors of the traditional hospital. Patients did better and regained some independence outside the bureaucratic control of the hospital. The worst kind of administrative behaviour restricts initiative. The danger is that the fear that things may go wrong in mental health services distracts us from the task of how to make things better for people.[29] We may become too defensive in protecting ourselves from litigation and other threats of blame. We are in danger of repeating the worst institutionalising excesses of the asylum in the community.

We need to recognise the inherent uncertainty in clinical practice. However much we may wish it were the case, guidelines and procedures cannot eliminate clinical judgement in the management of patients. We need to be able to trust professionals to act ethically to obtain the best quality care based on our own expertise as patients.

In these circumstances, it is important that doctors do not abuse their authority. This applies in relation to other professional groups, as much as patients, in that medical attitudes should not dominate over the validity of other professional views. Sometimes, defensiveness about bio-medical attitudes can create an authoritarianism that can cause harm to practice. Psychiatrists need to encourage an open culture where problems are discussed in a fair manner.

Conclusion

I have outlined the practice of psychiatry looking at it from an ethical point of view. Psychiatry may believe that it is based on scientific principles, but it cannot escape its basis in values (see Chapter 1). Making decisions about how mentally ill people should be treated is inevitably an ethical matter.

The history of psychiatry demonstrates that the mentally ill have not always been well treated. Their rights and dignity need to be defended. This applies as much in modern community practice as it ever did in the asylums.

Notes

1   Bewley, T. (2008) *Madness to Mental Illness: A History of the Royal College of Psychiatrists.* London: RCPsych Publications.
2   Peters, T. (2009) Thomas Wakley, King George II and acute porphyria. *Journal of the Royal Society of Medicine* 102: 505.
3   British Medical Journal (1914) Francis Willis and George III. *British Medical Journal* 1: 213–14.
4   Bartlett, P. and Wright, D. (1999) *Outside the Walls of the Asylum: The History of Care in the Community 1750–2000.* London: Athlone Press.
5   Tuke, S. (1996) *Description of the Retreat, an Institution near York for Insane Personas of the Society of Friends. Containing an Account of Its Origin and Progress, the Modes of Treatment and a Statement of Case.* (First published in 1813). London: Process Press.
6   Clark, D.H. (2005) *Therapeutic Community Memories: How We Learned to Operate the Therapeutic Communities.* The Planned Environment Therapy Trust Archive and Study Centre Publications, Series 2, Essay 1 http://www.pettarchiv.org.uk/pubs-dhclark-howwelearned.htm (accessed 10 February 2010).
7   Martin, J.P. (1984) *Hospitals in Trouble.* Oxford: Blackwell.
8   Goodwin, S. (1993) *Community Care and the Future of Mental Health Service Provision.* Aldershot: Avebury.
9   World Health Organisation. (1953) *Expert committee on mental health* (third report. Technical report series no. 73). Geneva: WHO.
10 Gartrell, N., Herman, J., Olarte, S., Feldstein, M., and Localio, R. (1986) Psychiatrist–patient sexual contact: Results of a national survey. I: Prevalence. *American Journal of Psychiatry* 143: 1126–31.
11 Kardener, S.H. (1974) Sex and the physician-patient relationship. *American Journal of Psychiatry* 131: 1134–6.
12 Angell, M. (2009) Drug Companies and Doctors: A Story of Corruption. *New York Review of Books,* January 15th http://www.nybooks.com/articles/22237
13 Sharaf, M.R. and Levinson, D. (1967) The quest for omnipotence in professional training: The case of the psychiatric resident. *International Journal of Psychiatry* 4: 426–42.
14 Glannon, W. (2008) The blessing and burden of biological psychiatry. *Journal of Ethics in Mental Health* 3: 1–3.
15 Jenner, F. and Kendall, T. (1991) The French revolution and the origins of psychiatry. In: D. Williams (ed.) *1789: The Long and the Short of It.* Sheffield: Sheffield Academic Press (pp. 99–120).
16 Weiner, D.B. (1992) Philippe Pinel's 'Memoir on madness' of December 11, 1794: A fundamental text of modern psychiatry. *American Journal of Psychiatry* 149: 725–32.
17 Weiner, D.B. (1979) The apprenticeship of Philippe Pinel: A new document, 'Observations of citizen Pussin on the insane'. *American Journal of Psychiatry* 136: 1128–34.

18 Gerrard, D.L. (1997) Chiaguri and Pinel considered: Soul's brain/person's mind. *Journal of the History of the Behavioural Sciences* 33: 381–403.

19 Buck-Zerchin, D.S. (2007) Seventy years of coercion in psychiatric institutions, experienced and witnessed. In: P. Stastny and P. Lehmann (eds) *Alternatives beyond Psychiatry*. Shrewsbury: Peter Lehmann Publishing (pp. 19–28).

20 Bourne, H. (1953) The insulin myth. *Lancet* ii: 964–8.

21 Freeman, W. and Watts, J.W. (1950) *Psychosurgery in the Treatment of Mental Disorders and Intractable Pain.* Springfield, IL: C.C. Thomas.

22 El-Hai, J. (2005) *The Lobotomist: A Maverick Medical Genius and His Tragic Quest to Rid the World of Mental Illness.* Hoboken, NJ: John Wiley.

23 Scull, A. (2005) *Madhouse: A Tragic Tale of Megalomania and Modern Medicine.* New Haven, CT: Yale University Press.

24 Avery, A.J. and Pringle, M. (2005) Extended prescribing by UK nurses and pharmacists. *British Medical Journal* 331: 1154–5.

25 Fisher, S. and Greenberg, R.P. (2007) (eds) *From Placebo to Panacea. Putting Psychiatric Drugs to the Test.* Chichester: John Wiley.

26 Buchanan, A. (1999) Independent inquiries into homicide. *British Medical Journal* 318: 1089–90.

27 Szmukler, G. (2000) Homicide inquiries: What sense do they make? *Psychiatric Bulletin* 24: 6–10.

28 Beck, U. (1992) *Risk Society: Towards a New Modernity.* London: Sage.

29 Cooper, A. (2001) The state of mind we're in: Social anxiety, governance and the audit society. *Psychoanalytic Studies* 3: 349–62.

5 The mental health nurse

Tony Warne, Sue McAndrew and Dawn Gawthorpe

Introduction

Death sets limits on life. Death serves as a nexus of concerns about what counts as meaningful and about what makes life not just liveable but good. Death involves not just the dying but also those others who, in many different ways are, or become, part of the process. At one level there is a whole cohort of others (medical and pharmaceutical researchers, politicians, generals, etc.) who are concerned with preventing death, defending the need for the sacrifice of death and/or ameliorating the impact of death on wider society. At another, more intimate level, are to be found the individual's family, friends and professional caregivers. It is within this latter group that an individual's involvement with the dying process and the death of an other can give rise to moral distress, despair and ethical conflict.

For family and friends the emotionality of being with a loved one during such times of personal distress cannot be underestimated. There can often be a conflicting desire to ensure that everything is done to avoid death occurring whilst at the same time not wishing to see a loved one in pain or suffering.

These dilemmas and concerns are often mirrored in the emotionality generated in the provision of care found in nursing practice. Liaschenko[1] makes a poignant point about nursing ethics in a medical world, that for nurses, death is not seen as the enemy to be fought, whatever the cost. Rather, she suggests that most nurses view death as a fact of human life. It is when such a perceived reality is denied, perhaps through the 'heroic' application of medical interventions that can on one hand extend the physiological processes of living, but on the other, reduce the sense of a meaningful quality of life. In such situations harm to nurses often occurs. The conflict and harm arise from many aspects of the work of nursing practice. In the 'heroic' illustration used here both the conduct of treatments and procedures that contribute to the suffering of the patient (albeit in the name of prolonging life) and the emotionality evoked in those associated with the patient (friends and families) require the nurse to bear witness to the patient's suffering. Such incongruities can give rise to conflict and harm to nurses. To witness suffering is to suffer oneself.[2]

The emotionality inherent in mental health nursing is now well recognised.[3] The emotional nature of the work comes not only from hearing the stories of traumatic or dissolute lives, but also often from not knowing where resolution might lie. Across multi-disciplinary health care teams nurses are more likely to face ethical dilemmas due to the nature of their practice. These dilemmas will be explored at both the wider level of *being* a nurse; looking at how these issues transpose to the practice of mental health nursing. Arguably, the practice of contemporary mental health nursing is still characterised by a number of unresolved issues around the nature of how care is provided. For example, the care versus control role of nurses (see Chapters 23–27 for further discussion) or the care versus the treatment role noted above. Throughout their practice, all nurses will bear witness to suffering, distress and deterioration of people's lives. In attending to the resulting impact on the lived experience, nurses come to know the patient as a *person*. This knowing comes from watching, listening and being with their patients. It comes from the establishment and nurturing of therapeutic relationships. However, such knowing is almost impossible to be meaningful without nurses first knowing themselves, especially in relation to others. We take this as the starting point in our exploration of the ethical issues of contemporary mental health nursing practice.

Id and nurses moral identity

Many nurses 'identify' themselves within the context of a practice narrative. Gaining a sense of identity often involves the establishment of what and where a person might be in social terms. Where identity is socially situated there is both the tacit and explicit acceptance of the social actions performed and expected.[1] For nurses, there is of course, both a personal and a grand narrative of nursing; for example, the relationship between the intra-personal, inter-personal and extra-personal dynamics as enacted and encountered through therapeutic encounters.[3] These dynamics are often addressed in clinical supervision. As a platform for challenging attitudes and fears brought to the fore during therapeutic encounters, the value of supervision cannot be under-estimated. It offers the mental health nurse the opportunity to bring conscious awareness to aspects of the self that are hidden but none the less are present in the therapeutic encounter.

However, the inter-personal relationship states at play within these processes of self-development, identity formation and reinforcement can provide fertile ground for the growth (unconsciously) of moral distress and personal challenge. This is a state of being that often gives rise to what might be described as 'victim claims'. Here nurses maintain an identity of being ethical, caring and competent, but find themselves working in a situation of scarce resources and/or organisational prescriptions, which limit what they see to be appropriate nursing care. For example, on arriving at an acute admission ward recently we found that the front door was locked. When we asked why the door was locked, we were told that although the door shouldn't be locked, there was not enough staff on duty that morning and there were patients who, if they left the ward, might pose a risk to themselves and possibly to others. The nurse appeared to be speaking to us from the position of victim. She appeared to be saying: 'this is not my free choice, but in the circumstances this is my only choice'. Various organisations – from the Trust, which encourages staff to avoid litigation – to the more nebulous influences of media and society act as a 'persecutor', dictating the nurse's preferred course of action. In this instance the role of rescuer was enacted by the nurse's own defence structure, believing that the story she offered was an accurate reflection of her own beliefs.

It was that the grand narrative of a nurse providing 'contemporary and non-oppressive mental health nursing care' was conflicted by the personal decision-making of the nurse in charge. Perhaps with good intent, she was trying to protect others (and arguably herself) from harm, thus maintaining the principle of beneficence. However, the result was both an unsatisfactory practical situation *and* the 'moral distress' people experience when they make moral judgements about the 'right' course of action, but for whatever reason are unable to carry it out.[5] The 'rightness' or 'wrongness' of her decision to lock the door was replaced by what Tirrell[6] described as a kind of 'fittingness' of action and personal identity. This may be more familiar to mental health nurses as the use of the defence mechanism rationalisation. We *rationalise* why we behave in a certain way in a specific context to modify the internal conflict that would otherwise arise.

Few of us would think of the ethical nurse as someone who exercises a particular set of morals in one situation and a vastly different set in another. Most of us expect an honest and ethical person to be consistent in the values he/she use to make decisions. However, to understand how individuals make ethical decisions we first need to understand their cultural values and beliefs. We do not mean to infer that the nurse in our example intentionally sets out on this path of 'fittingness'. However, where such a path is not in keeping with one's personal culture, values and beliefs, it can create a process of dichotomous tension between the public self and the private self. The action of the nurse could be construed as *mimesis*: an instinctual defence mechanism whereby an attempt is made to make the inner world like the outer world by using mimicry to blend in and be more able to cope with the outer world.[7] The splitting of the 'public self' from the 'private self' can create fragmentation within the self; the consequence of which is likely to be the unacceptance of part of the self. This in turn can lead to a distorted perception whereby the part of the self that should be integrated – the caring, moral self and self as a professional – is separated, as a means of defending the self. Reaching this point usually allows the angst within the inner world to be projected onto the external world, in this case the organisation.

These concerns are heightened by Doane's[8] study of socially mediated processes of gaining a sense of identity in nursing. She noted that, ultimately, it was through the collective sense of belonging – having interdependent relationships with other nurses – that nurses come to view themselves, and their actions, as being ethical (or not). Interestingly, she noted that how nurses viewed themselves was also shaped by the values of the wider community of practice; and what that community agreed was 'the right action'. However, at the same time individual nurses' perception of how ethical the wider community of practice was arose through their personal view of what constituted the 'right action'. Clearly, our ethical identity and actions are shaped *not only* by our sense of professional self (the roles and obligations that come from being a member of a larger community of practice) *but also* by the prevailing health care discourse. This discourse is embedded and arises from a history, culture and tradition that *enculturates* the individual into a way of being and behaving. A responsible person can be defined as a rational being who understands that he or she has both legal and moral obligations, can make decisions, and is competent to perform the task in hand and can also justify his or her actions.[9] However, the responsibility for ethical practice probably goes far beyond the individual nurse. How individual nurses behave and the actions they take are likely to be profoundly influenced by contextual and relational forces. Such forces will include role expectations, hierarchical relationships, political policy, limited resources, conflicting values, organisational expediencies and cultural norms. Whilst such influences, whether conscious or unconscious, may lead to an interpretation of what was described earlier as 'victim claims', the nurse as an individual remains culpable for her actions (see Chapter 2 and the 'Nuremberg defence'). In light of this we turn to a further exploration of these shaping forces in the next section of this chapter.

The shape of things as they are

The goals of effective mental health nursing care should be to promote health and enable individuals to cope with their illness. As with many ideas, this simple statement can mean different things to different individuals and groups. In mental health, such objectivity forms the backbone of many models of practice. For example, recovery is an approach that has been around for some 70 years in addiction services and, in the last decade, has gained wider political, professional and patient approval (see Chapter 28). In 2004 the *National Institute for Mental Health in England* (NIMHE)[10] published a definition of recovery which includes the following meanings:

1   a return to a state of wellness;
2   achievement of a quality of life acceptable to the person;
3   a process or period of recovering;
4   a process of gaining or restoring something;
5   an act of obtaining usable resources from apparently unusable sources; and
6   recovering an optimum quality and satisfaction with life in disconnected circumstances.

As a basis for the development of this model and emerging best practices, NIMHE defined recovery as: '*a personal process of overcoming the negative impact of diagnosed mental illness/distress despite its continued presence*'.

However, the notion of recovery conveys a number of different meanings to those working within the mental health care services. There is no one definition of the term acceptable to all parties involved. For example, some mental health nurses conceptualise recovery as being concerned with those clinical approaches that focus on achieving improvement in particular symptoms and functions and on the role of treatments; whereas consumer/survivor models tend to put more emphasis on peer support, empowerment and real-world personal experience. Unusually, however, across these different conceptual views of what recovery might mean, a number of qualities, which are said to be inherent in each, are generally agreed:

- Recovery can occur *without* professional intervention.
- Those who *believe in* and *stand by* the person in recovery best facilitate recovery.
- Recovery is possible *even if* symptoms of mental illness *reoccur*.
- Recovery from the *personal consequences* of a psychiatric diagnosis is often far more difficult than from the illness.
- Recovery is best thought of as being a series of *small steps*.
- Recovery focuses on *wellness* not illness.

Indeed, some authors advocate an approach to recovery predicated on the notion of finding ways of tapping into the continuous process of change inherent in all people and in so doing, finding individual ways of capturing and communicating the meaning of personal experience as they apply to self and relationships with others. Interestingly mental health nurses and service users first developed this approach to recovery. Recovery is an approach that is based on research as well as values. Within this approach the importance of each individual voice, resourcefulness and wisdom is valued.

But recovery is also a contested issue for professionals, politicians and patients. It will be no surprise that mental health nurses experience ethical conflicts while providing care within this rubric of therapeutic encounters. For some mental health nurses ensuring that service users have a voice and are enabled to articulate this will bring them into conflict with not only the organisations that employ them, but also the policy makers that shape and performance manage these organisations. Such occurrences have been described as professional obligations: where the mental health nurse is bound by policies, norms and organisational directives that are counter-productive to the obligations they have towards the individual.[11]

Mental health nurses are often faced not with *big* ethical dilemmas requiring the convening of ethics committees to resolve issues, but with the ethics of the *ordinary*.[12] As noted above, the stated goals of the mental health nursing profession are demonstrably ethical: to protect the patient from harm; to provide care that reduces or prevents complications; and to maintain a healing psychological environment for service users and their families. Such goals can be regarded as common morality and the upholding of the moral principles of beneficence, non-maleficence, and the consideration of autonomy and justice (see Chapter 1). There are also moral rules in regard to veracity, fidelity, privacy and confidentiality. Because many people with mental health problems are vulnerable as well as requiring competent and timely care they often need protection and advocacy.

The notion of advocacy has long presented mental health nurses with dilemmas that characterise the '*ethics of the ordinary*'. For example, the Royal College of Nursing (RCN)[13] noted that nurses should '*understand the difference between acting in the person's best interest and acting to enable the person to say what they want*'. For mental health nurses working with individuals detained against their will or in receipt of interventions that they don't understand or want, this is an important distinction. By representing the individual rather than trying to work in their best interests, or mediating between staff and service users, nurses as advocates, are combating the '*dangers of unchecked medical paternalism in psychiatry*'.[14]

To advocate is to speak on behalf of someone else. However, until recently, anyone with a mental illness and in contact with services only had access to advocacy if they specifically requested it. Such arrangements clearly reinforced the paternalism of mental health services, which advocacy exists to challenge.

The new Mental Health Act (2007) for England and Wales created a 'statutory right to advocacy' (see Chapter 23). This new system is independent of existing professional and organisational structures. Only someone who is formally employed as an advocate by either a commissioner (NHS PCT or Local Authority) or an organisation that has a contract with a commissioner for Independent Mental Health Advocacy (IMHA) services can act as an advocate under the Mental Health Act. An advocate must:

- have appropriate training or experience, or a combination of both;
- be a person of integrity and good character;
- be able to act independently of any person who requests an advocate to visit and interview the patient; and
- be able to act independently of any person who is professionally concerned with a patient's medical treatment.

Mental health professionals (including mental health nurses) now have a responsibility to inform detained patients of their entitlement to an IMHA service and make relevant parts of their records available to the advocate. They may also find that the patient wishes an advocate to represent them at decision-making meetings. For many mental health nurses taking on such responsibility has long been seen as part of what being an effective nurse entailed. For example, it was Conlan and colleagues[15] who, in developing the Code of Conduct for Advocates, described the role of advocates in a way that many mental health nurses would perhaps want to describe the approach they adopt in working with others experiencing mental health problems:

> Advocates will only act or speak on the user's behalf as the user wishes. The key aim is to help people regain their own power and speak for themselves . . .. Advocates are there to speak with, rather than for, people whenever possible. . ... The advocate should make no decisions or choices on behalf of the service user . . ..

It is possible to see how the word nurse might be exchanged for the word advocate used here. Likewise it is easy to see why there might be a need to clarify the attitude of mental health nurses towards advocacy in order to avoid the perpetuation of beliefs that advocates are in some way '*anti-psychiatry*' and undermine the work of mental health professionals.[16] Such clarification can be difficult to achieve particularly as mental health nurses and patients can both inhabit a world that has an organisational and administrative approach that has been constructed for the benefit of others. For example, many services rely upon the administrative use of DSM-IV or ICD-10 diagnoses to manage people, processes and payment for services provided. Many service users dislike the personal consequences of such diagnostic labels.[17] The consequence for many service users can include continued stigma, prejudice and an unhealthy dependence on a self-serving system rather than a patient or person-centred system.

Similarly, the mental health nurse needs to recognise the individual nature of a person's problem. *Schizophrenia* may have discernible and common symptoms, but as an illness individuals will experience it differently. If the individual experience is different, it follows that the treatment and intervention need to be an approach that is defined by the patient, nurse, doctor and others collaboratively and specific for that person. Unfortunately, the choice of what is good for that patient may conflict with what is best for the organisation, the doctor, the family and or other patients. It might also conflict with what is thought to be best for the wider society.

Christopher Clunis, who stabbed and killed Jonathan Zito in the London Underground, had been diagnosed as suffering from schizophrenia but had 'fallen through the net' by not having had his prescribed medication when the killing took place. Jonathan Zito's widow, supported by the media, launched a campaign to raise awareness of the dangers of people diagnosed with schizophrenia not taking their prescribed medication; demanding that mental health services protect the public by ensuring this would not happen in the future. From a consequentialist point of view this would be to apply the maxim the *greatest good for the greatest number*. However, this often results in society's need for safety polarising opinion to groups of people and away from individuals, thus negating or discarding personal autonomy. For those diagnosed with schizophrenia the consequence of such polarisations can be stigma, discrimination and exclusion.

If the nurse comes to know what is best for the patient and yet cannot provide this, the nurse (and the patient) is likely to suffer moral distress. Moral distress moves the nurse from the virtuous circle of the ethical work environment (practice) to the vicious circle of ineffective and poor nursing care and patient experience. Jameton[18] defined the moral distress experienced by nurses in the context of organisational and political turbulence and constraint. This involved the painful feelings and psychological disequilibria that occur when nurses are conscious of the morally appropriate action a situation requires but cannot carry out that action because of institutionalised obstacles. These obstacles can be inadequate staffing, medical hegemony, organisational policy and focus, and so on.

Jameton's model involved two levels of moral distress: (1) the immediate or initial, characterised by frustration, anger, anxiety and interpersonal conflict about values; and (2) second, reactive distress, which is perhaps the more pernicious of the two. Here the distress is caused by a failure on the part of the nurse to act upon her initial distress. Whilst stress can be a motivator for change, moral distress reflects a negative response to the types of problems and obstacles described above. Corley and colleagues[19] reported that moderate-to-high numbers of all nursing staff experience moral distress leading to burnout, high staff attrition and poor patient care. Their work resonates with the outcomes of studies concerned with acute mental health care in-patient environments.[20,21] It is possible to see both the grand narrative and the personal stories in this work.

For example, acute nursing has become less attractive primarily as a consequence of the community care agenda: if the community is the 'right' place for mentally ill people, then the hospital is the wrong place.[20] Acute care is accused of 'failing', leading to staff leaving for more attractive posts in the community. This then is the negative backdrop against which specifically unappealing nursing issues get played out. These include the persistent criticism that acute wards are not therapeutic, and therefore, by association acute mental health nursing is not therapeutic either (see Chapter 16). This narrative has a familiar refrain; for example, there are claims that acute nurses work within a culture of observation rather than one of engaging with patients[21] and that the focus of acute mental health nursing is not based on caring relationships but rather on authority and control.[22] The assumption that these perspectives are incompatible is part of the disapproval of acute care, yet clearly the containment of disturbed behaviour is a routine component of this setting.[23] In summary, the grand narrative would suggest that acute mental health nursing may be considered unattractive because, fundamentally, it is regarded as being incongruent with current mental health nursing ideals. For those working in such settings, this narrative simply reinforces an unhelpful backdrop to practice. Against this backdrop, if the individual nurse experiences inadequate support or poor staffing the resolution of the ethics of the ordinary can become almost impossible.

The resolution of inappropriate staffing levels and skill mix should rightly be the employing organisations' concern. However, the NMC Code[21] (of Standards of conduct, performance and ethics for nurses and midwives) explicitly makes it the responsibility of the individual nurse to put in writing any concerns they may have about the environment they work in where they believe people are being put at risk. However, the situation may involve more than simply committing one's concerns to paper as the NMC Code suggests.

In late 2007, the community nurse and union official Karen Reissmann was sacked after 25 years as a qualified mental health nurse. Her *'alleged offence'* was speaking out about the proposed service cuts and privatisation plans her employer, a large NHS Mental Health Trust, was planning. The case took two years to resolve. Part way through an employment tribunal hearing an out-of-court settlement was reached. Karen was not reinstated by her employer. Even as this case was being resolved, another and perhaps more troubling case was brought to the British public's attention through the BBC *Panorama* programme. This was the case of Margaret Haywood, who was subsequently struck off the register by the NMC for secret filming of the neglect of elderly people in the hospital she worked at. This act was described[25] as a *'major breach'* of the NMC Code of Conduct. However, to ignore 'patient neglect' would equally have been a breach of professional conduct. Blind compliance with what might be a rather uncomplicated sense of protecting the confidentiality of another is clearly wrong. As professionals we should be aware of when such protection has to be placed to one side. For example, where information with legal, ethical and/or moral implications becomes available which transcend the individual's right to confidentiality; or which places oneself or others at risk. In Haywood's defence it was claimed that she had tried every formal procedure to bring these concerns to the attention of her employing organisation, all of which were ignored.

Although both these cases have features that are unknown to the public, even a naive reading of these events is likely to inhibit most nurses in bringing their employers attention to the ethical dilemmas encountered in their ordinary practice. The cumulative consequence of being unable to resolve such moral distress is likely to be what Webster and Baylis[26] refer to as a 'moral residue': an intensity of feeling and emotion that over time becomes corrosive and damaging to the individual's sense of self. How might the individual learn to deal with these challenges?

The shape of things to come

As mental health nursing has changed, albeit slowly[27] the number and type of ethical issues nurses face have also changed. As mental health nurses, we have choices and responsibilities in dealing with the moral distress, emotional pain and suffering from which we ourselves are not immune. We have a deep and true responsibility to care for ourselves and to support one another. It may be unreasonable to expect regulatory councils like the NMC to create opportunities for such professional support and help, despite, their main concern being to protect the public from unethical professionals. Similarly, until relatively recently, health and social care employer organisations were largely rhetorical in their approaches to the provision of such support having any kind of organisational priority. Indeed, Menzies Lyth's[28] famous work described the hospital environment as characterised by high levels of stress and anxiety. She noted that socially structured defence mechanisms are used as a response to such anxiety. These include: ritual task performance; highly bureaucratic decision-making, involving checking and re-checking processes; encouraging psychological detachment; and so on. Such approaches usually typify a negative and unsupportive organisational culture. By contrast, there is evidence of positive correlations between ethical work satisfaction (being able to deal with the ethics of the ordinary) and constructive organisational cultures.[29] The mental health nurse as an *individual*, rather than the representative of an anonymous organisation, will have opportunities in carrying out her daily practice to contribute to a constructive culture. Indeed, the many classic works describing psychiatric institutions as coercive, regimented, restricting and hostile recognise that nurses can do much to reduce these aspects of hospital care.[30-32]

At the beginning of this chapter we asked the reader to consider moral distress in terms of death, but throughout we have tried to explicate how such distress, and the associated ethical conflict, can transcend all aspects of mental health nursing. We draw upon the ethical work of the late philosopher Paul Ricoeur,[33] who established three components of the ethical aim which resonate with the notion of good mental nursing practice: the individual; the inter-personal; and societal. These three components can be applied to both the nurse and the patient, and to the interactions they have as therapeutic relationships are formed, taken forward and dissolved. For example, in considering self-esteem, Ricoeur concludes this is not esteem for a '*myself*', but for a universal self that more properly becomes an acceptance of and a respect for '*selves*'. The nurse as self and a self in relation to an other and in turn, in relation to many others. It becomes important for the mental health nurse to recognise that in this inter-personal relationship the person suffering distress is not *solely* receiving and the care giver is not only *giving*. Gaining such recognition requires a constant re-evaluation and interpretation of self. These processes of re-evaluation and interpretation will in turn help enable the mental health nurse to both respect and take responsibility for his/her relationships with patients. Where this is achieved, then the mental nurse will truly inhabit a relational position of '*being with*' their patient and be better equipped to deal not only with the ethics of the ordinary but also with the ethics of caring.

Notes

1 Liaschenko J. (1995) Artificial person hood: Nursing ethics in a medical world. *Nursing Ethics* 2 (3), 183–96.
2 Ricoeur P. (1992) *Oneself as Another.* Chicago, IL: University of Chicago Press.
3 Warne T. and McAndrew S. (2008) Painting the landscape of emotionality: Colouring in the emotional gaps between the theory and practice of mental health nursing. *International Journal of Mental Health Nursing* 17 (2), 108–15.
4 Altheide D. (2000) Identity and the definition of the situation in a mass-mediated context. *Symbolic Interaction* 23, 1–18.
5 McCarthy J. and Deady R. (2008) Moral distress reconsidered. *Nursing Ethics* 15 (2), 254–62.

6 Tirrell L. (1999) Story telling and moral agency. *Journal of Aesthetics and Art Criticism* 48, 115–26.
7 Horkheimer M. and Adorno T. (1994) *Dialectic of Enlightenment.* New York, NY: Continuum.
8 Doane G. (2002) Am I still ethical? The socially mediated process of nurses' moral identity. *Nursing Ethics* 9 (6), 623–35.
9 Thompson I., Melia K., and Boyd K. (2000) *Nursing Ethics* (4th ed.). Edinburgh: Churchill Livingstone.
10 NIMHE (2004) *Emergent Best Practices in Mental Health Recovery.* London: National Institute for Mental Health in England, University of Wolverhampton.
11 Povis C. and Stack S. (2004) Caring work, personal obligations and collective responsibility. *Nursing Ethics* 11(1), 5–14.
12 Worthley J. (1997) *The Ethics of the Ordinary in Health Care.* Chicago, IL: Health Administration Press.
13 Campbell P. and Lindow V. (1997) *Changing Practice. Mental Health Nursing and User Empowerment.* London: Royal College of Nursing Learning Materials on Mental Health, RCN.
14 Thomas P. F. and Bracken P. (1999) The value of advocacy: Putting ethics into practice. *Psychiatric Bulletin* 23, 327–9.
15 Conlan E., Gell C., and Graley R. (UKAN) (1997) *Advocacy – A Code of Practice.* London: NHS Executive Mental Health Task Force User Group.
16 Gamble D. (1999) The value of advocacy: Putting ethics into practice. *Psychiatric Bulletin* 23, 569–70.
17 Warne T. and McAndrew S. (2007) Bordering on insanity: Mis Nomer, reviewing the case of the condemned women. *Journal of Psychiatric and Mental Health Nursing* 14, 155–62.
18 Jameton A. (1984) *Nursing Practice: The Ethical Issues.* Upper Saddle River, NJ: Prentice Hall.
19 Corley M., Minick P., Elswick R., and Jacobs M. (2005) Nurse moral distress and ethical work environment. *Nursing Ethics* 12, 382–90.
20 Deacon M., Warne T., and McAndrew S. (2006) Closeness, chaos, and crisis: The attractions of working in acute mental health care. *Journal of Psychiatric and Mental Health Nursing* 13, 750–7.
21 Barker P. and Cutliffe J. (1999) Clinical risk: A need for engagement not observation. *Mental Health Practice* 2, 8–12.
22 Bowles A. (2000) Therapeutic nursing care in acute psychiatric wards: Engagement over control. *Journal of Psychiatric and Mental Health Nursing* 7, 179–84.
23 Bowers L., Alexander J., Simpson A., *et al.* (2004) Cultures of psychiatry and the professional socialization process: The case of containment methods for disturbed patients. *Nurse Education Today* 24, 435–42.
24 Nursing and Midwifery Council (2008) *The Code: Standards of Conduct, Performance and Ethics for Nurses and Midwives.* London: NMC.
25 Higginson R. (2009) Haywood Case shows NMC out of touch. *British Journal of Nursing* 18 (9), 522–3.
26 Webster G. and Baylis F. (2000) Moral residue. In Rubin S. and Zoloth L. (Eds.) *Margin of Error: The Ethics of Mistakes in the Practice of Medicine.* Hagerstown, MD: University Publishing.
27 Gourney K. (2005) The changing face of psychiatric nursing. *Advances in Psychiatric Treatment* 11, 6–11.
28 Menzies Lyth I. (1988) *Containing Anxiety in Institutions: Selected Essays.* London: Free Association Books.
29 McDaniel C. (1995) Organisational culture and ethics work satisfaction. *Journal of Nursing Administration* 25, 15–21.
30 Goffman E. (1961) *Asylums: Essays on the Social Situation of Mental Patients and Other Inmates.* Garden City, NY: Anchor Books.
31 Rosenhan D.L. (1973) On being sane in insane places. *Science* 179, 249–58.
32 Eizenberg M., Desiviya H., and Hirschfeld M. (2009) Moral distress questionnaire for clinical nurses: Instrument development. *Journal of Advanced Nursing* 65 (4), 885–92.
33 Ricoeur P. op. cit.

6 The social worker

Shulamit Ramon

The historical development of mental health social work

Social work was formally established in the United Kingdom at the end of the nineteenth century. It developed out of charitable work focused on financial support for poor families. The second main strand in social work was represented by the *Settlement Movement*, which concentrated on improving the communal life of poor people by living with them, using community work methods to support and empower.

The major impetus to developing mental health social work at the beginning of the twentieth century was related to the work of leading psychiatrists and psychologists with 'shell-shocked' soldiers during the First World War.[1,2] This approach led to the establishment of the psychodynamically oriented Tavistock Clinic in London, where the first British psychiatric social worker was appointed in 1920.[3] The second such appointment took place only in 1927, to the Hackney Jewish Child guidance clinic.

Social workers in both the children and the adults outpatient services provided comprehensive psychosocial history of the child/adult and their family, enabled parents, teachers and partners of adult clients to understand the underlying psychological reasons for the index client's mental ill health, and guided them as to how they could actively support that family member.

The first course leading to the qualification of mental health social workers (originally titled 'psychiatric social workers') took place in 1929, at the London School of Economics, with an American grant.

Duly Authorised Officers without social work qualification have been employed in psychiatric hospitals since 1935, to provide a mixture of administrative and support functions to inpatients. This title was changed in the 1959 Mental Health Act to that of *Mental Welfare Officers*, who were recruited mostly from among qualified psychiatric social workers, though the Act did not stipulate such a qualification.

Until 1972 mental health social work existed as a separate service unit within social services departments. With the acceptance of the recommendations of the Seebohm report in 1968, generic social services departments came into being, strongly opposed by most psychiatric social workers afraid of being squeezed by child protection workers.

All English-speaking countries have also opted in the last quarter of the twentieth century for de-institutionalization as their core mental health policy, leading to the closure of many of their psychiatric hospitals, replacing them by community-based services and by small psychiatric wards in general hospitals.[4] This fundamental change has led to the relocation of Mental Health Social Workers (MHSWs) away from institutions into community services, to a renewed interest in rehabilitation, and more recently also in the newly defined recovery approach.[5] This trend suited MHSWs, who were more in favour of both de-institutionalization and community mental health than other members of the multi-disciplinary mental health teams.[6]

Furthermore, since the 1990s we have witnessed a considerable increase in user involvement in mental health education, in research and in advisory capacity in services,[7] some of which have been initiated by social workers (such as the *Camden Mind Users Policy Group*, initiated by Iris Nutting, then team leader of Camden mental health social workers at Friern hospital, North London).

Since the mid-1990s social workers have been seconded to mental health trusts, though they remain formally members of social services departments. They are to be found in most service teams of the trusts (e.g. crisis and home treatment teams, early intervention, rehabilitation), though usually there would be only one or at most two of them per team.

Underpinning values

Social work, including its mental health branch, is ethically governed by a set of values which are expected to be universal and adhered to in everyday practice,[8] even though their implementation may prove at times to be problematic in terms of balancing care and control and in terms of professional authority and power.

The values are derived from the liberal collectivist, humanistic, tradition of the twentieth century within which social work developed.

The core values are social justice; respect for people who social workers meet at their most vulnerable state; readiness to help in a way which will enable the client to retain dignity; self-determination; and enhancement of their problem-solving abilities. Social workers are expected to take an active stance against any type of discrimination. Furthermore, social workers are committed to pursuing a psychosocial approach in any area of their practice, and believe that most clients have the potential to grow and positively change.

The usual ethical rules of any helping profession also apply to MHSWs, such as maintaining confidentiality and a non-judgemental approach towards clients' behaviour.

Several elements stand out as central to MHSW:

1   The right to fail – this comes as part of the right to self-determination, in that social workers are aware that risk needs to be taken at times to enable people to grow and develop, or as a basic human right of making a mistake. When social workers take this right seriously, they are able to have a genuine discussion with clients as to the pros and cons of risk taking, of learning from success as much as of learning from failure.[9]

2   The wish to take an active stance against discrimination applies to working well with clients who come from ethnic minorities, from sexual orientation minorities, and to combating stigma against mental illness in one's practice.

3   The adherence to a psychosocial approach entails ensuring that both the psychological and the social aspects of users' lives are attended to, an issue of importance in mental health where often biological aspects are attended to, but the psychosocial ones are not getting the same priority.[10]

Conceptual frameworks

Conceptually social workers have been influenced by psychodynamic as well as learning theories,[11-14] but have not embraced any given method of work coming out of these approaches in its pure form. The social dimension of their work is at times perceived to be more important than the psychological aspects.[15] In addition to accepting that structural issues prevent people from having the social place they deserve,[16] and being critical of the medical model, social workers developed the strengths approach in its application to mental health,[17] though this is not acknowledged by other mental health disciplines.

Ways of working

Social workers in the United Kingdom use mainly casework methods, namely working with individuals affected by mental ill health and their families; seeking to find solutions to the psychosocial difficulties they face, such as inability to work, family relationships, financial and housing needs.[18] They often act as advocates and intermediaries between social security, housing, education services, the clients and their family; initiate direct payments/individual-ized budgets schemes, acting as care co-ordinators of the care programme approach (CPA), social supervisors and an appropriate adult in addition to being an Approved Social Worker (ASW).

An important component of their work presently focuses on their legal role. In place since 1983, ASWs have to provide their view as to whether such an admission is warranted along-side the views of psychiatrists and general practitioners (GPs).

In England and Wales, but not in Scotland or Northern Ireland, other mental health professionals, such as nurses, occupational therapists and psychologists, can also be trained to become Approved Mental Health Practitioners (AMHPs) alongside existing ASWs as from 2009.[19]

The role requires them to:

- assess people when an application has been made for a compulsory admission to a psychiatric unit;
- arrange the follow-up to such an admission;
- prepare reports on individual service users for mental health review tribunals (estab-lished within the 1959 Mental Health Act);
- work with the nearest relative;[20]
- co-ordinate the multi-disciplinary assessment, which has to be carried out by a psychia-trist and a GP in addition to the social worker, within a specified limited period of time;
- co-ordinate the transfer of the client to a safe facility as agreed in the assessment; and
- initiate a guardianship order.

Each of these tasks calls for somewhat different knowledge and skills, as well as emphasis and use of a range of more generic skills.[21-23] In each task social workers are asked not to replicate the psychiatric assessment but to complement it. For example, they have to look for the least restrictive alternative to hospitalization before they can recommend a hospital admission, rather than diagnose mental illness. Social workers have an autonomous position as they can disagree with the views of the other professions. The role requires exercising more social control than care, a contested issue within social work.

Training to become an approved social worker requires 60 days of academic input and supervised practice initially, followed by 5 days refresher training annually. Individual social workers can take it up after 2 years of post-qualification work experience. This compares with 2 days training for GPs and 1 day for psychiatrists.

ASWs are unhappy and unsure about the move to AMHPs, mainly due to the fear of further dilution of the social perspective by people coming from a non-social work background who have not been trained to know and apply such a perspective in practice.[21] Workforce research has highlighted that there were 4,500 ASWs in the United Kingdom in 2004 out of 46,000 qualified social workers, a large proportion of them over 50 years of age. As a group they were demoralized due to high caseloads, lack of support from other stakeholders (chiefly the police and the ambulance service) and the high level of risk to themselves that the role entails.[25]

Ethical dilemmas

The role of mental health social worker brings with it some inherent ethical dilemmas unrelated to the legal role, and some which are more focused within the legal function.

Ethical dilemmas inherent to the role

1   MHSWs in the United Kingdom tend to work in the statutory sector, where they have a dual social mandate to provide both care and control to their clients and the general public. Straddling these two poles inevitably leads to experiencing ethical dilemmas. Most of the dilemmas looked at below demonstrate an aspect of the care and control unresolved tension.[26,27] Research on inquiries in health and social care[28] and of mental health inquiries specifically[29] highlights this tension, as well as the difficulties which MHSWs have in defining their precise contribution *vis-à-vis* that of other professions.

Furthermore, in her analysis of the lessons from mental health inquiries for social workers, Reith[30] outlined the obstacle of underplaying or overplaying the role of social factors in mental health work, and suggested that it is necessary to balance the social perspective with the medical one. I would argue that the issue is not one of balance, but of what is more pertinent to a specific case/person, and that attempts at forcing a balance would only lead to an artificial construction of reality. The reality of mental health services is one in which psychiatrists are the most dominating group, who by and large opt for the medical model even when they are ready to consider social perspectives. Social workers are in a minority position, and though they may be listened to within their team due to shared experience and respect, this is insufficient to swing the power imbalance presently in existence in our mental health services.

2   Working with adults experiencing mental health problems often brings to focus the likely negative impact their ill health has on other family members, especially children. However, often the parents – usually mothers – are keen to continue to function in their parenting role, which can act as an important motivator in enabling them to recover earlier. The removal of a child is often experienced by the parent clients as a confirmation of their failure as human beings, at a time when they need to feel that there is a purpose to their lives and that they have abilities, and not only disabilities.

For the social worker working with adults this is a difficult ethical dilemma. Often child protection workers are keen on the early removal of the child to ensure that she/he is neither neglected nor abused, failing to see the perspective of the parent. While the social worker of the parent is often able to see the value of the child remaining with the parent, they too are committed to ensuring that the child will not suffer unduly. We are also aware of the damage that removal from home carries with it for the child and the family as a whole.

A creative and constructive way of addressing this issue was established by a social worker in the early 1990s.[31] Marie Diggins, then working as a senior mental health social worker in Lambeth, having won a Community Care Award, began taking children from such families away on outings with a colleague in her own time. She then created a specialized project, titled 'Building Bridges', dedicated to working jointly with parents experiencing mental illness, their partners and children, where the needs of each family member were addressed too. The initial scheme was funded by the Department of Health (England) and Joint Health and Social Care funding; nine such services exist today within the Family Welfare Association, and a national network of more than 200 organizations has been established, led by the Social Psychiatry Network (www.spn.org.uk).

While this seminal work cannot ensure that children of parents experiencing mental illness will not be removed from home ever, it highlights the need for thinking creatively 'outside of the box' when an ethical dilemma of this magnitude is met.

Ethical dilemmas related to the legal role of ASWs and AMHPs

A number of such dilemmas relate to risk issues inherent in mental health work for any discipline. These include the need to avoid harm to others by the client as well as to avoid self-harm; and self-harm is much more prevalent than harm to others in the field of mental health, even though UK media and politicians would lead one to believe that this is not the case.[32,33] The professional and government-led literature is full of references to risk avoidance.

However, risk taking is hardly ever mentioned, while it is an essential component to any work with mental health clients which focuses on their growth – as it is for all human beings. Elsewhere[34] I have attempted to look at the cost of focusing only on risk avoidance and what calculated risk taking in mental health might mean. The value of the right to fail, the development of the 'strengths approach' mentioned above and of the recovery approach which has come to the fore in the 1990s[35] highlight the necessity to develop risk-taking thinking and practice within mental health.

Specific dilemmas related to the role of the ASW (and now of the AMHP) entail:

1   The decision to recommend the removal of a person from his/her home, and against his/her will, due to being at risk to himself/herself or to others, or to the inability to function because of mental illness, implies the temporary suspension of his/her basic citizens' right for the duration of the hospitalization. This cannot be taken lightly, as ASWs are made aware of the implications of such a deprivation, the risks of hospitalization itself in terms of self and social esteem and at times of safety too.

In addition, the ASWs are specifically asked to look for the least restrictive alternative to hospitalization when they recommend the removal of the person from their home. However, very few such alternatives exist in the United Kingdom, making a mockery of this requirement, and putting ASWs in an untenable position.

2   If the ASWs disagree with the psychiatrist and the GP's recommendation at the end of an assessment, they have the right to say so and to refuse to follow the recommendations made by the non-social workers assessors. While this is rare, it does happen. One can imagine the pressure put on the social worker to change their mind.

The analysis of mental health inquiries[36,37] highlights that often ASWs have been accused of ill judgement and negligence, either when people were not hospitalized or allowed to leave a hospital too early to prevent a killing by a person experiencing severe mental illness. While such accusations were not attributed *only* to ASWs, the personal, and often the professional, cost to any mental health professional of being involved in such an inquiry is extremely high. Under these circumstances most mental health professionals, including social workers, would succumb to the pressure and tend to opt for hospitalization and deprivation of liberty than otherwise.

The same dilemma of deprivation of liberties applies also to guardianship, though to a lesser extent. A guardianship order is usually initiated by social workers, and requires the person to present himself/herself to a mental health facility as well as to live in a sheltered accommodation. Similar issues arise in regard to the existing community supervision order.[38]

The community treatment order (CTO), used in Australia, Canada and the United States, is currently being experimented with in Scotland[39] (see Chapter 25). It makes more mandatory demands on the person than guardianship does. If social workers are asked to be involved in supervising people on CTO – as is the case in Australia, then they will be presented with similar dilemmas to those highlighted in relation to guardianship.

Until now it has been straightforward to limit the issue of deprivation of liberty to hospital/secure unit admissions, but this is increasingly not the case, raising the issue of the justification of imposing restrictions on people judged to be able to live in the community.

3   In working with the Nearest Relative (NR) ASWs encounter more than one ethical dilemma. The NR has the right to initiate an assessment and to oppose the decision to compulsorily admit a family member; the ASW's duty is to provide the NR with the information as to how to initiate an assessment and how to oppose decisions taken by professionals. The information and the procedure are complicated, and require sensitive handling, especially given that the NR is likely to be upset. When the ASW disagrees with the NR's decision it is less likely that the right information will be delivered in the right way.

4   Confidentiality presents a major challenge in terms of the potential ethical dilemmas it raises for social workers. It is often an issue in the relationships between social workers and their colleagues from other professions, in the relationships between social workers and their clients and in the relationships between social workers and NRs. Unless users are happy for ASWs to disclose information to their NR and other professional figures, the social worker should not do so, *in principle*. However, this principle is called into question if disclosing the information could be essential to risk avoidance. Furthermore, if the disclosure could lead to a more shared way of working among all of the relevant partners, it should at least merit a re-consideration.

A thorough attempt to put these considerations into a working policy was made by a service coalition in Surrey, England in 2001 (Surrey-Wide Operational Partnership Group), followed by research work carried out by Rapaport, Pinfold and Bellringer at the Institute of Psychiatry.[40]

Conclusions

This chapter has highlighted ethical dilemmas inherent in the role of mental health social workers in the United Kingdom, as well as the dilemmas which arise out of their legal role. The dilemmas relate closely to the tension derived from the dual social mandate this group has, to both care for *and* control people experiencing mental ill health. The tension relates also to the wish and need to reduce harm to self and to others within this population (risk avoidance), side by side with the wish and need to support clients who have been institution-alized for a long time on their journey to a more dignified life in the community and towards a greater control over their own lives (risk taking). The co-existence of these trends is con-flictual and is often resolved by opting for the more controlling option in the name of risk avoidance, reinforced by the cultural and political climate of living in a risk-oriented society.[11,12] Although MHSWs continue to support non-institutionalized options as well as user involvement, this seems insufficient to lead to less controlling solutions, especially given the general trend to introduce more controlling measures in the community.

It is rare to find resolutions which focus on shared work and giving clients more say, but these do exist as the case of the Building Bridges project highlighted earlier, and need to be fostered further. However, the weak power position of MHSWs within the multi-disciplinary network of mental health services militates against the search for such solutions.

Notes

1 Timms, N. *Social Casework*. London: Routledge and Kegan Paul, 1964.
2 Ramon, S. *Psychiatry in Britain: Meaning and Policy*. London: Croom Helm, 1985.
3 Dicks, H. *Fifty Years of the Tavistock*. London: Tavistock Publications, 1970.
4 Shera, W., Aviram, U., Healy, B., and Ramon, S. Mental health systems reform: A multi country comparison. *Social Work in Health Care*, 2002, 35, 1–2, 547–75.
5 Ramon, S., Healy, B., and Renouf, N. Recovery from mental illness as an emergent concept and practice in Australia and the UK. *International Journal of Social Psychiatry*, 2007, 53, 2, 108–22.
6 Ramon, S. (eds.) *Psychiatric Hospital Closure: Myths and Realities*. London: Chapman Hall, 1992.
7 Beresford, P. The right for self determination of Mental Health Service Users. In: Ramon, S., and Williams, J.E. (eds) *Mental Health at the Crossroads: The Promise of the Psychosocial Approach*. Aldershot: Ashgate Publishing, 2005.
8 Beckett, C. and Maynard, A. *Values and Ethics in Social Work*. London: Sage, 2006.
9 McDermott, R. (ed.) *Self Determination in Social Work*. London: Routledge and Kegan Paul, 1975.
10 Tew, J. (ed.) *Social Perspectives of Mental Health*. London: Jessica Kingsley, 2005.
11 Howe, D. *Attachment Theory for Social Work Practice*. London: Macmillan, 1995.
12 Hutton, J.M. (ed.) *Short-Term Contracts in Social Work*. London: Routledge and Kegan Paul, 1977.
13 Marsh, P. and Doel, M. *Task-Centred Social Work*. Aldershot: Ashgate Publishing, 1993.
14 Hudson, B. and Macdonald, E. *Behavioural Social Work: An Introduction*. London: Macmillan, 1986.
15 Tew 2005 op. cit.
16 Pilgrim, D. and Rogers, A. *Mental Health and Inequality*. Basingstoke: Palgrave Macmillan, 2003.
17 Rapp, C. *The Strengths Perspective of Case Management with Persons Suffering from Severe Mental Illness*. Oxford: Oxford University Press, 1998.
18 Golightly, M. *Social Work and Mental Health: Transforming Social Work Practice*. Exeter: Learning Matters, 2008.
19 Rapaport, J. New roles in mental health: The creation of the approved mental health practitioner. *Journal of Integrated Care*, 2006, 14, 5, 37–46.
20 Rapaport, J. The informal caring experience: Issues and dilemmas. In: Ramon, S. and Williams, J.E. (eds.) *Mental Health at the Crossroads: The Promise of the Psychosocial Approach*. Aldershot: Ashgate Publishing, 2005, pp. 155–70.
21 Barnes, M., Bowl, R., and Fisher, M. *Sectioned: Social Services and the 1983 Mental Health Act*. Routledge: London, 1990.
22 Rapaport 2005 op. cit.
23 Hatfield, B. Powers to detain under mental health legislation in England and the role of the approved social worker: An analysis of patterns and trends under the 1983 Mental Health Act in six local authorities. *British Journal of Social Work*, 2008, 38, 8, 1553–71.

24 Rapaport op. cit. pp. 155–70.

25 Huxley, P., Evans, S., Webber, M., and Gately, C. Staff shortages in the mental health workforce: The case of the disappearing social worker. *Health and Social Care in the Community*, 2005, 13, 6, 504–13.

26 Bainbridge, L. Competing paradigms in mental health practice and education. In: Pease, B. and Fook, J. (eds.) *Transforming Social Work Practice: Postmodern Critical Perspective*. London: Routledge, 1999, pp. 179–94.

27 Thompson, P. Devils and deep blue seas: The social worker in-between. *Journal of Social Work Practice*, 2003, 17, 1, 35–47.

28 Stanley, N. and Manthorpe, J. *The Age of the Inquiry: Learning and Blaming in Health and Social Care*. London: Routledge, 2004.

29 Reith, M. *Community Care Tragedies: A Practice Guide to Mental Health Inquiries*. Birmingham: Venture Press, 1998.

30 Reith ibid. pp. 180–6.

31 Diggins, M. Innovation as a professional way of life – the Building Bridges Project for Parents-Users of mental health services and their children. In: Ramon, S. (ed.) *A Stakeholder Approach to Innovation in Mental Health Services*. Brighton: Pavilion Publishers, 2000, pp. 77–93.

32 Taylor, J.P. and Gunn, J. Homicides by people with mental illness: Myth and reality. *British Journal of Psychiatry*, 1999, 174, 9–14.

33 Ramon, S. and Savio, M. *A Scandal of the 80s and 90s: Media Representations of Mental Illness Issues in Britain and Italy*. Brighton: Pavilion Publishers, 2000.

34 Ramon, S. Risk avoidance and risk taking in mental health social work. In: Sapouna, L. and Hermann, P. (eds.) *Knowledge in Mental Health: Reclaiming the Social*. New York, NY: Nova Publications 2006, pp. 39–56.

35 Repper, J. and Perkins, R. *Social Inclusion and Recovery: A Model for Mental Health Practice*. Edinburgh: Balliere Tindall, 2003.

36 Reith 1998, op. cit.

37 Stanley and Manthorpe 2004, op. cit.

38 Canvin, K., Bartlett, A., and Pinfold, V. A bittersweet pill to swallow: Learning from mental health service users' responses to compulsory community care in England. *Health and Social Care in the Community*, 2002, 10, 5, 361–9.

39 Campbell, J., Brophy, L., Healy, B., and O'Brien, A.M. International perspectives on the use of community treatment orders: Implications for mental health social workers. *British Journal of Social Work*, 2006, 36, 1101–18.

40 Slade, M., Pinfold. V., Rapaport, J., and Bellringer, C. Best practice when service users do not consent to sharing information with carers. *British Journal of Psychiatry*, 2007, 190, 148–55.

41 Beck, A. *The Risk Society*. London: Sage, 1992.

42 Rose, N. *Powers of Freedom: Reframing Political Thought*. Cambridge: Cambridge University Press, 2002.

7   The clinical psychologist

Lucy Johnstone

Introduction

Clinical psychology is a popular career route for psychology graduates, who gain their professional qualification by following a 3-year postgraduate course which covers clinical, academic and research skills. The majority work in Adult Mental Health, in a variety of settings such as wards, clinics and community teams. Clinical psychologists are perhaps most strongly associated with individual therapy, especially cognitive behavioural therapy (CBT). However, they also work with families and groups, offer supervision to individuals, teams and, organisations, carry out research and evaluation into services, and, increasingly, take on consultancy and leadership roles now that other professions may be able to offer psychological therapy more cheaply.

Here I explore clinical psychology's dilemma about how to position itself in relation to psychiatry. Of course, whether or not this is seen as an ethical issue depends on one's views about the nature and purpose of psychiatry (see also Chapters 2 and 3). Biomedical models of mental distress are not necessarily problematic if psychiatry is seen as sound in its basic principles, working steadily towards more effective 'treatments' for those who are unfortunately stricken by 'mental illness'. If this is accepted, disputes will mainly arise about the most effective or efficient ways of achieving this worthy aim. In the words of one psychologist, 'There have never been any anti-oncologists, anti-cardiologists, (or) anti-gastroenterologists' (p xiv).[1] In psychiatry this is not the case; fundamental disagreements about the validity, nature and purpose of traditional psychiatry date back to its origins in the early nineteenth century and have continued ever since, surfacing most powerfully in the so-called 'anti-psychiatry' movement of the1960s and in today's service user/survivor movement. The issues have also been extensively debated within the profession of clinical psychology.

Clinical psychologists who accept these critiques are faced with unavoidable ethical dilemmas about their role and work. The key question becomes not 'How can we best use our scientific expertise to help the sick?' but 'How ought we to help the most disadvantaged members of our society when they are emotionally distressed?' This quickly leads to other questions:

- How do we understand the reasons for people's distress?
- What role ought we to play in alleviating these causes?
- What are our professional and moral obligations as members of a society in which this kind of suffering occurs?

Psychologists who believe that service users' distress is nearly always an understandable response to trauma, abuse and social deprivation, see the answers in terms of an explicit commitment to social justice which must inform all aspects of our theories and practice.

My main references in this chapter come from the two publications in which the profession has debated these issues, *Clinical Psychology Forum* and *The Psychologist*. The strength of feeling on both sides is evident in the language, which is often passionate and forthright.

Brief history of clinical psychology

The dilemma of how to position itself in relation to psychiatry dates back to the origins of clinical psychology in the 1950s (see Pilgrim and Treacher[2]).

In the early years, the political imperative was to carve out a separate area of expertise from psychiatry, rather than simply carrying out tests at the request of the psychiatrist. This involved a challenge to the status quo which at the time consisted of the two extremes of biomedical and psychoanalytic tenets. Psychiatry was seen by early behaviourists as failing to lead to behaviour change, whereas psychoanalysis was criticised for its reliance on unscientific and unobservable concepts; clinical psychologists argued that their theories offered a credible alternative to both. A defining moment was the inauguration of the core identity of 'scientist-practitioner', skilled in research-based therapy, at the Boulder Conference, Colorado, in 1949. This provided the foundation for clinical psychologists to develop independent expertise in the empirically-based approach of behaviour therapy, supplemented by cognitive therapy in the 1970s.

During the 1980s many psychologists withdrew from the professional conflicts inherent in in-patient work to carve out a more autonomous role in the community. This usually consisted of offering individual therapy, generally CBT, to out-patients. This trend has recently been reversed and there has been a revival of interest in psychological approaches to psychosis, 'personality disorders' and so on. While CBT is still a core skill, most psychologists now describe themselves as 'integrative' in orientation, and many training courses claim to offer a hybrid 'reflective scientist-practitioner' model which acknowledges that working with people draws on intuition and personal qualities as well as empirical data, and encourages awareness of the impact of one's own feelings and social identity.

The biomedical perspective, based on the assumption that most psychiatric patients are suffering from disease processes with primarily biological causes, is alive and well, despite various recent modifications. Clinical psychologists are, by virtue of their training and status, particularly well-placed to reflect on and raise questions about these assumptions and argue for better answers. However, while the relationship between clinical psychology and psychiatry has often been strained, this has usually been because of professional issues of boundaries, status and ownership of particular privileges and skills – 'turf wars', as such tussles are sometimes termed. Much more rarely have the conflicts arisen from ethical concerns about the nature and purpose of psychiatry – indeed many, perhaps most, clinical psychologists seem to regard this as unproblematic. This is one consequence of an uncritical acceptance of the assumption that as applied scientist-practitioners drawing on empirical evidence, our theory and practice are objective and value-free.

At the same time, a vocal minority of clinical psychologists has, over the few decades, protested loudly and clearly about what they see as unjustified collusion with biomedical psychiatry. Mary Boyle, a senior member of the profession, phrases it thus:

> We work in service systems largely based on a theoretical model which is more or less completely incompatible with ours. Heaven knows, we have bent over backwards to disguise this fact, not to give offence. We have extensively adopted the language of medicine, calling our clients' problems symptoms, illnesses and disorders; we have searched assiduously for the 'psychopathology' which would explain them. . . . Why are

we so timid in taking the lead? Why are we not producing high-profile reports with titles like 'Social causes of psychological problems'. . .. or 'The psychological impact of domestic violence'?. . .. Which (are the) truths we are still not speaking? (pp 4, 6).[3]

Similarly, David Pilgrim sees collusion in the profession's 'ambivalent position towards psychiatry – wanting full professional independence but, at times of selective convenience, co-opting a medical knowledge base' (p 304),[4] an on-the-fence position that has been criticised by other psychologists as well.[5,6]

Clinical psychologists who disagree with the tenets of biomedical psychiatry, sometimes loosely known as 'critical psychologists', are faced with three possible options in how they respond: challenge, compromise or avoidance. The challenge/compromise debate can be illustrated through discussion of diagnosis and biomedical models. The development of individual therapy perhaps gains its impetus from a desire to avoid such conflicts, but arguably it simply reproduces dilemmas about the 'psychologisation of distress' in a different setting, as described below. All these possible responses need to be considered in the light of the profession's views on the role of social inequality as the context for individual distress.

Clinical psychology and psychiatric diagnosis

Psychiatric diagnosis (see Chapter11) has been subjected to extensive criticism by clinical psychologists (and others) for being unreliable, non-valid, stigmatising and so on.[7-10] However, the profession is deeply divided on this issue, as was apparent after *The Psychologist* published a collection of scholarly articles arguing against the use of diagnosis in May 2007. Responses varied from moderate wishes 'not to abandon a procedure which has served us well' (p 346)[11] to the accusation that critics are 'the new totalitarians'[12] who use 'defensive rhetoric, ad hominem argument and sneer quotes' to advance their case.[13]

Clearly, where such passions are aroused, there must be more at stake than a disinterested scientific debate about the evidence. Pilgrim[1] suggests that this can only be fully understood by examining the related social, economic and professional issues, among them the role of the pharmaceutical companies. The hub of the argument for psychologists can perhaps be summarised as whether we see ourselves as dealing with people with problems, or patients with illnesses. If the former (as a great deal of recent evidence suggests), it does not make sense to expect service users' distress to fall into neat parcels along the lines of categorisation in the natural sciences, and nor should we expect anything other than superficial and temporary solutions from medical interventions.

Adherence to diagnosis despite its known limitations is particularly puzzling given that, as I and other critical psychologists have argued, our own core skill of formulation – a hypothesis about a person's difficulties, drawing on psychological theory – does in principle provide a valid, though not unproblematic, alternative which sets the scene for psychosocial rather than medical interventions.[14,15]

Clinical psychology and the biomedical model

Since diagnosis is the foundation stone of traditional psychiatry, the above critiques have been extended to the whole biomedical disease model and its associated theories, language and interventions. Psychologists have argued that this model is not only not evidence-based, but is actively damaging, medicalising the consequences of abuse and deprivation and creating life-long 'patients' in the process.[16,17] John Read in particular has argued strongly that much, perhaps most, of what is conceptualised as 'schizophrenia' or 'bipolar disorder' is in fact a psychological response to unresolved trauma.[18]

A kind of compromise has been reached by those psychologists, probably the majority, who now subscribe to the new orthodoxy of the 'vulnerability-stress' or 'biopsychosocial' model of mental distress. While this does at least put psychological and social factors on the map, it contains conceptual traps for the unwary. Sophisticated versions of the mixed model include Read's 'traumagenic neurodevelopmental' model[18] which acknowledges that abuse and emotional deprivation can have physiological effects on the brain and nervous system. In other words, there is a complex circular relationship between psychosocial events and our brains and bodies, not a simple one-way causal link which starts with biology. Critical psychologists argue that less sophisticated versions can simply serve to perpetuate the old assumptions under a new guise:

> The vulnerability-stress hypothesis . . . has proved to be an extraordinarily useful and effective mechanism for managing the potential threat to biological models. . . . Its usefulness lies in its seeming reasonableness (who could deny that biological and psychological and social factors interact?) and its inclusiveness (it encompasses both the biological and the social – surely better than focusing on only one?) while at the same time it firmly maintains the primacy of biology . . . by making it look as if the 'stress' of the model consists of ordinary stresses which most of us would cope with, but which overwhelm only 'vulnerable' people. We are thus excused from examining too closely either the events themselves or their meaning to the 'vulnerable' person (p 13).[19]

Read agrees: 'This is not an integration of models, it is a colonisation of the psychological and social by the biological. . . . The war is far from over. . . . Many of us still feel we are living in occupied territory' (p 596).[20]

Clinical psychology and psychological therapy

As already described, clinical psychologists have managed to avoid some of the more direct conflicts inherent in working within the mental health system by developing their own special skills such as individual therapy, traditionally CBT. However, this is not free of ethical dilemmas. Recently, clinical psychologists have been in the forefront of designing and delivering the new CBT training courses and interventions which constitute the first wave of the national *Improving Access to Psychological Therapies* (IAPT) project. Based on the arguments of Richard Layard, a Labour peer and health economist, IAPT is intended to treat less severe forms of anxiety and depression which prevent people from working, and thus pay for itself in terms of increased productivity and reduced uptake of benefits.

The explicitly economic justification for the IAPT programme raises, in a very stark form, the general ethical question of whose agent the clinical psychologist is, when working therapeutically. Is she/he primarily representing the interests of the state or the client? In the case of IAPT, is her/his main aim to help the clients makes sense of their distress, or to get them back to work, and what if these aims conflict? ('Do psychologists really want to get involved in . . . "therapy" as one means of cajoling the unwell and the impoverished into jobs that, for many, will be poorly paid, unrewarding and, indeed, unhealthy?').[21]

The roll-out of IAPT represents very specific opportunities (or perhaps temptations, in a moral sense) for clinical psychologists as trainers and deliverers of the new service. As David Smail puts it in an article titled 'Is clinical psychology selling its soul (again)?', 'As a clinical psychologist, one would have to be phenomenally incorruptible not to experience just a tiny frisson of interest at contemplating such inducements as those dangled by Layard before one's eyes' (p 18).[22] There are certainly those who feel that the profession has jumped onto a bandwagon without paying sufficient attention to practical or ethical issues, let alone the lack of evidence for the grand claims made for CBT.[23] However, such criticisms have been forcefully dismissed by senior members of the profession ('It is impossible to itemise all the misleading statements in Marzillier and Hall's seven pages of opinion . . . .'[24]).

Clinical psychologists have debated these issues extensively in relation to individual therapy in general. David Smail is well-known for his argument that psychotherapies are concerned with individual internal psychological states viewed in isolation from the social contexts which make them understandable and even rational responses.[25] This may be more of a danger for clinical psychologists than other therapists, since their chosen therapy specialism of CBT is arguably more directive and individualising, with the consequent danger of re-defining social problems as personal failings to be adjusted – negative cognitions to be challenged, core schema to be replaced by more 'adaptive' ones, and so on.[26] In this respect, CBT is a good fit with psychiatry, which may partly explain the foothold it has gained in services. (Some of the most lauded recent developments consist of exactly this kind of medical/CBT hybrid – for example cognitive therapy for depression, family management in psychosis[27]) (see also Chapter 8).

The middle ground should perhaps be an acknowledgement that therapy is not intrinsically individualising or unhelpful; it depends on how it is done.[28] All types of therapy should be practised within a reflexive, politically informed awareness of the impact of personal and social contexts on both therapist and client. Such a stance might have encouraged psychologists to be more outspoken about some aspects of IAPT while not denigrating the whole project. Some psychologists have played a part in the development of approaches (narrative, social inequalities and some systemic therapies) that explicitly start from this standpoint.[29]

Clinical psychology and social justice

Critical psychologists see a close link between adopting a perspective based on social injustice, and the need to challenge biomedical psychiatry. For example, they argue that psychiatric diagnosis, despite (or because of) its claims to be objective and value-free, can be used for the ultimately political purpose of re-defining understandable emotional reactions as illnesses, thus mystifying individuals about the true origins of their difficulties and allowing society as a whole to avoid painful truths about the way we live (see also Chapter 23). As described above, the arguments can also apply to the practice of therapy, and to the general 'psychologisation of distress' which means that 'deprivation, abuse, oppression and the social and political contexts of distress can largely be ignored' (Proctor cited on p 429).[30] This inevitably raises the question of whether, and how, clinical psychologists should be involved in wider moral and political problems and debates. Should the profession be expressing a view on such issues? Or should we shelter behind the traditional defence that these are 'political' matters beyond our remit as applied scientists?

The sub-group of clinical psychologists who describe themselves as community psychologists has developed the clearest response to these issues. Their core values are to do with seeing people holistically in their social settings. Rather than working primarily with individuals or families, community psychologists work in consultation with organisations and communities, supporting people to gain more control and influence over their lives through social action at a local level. Community psychologists do not see people's difficulties as a sign of individual failure to manage your life (by, for e.g. developing 'mental illnesses' or 'faulty cognitions'). Instead, they see distress as arising primarily from people's struggle to cope within a complex society that exerts many pressures on them. Hence, people do not need 'diagnosis' or 'treatment', but to build on the strengths they have developed in order to survive. The main role of individual therapy, if any, is to provide comfort, clarification about the social causes of distress and encouragement to use whatever resources are available to the client.[31]

The community psychology perspective receives strong support from two recent epidemiological summaries which put the case for the causal role of social inequality in a whole range of ills, including mental health problems, beyond reasonable doubt. Wilkinson and Pickett[32] present an overwhelming set of data in support of the hypothesis that above a certain level of material wealth, more equal societies do best on almost every measure – mental and physical health, violence, crime, obesity, education, community life and so on. The crucial factor here turns out not to be absolute material deprivation, harmful although that can be, but relative inequality within societies, which ultimately affects the security and social cohesion of the whole community.

This work is given added impetus from a recent World Health Organisation report[33] which found that as countries get richer, rates of mental illness increase, and that this needs to be understood and treated less in terms of individual pathology and more as a response to the complex consequences of inequality and injustice. The main author summarised the findings as: 'Injustice and inequality are deeply toxic to us' (Friedli[34]). The implication is that the narrow focus on individual solutions to mental health problems should be replaced by a 'social solution'.[33]

The challenge in this research is to all mental health professionals, not just psychologists. However, as psychologists our extra privileges (high status and pay, minimal statutory duties, doctoral-level training) perhaps bring extra responsibility to use our position wisely and ethically.

Summary: challenge, compromise or avoidance

The common thread running through these issues is the dilemma, for critical psychologists, about challenge, compromise or avoidance as a response to traditional psychiatric practice. There are no clear guidelines for indicating when compromise turns into collusion. It is impossible to work as a critical psychologist on, for example, an in-patient ward and not collude to some extent; if you object to every use of psychiatric labelling, your role will be impossible. Hence one psychologist's conclusion that 'Many psychologists have spent enormous amounts of energy (sometimes whole careers) trying to change intransigent systems and institutions such as hospitals; I believe that our energies are best spent working where we can be most effective and taking a critical stance on things from the outside which we feel are harmful and unethical' (p 42).[35] Others have described such attitudes as 'misplaced preciousness about the lofty and unsullied role that the profession should have in the field of mental health' (p 35).[36] For some, the answer is avoidance, although Pilgrim argues that you cannot resolve the dilemma by 'leav(ing) the dirty work to others for reasons of convenience or conscience' (p 6).[37]

> Relocating activity does not mean that psychologists are outsiders . . .. Those working in voluntary settings are still backed up by, and refer to, more coercive parts of the system . . . . We cannot opt about and climb some moral high ground. We are all implicated.

The dilemmas surface in a particularly acute form in the debate about the possible role of clinical psychologists as prescribers, and their recent new roles as Clinical Supervisors and Approved Mental Health Professionals, making decisions about compulsory treatment and detention. Some critical psychologists argue that the profession's involvement could lead to opportunities to 'unprescribe', or resist the overuse of medication.[1,38] Similarly, Pilgrim (p 5)[37] argues that psychologists' inclusion in decisions about compulsory treatment could create 'new possibilities to break the medical mould of the past. For example, diagnosis could be replaced by formulation'. Others are more sceptical: 'Perhaps we need more humility regarding how much better or more humane we would be in comparison to our colleagues' (p 41).[35]

Gelsthorpe notes that 'stayers believe they have done the right thing in remaining in the service. Conversely leavers believe they themselves have done the right thing by leaving' (p 34).[39] He suggests that this is an unhelpful polarisation, and that both groups need to find 'the opportunity to dissent in an appropriate way without feeling obliged to defend themselves from the criticisms of people who have chosen another course' (p 38). It must be acknowledged that trying to bring about change in systems by working within them can be exhausting, demoralising and frustrating; an article in which I explored these pressures elicited many heartfelt responses from other psychologists.[40] Perhaps a middle ground is to acknowledge that individuals may need to adopt different strategies at different points in their lives and careers, but to hope that they retain their commitment to change wherever they work.

The collective noun for a group of clinical psychologists, as the joke goes, is 'a disagreement'. It sometimes seems as if we are happier to fight among ourselves than to direct our anger where it is most needed. There are some shining exceptions, of course; Sue Holland's work in deprived communities,[11] the STEPS Primary Care Project in Glasgow;[12] and the West Dunbartonshire Literacy Project[13] to take just three examples. Other psychologists choose to work with refugee survivors of torture[14] or bring a psychological perspective to nuclear weapons, apartheid and the Iraq war.[45] It is not a coincidence that all of these pioneers frame their inspiration in explicitly value-based and social equalities terms, while also retaining a strong commitment to scientific endeavour in order to improve human welfare, or, to put it at its simplest, 'make the world a better place' and 'tackle oppression and injustice in our world' (p 930).[13] This implies a need for psychologists who are 'not precious' and 'are happy to challenge the dominant ideas and sacred cows' (p 847).[12] For critical psychologists,

> whether we like it or not, psychology, like any discipline, contains an implicit political ideology; and silence or denial of our involvement is no less a political act than explicit political action . . . .. The choice we have to make, therefore, is not between involvement and non-involvement, but between awareness of our involvement or denial.
>
> Kidner, cited on (p 430)[30]

The problem is, as we have seen, that these are not the convictions of the profession as a whole. 'It is as if the profession still is uncertain about whether to critique or emulate the medical framing of distress and difference' (p 4).[16] We urgently need to develop a clear and coherent position on these matters. 'We see it as essential that psychologists working in psychiatric systems have a critical and questioning perspective on the values and practice that dominate mental health services and psychology. . . . Whilst we believe that our profession can contribute to obscuring and individualising people's experiences, we also believe it has much to offer in terms of explanations of human despair' (p 8).[17] For critical psychologists, this includes 'a satisfactory analysis of the structure and functioning of social power', (p 6),[18] a position which has been explored elsewhere.[19]

One obvious way of meeting these aims is, as many clinical psychologists are doing, to work alongside the increasingly sophisticated service user/survivor movement in its campaign for more humane mental health services which offer an alternative to the current theories and practices. The *Hearing Voices Network* is a prime example of this kind of collaboration.[50]

Finally, clinical psychologists should not forget the nearest thing they have to a unique skill – psychological formulation. Depending on how it is carried out, this 'process of ongoing collaborative sense-making' (p 8)[51] can be a way of reintroducing personal meaning, relationship and social contexts and mutual collaboration into the understanding of mental distress. In this way, formulation can provide an antidote to the expert-driven, individualising, disempowering process of psychiatric diagnosis and the practice which is based on it.[9,14,15]

Conclusion

An overwhelming amount of evidence tells us that as clinical psychologists we cannot afford to ignore the context of social inequality and injustice in our work, for scientific as well as ethical reasons. This will inevitably also involve us in challenging, not colluding with, some of the core tenets of biomedical psychiatry. In this way we will be facing ethical dilemmas head on, wherever we work, and fulfilling our moral and professional responsibilities as clinical psychologists.

Notes

 1 Bentall, R (2009) *Doctoring the mind: Why psychiatric treatments fail.* London: Allen Lane.
 2 Pilgrim, D and Treacher, A (1992) *Clinical psychology observed.* London: Routledge.
 3 Boyle, M (2006) Speaking the truth about ourselves. *Clinical Psychology Forum*, 168, 4–6.
 4 Pilgrim, D (2000) Psychiatric diagnosis: More questions than answers. *The Psychologist*, 13, 6, 302–5.
 5 Diamond, B (2001) Clinical psychologists' responses to the Mental Health Act Reforms. *Clinical Psychology*, 19, 9–12.
 6 Harper, D (2001) Psychiatric and psychological concepts in understanding psychotic experiences. *Clinical Psychology*, 7, 21–7.
 7 Boyle, M (2002) *Schizophrenia: A scientific delusion?* (2nd edn). Hove: Routledge.
 8 Boyle, M (2007) The problem with diagnosis. *The Psychologist*, 20, 5, 290–2.
 9 Johnstone, L (2008) Psychiatric diagnosis. In R Tummey and T Turner (eds.) *Critical issues in mental health*. Basingstoke: Palgrave Macmillan.
10 May, R (2007) Working outside the diagnostic framework. *The Psychologist*, 20, 5, 300–1.
11 Congdon, P (2007) Correspondence. *The Psychologist*, 20, 6, 346–7.
12 Scott, M (2007) Correspondence. *The Psychologist*, 20, 6, 346.
13 Egan, V (2007) Correspondence. *The Psychologist*, 20, 8, 468.
14 Boyle, M (2001) *Abandoning diagnosis and (cautiously) adopting formulation.* Paper presented at British Psychological Society Centenary Conference, Glasgow.
15 Johnstone, L (2006) Controversies and debates about formulation. In L Johnstone and R Dallos (eds.) *Formulation in psychology and psychotherapy: Making sense of people's problems.* London: Routledge.
16 Johnstone, L (2000) *Users and abusers of psychiatry: A critical look at psychiatric practice* (2nd edn). Hove: Brunner-Routledge.
17 Read, J (1997) Child abuse and psychosis: A literature review and implications for professional practice. *Professional Psychology: Research and Practice*, 28, 4, 448–56.
18 Read, J, Rudegeair, T, and Farrelly, S (2006) Relationship between child abuse and psychosis. In W Larkin and AP Morrison (eds.) *Trauma and psychosis: New directions for theory and therapy*. London: Routledge.

19 Boyle, M (2002) It's all done with smoke and mirrors. Or, how to create the illusion of a schizophrenic brain disease. *Clinical Psychology*, 12, 9–16.

20 Read, J (2005) The bio-bio-bio model of madness. *The Psychologist*, 18, 10, 596–7.

21 Moloney, P and Priest, P (2009) Correspondence, *The Psychologist*, 22, 2, 96.

22 Smail, D (2006) Is clinical psychology selling its soul (again)? *Clinical Psychology Forum*, 168, 17–20.

23 Marzillier, J and Hall, J (2009) The challenge of the Layard initiative. *The Psychologist*, 22, 5, 396–9.

24 Clark, D, Fonagy, P, Turpin, G, Pilling, S, Adams, M, Burke, M, Cape, J, Cate, T, Ehlers, A, Garety, P, Holland, R, Liebowitz, J, MacDonald, K, Roth, T, and Shafran, R (2009) Correspondence. *The Psychologist*, 22, 6, 466.

25 Smail, D (1996) *How to survive without psychotherapy*. London: Constable.

26 Proctor, G (2002) *The dynamics of power in counselling and psychotherapy*. Ross-on-Wye: PCCS Books.

27 Johnstone, L (1993) Family management in 'schizophrenia': Its assumptions and contradictions. *Journal of Mental Health*, 2, 255–69.

28 Roy-Chowdhury, S (2003) What is this thing called psychotherapy? *Clinical Psychology*, 29, 7–11.

29 Johnstone, L and Dallos, R (2006) (eds.) *Formulation in psychology and psychotherapy: Making sense of people's problems*. London: Routledge.

30 Joseph, S (2007) Agents of social control? *The Psychologist*, 20, 7, 429–31.

31 Orford, J (1994) *Community psychology: Theory and practice*. Chichester: Wiley.

32 Wilkinson, R and Pickett, K (2009) *The spirit level: Why more equal societies almost always do better*. London: Allen Lane.

33 World Health Organisation (2009) *Mental health, resilience and inequalities*. Copenhagen: WHO Regional Office for Europe.

34 Friedli, L quoted in O'Hara (2009) Inequality is bad for your health. *The Guardian*, 11th March, p 3.

35 Holmes, G (2002) Some thoughts on why clinical psychologists should not have formal powers under the new mental health act. *Clinical Psychology*, 12, 40–3.

36 Taylor, JL, Gillmer, BT and Robertson, A (2003) An alternative perspective on the proposed Mental Health Act reforms. *Clinical Psychology*, 22, 35–7.

37 Pilgrim, D (2005) A case for clinical psychologists becoming clinical supervisors. *Clinical Psychology Forum*, 155, 4–7.

38 Resnick, R (2003) To prescribe or not to prescribe: Is that the question? *The Psychologist*, 16, 4, 184–6.

39 Gelsthorpe, S (1997) Conflict, collusion, co-operation and trying to be constructive. *Clinical Psychology Forum*, 103, 34–8.

40 Johnstone, L (1993) Psychiatry: Are we allowed to disagree? *Clinical Psychology Forum*, 56, 30–2.

41 Holland, S (1992) From social abuse to social action: A neighbourhood psychotherapy and social action project for women. In J Ussher and P Nicholson (eds.) *Gender issues in clinical psychology*. London: Routledge.

42 White, J (2007) Stepping up primary care. *The Psychologist*, 21, 10, 844–7.

43 MacKay, T (2008) Can psychology change the world? *The Psychologist*, 21, 11, 928–31.

44 Patel, N and Mahtani, A (2007) The politics of working with refugee survivors of torture. *The Psychologist*, 20, 3, 164–6.

45 Roberts, R (ed.) (2007) *Just war: A psychology for peace*. Ross-on-Wye: PCCS Books.

46 Pilgrim, D (1997) Clinical psychology observed (reprise and remix). *Clinical Psychology Forum*, 107, 3–6.

47 Coles, S, Diamond, B, and Keenan, S (2009) Clinical psychology in psychiatric services: The magician's assistant? *Clinical Psychology Forum*, 198, 5–10.

48 Smail, D (1995) Clinical psychology: Liberatory practice or discourse of power? *Clinical Psychology Forum*, 80, 3–6.

49 Prilleltensky, I and Nelson, G (2002) *Doing psychology critically: Making a difference in diverse settings*. Basingstoke: Palgrave Macmillan.

50 Romme, M and Escher, S (1993) (eds.) *Accepting voices*. London: MIND.

51 Harper, D and Moss, D (2003) A different kind of chemistry? Reformulating 'formulation'. *Clinical Psychology*, 25, 6–10.

8 The therapist

Phil Barker

Introduction

Dramatic language

Psychotherapy and counselling are best known, at least to the general public, through films and television. However slow paced and awkward, these encounters have been central to many dramatic story lines – from Ingrid Bergman's probing analyst in Hitchcock's *Spellbound*[1] to the conflicted relationship between Dr Melfi and Tony in the *Sopranos*.[2] Arguably, it is the *confessional* heart of psychotherapy and counselling that intrigues us most: people baring their souls; seeking redemption; or the means of easing their guilt or anguish. The parallel between the therapeutic encounter and Catholic confession was first discussed by Jung[3] and continues to intrigue scholars of religion[4] and psychotherapy alike.[5]

The similarities between confession and therapy are well noted: the experience of a state of heightened self-awareness; the realisation that our predicament means something beyond itself; the need to do something to respond to our present difficulties or dilemmas; and the potential for a spiritual encounter.[6] The atheist or agnostic might baulk at the mention of therapy as a 'spiritual' encounter. However, for most people, the need to address the notion of our 'inner selves', if not actually our 'souls', is so mercurial, intangible and formless, that it has all the appearances of 'spirit'. Despite the secular nature of most therapy, in an increasingly secular society, most people acknowledge that psychotherapy – at least originally – dealt with the 'soul' (or *psyche*) and its influence in our everyday lives, across all societies and cultures.[7,8]

Psychotherapy's history – especially psychoanalysis – is peppered with squabbling and internecine feuds, between different 'schools' and within specific 'movements'. This undistinguished history dates back to Freud, with different therapy systems, like siblings, competing for attention and affection in a 'dogma eat dogma' environment.[9] The founders and early advocates of many therapies had a limited grasp of ethics.

Freud believed that the psychoanalyst was a 'secular pastoral worker' and that psychoanalysis was 'pastoral work in the best sense of the word'.[10] This reference to 'shepherding' is unashamedly biblical in character, anticipating Jung's declaration that the psychotherapist fulfils a role once associated with the priest[11] (see Chapter 10). Given that all therapies involve nothing more than talking and listening, all talk of 'treatment' and 'therapeutic methods' seems fanciful, if not disingenuous. Long before Freud, *Johann Christian Heinroth* (1773–1843) proposed that 'disturbances of the soul' should be the preserve of medicine: 'Since we are speaking of medical art and science, we should think that nobody but a doctor should have a right to make mental disturbance the object of his studies and treatment'.[12]

Over the years, the role of doctors in the delivery of psychotherapy has diminished, with other professionals and lay therapists taking precedence. However, many therapists maintain the connection with medicine, and for most governments, therapy remains a 'health' service. Even lay therapists talk about 'treatment' and the popular understanding of 'therapy' is as a synonym for treatment. However, it would be more honest – and ethical – to acknowledge that the original meaning of therapy was: 'an attendance or service', implying the essentials of the act: '*I wait upon*'.[13] In the same vein, a more honest definition of 'treatment' is the *conduct* of the therapist towards the person: how the person is *treated*. Indeed, how the therapist and the person use language to explore and manipulate their ideas about 'problems', owes more to the aesthetic definition of treatment, than to medicine.

In this context Szasz reminded us that if we are to: 'rescue the cure of souls from the medical morass in which it is now mired, we must call psychotherapy by its proper name'.[14] He noted that: 'Aeschylus had a name for what we now call psychotherapy. He called it the employment of *iatroi logoi*, or "healing words". In those ancient roots, then, lies our proper term for the modern, secular cure of souls: *iatrologic*'[15] – involving the use of rhetoric and logic.[16]

However, it is highly unlikely that therapists will decide to 'rebrand' their practice. The shelter afforded by medicine, and the false definition of problems in living as 'psychological disorders' or forms of 'mental illness', provides a status for therapists, which most will be reluctant to abandon. However, the search for an honest, accurate name for the practice of 'therapy' must represent the primary ethical dilemma for all who wish to dispense 'healing words'.

Psychotherapy and counselling

Despite the diversity of practice psychotherapy and counselling are simply ways of helping people deal with problems in their lives. These might involve their relationship with themselves, whether actual or idealised; relationships with others, whether friends, lovers or strangers; or relationships with abstract ideas, such as luck, misfortune or death. The difference between psychotherapy and counselling is unclear if not intentionally confusing. Whereas some practitioners call themselves counsellors, others with identical qualifications call themselves psychotherapists, perhaps as part of a struggle for status or authority. Ever since Freud launched his psychoanalytic method in 1900 it has been assumed that psychotherapy (especially psychoanalysis) is more demanding than counselling; involving deeper exploration of a person's experience. Today, there is less concern with making such distinctions.

Traditionally, people who offered *short-term* help called themselves counsellors – especially those working in the voluntary sector, addressing bereavement,[17] relationship or sexual problems.[18] Those who had completed longer training (usually over two years) would describe themselves as psychotherapists. However, the general view is that counselling might appear less intimidating to the general public. As a result many practitioners redefine themselves as counsellors, to attract more clients.[19] However trivial, some practitioners use 'counselling' so that their name comes up sooner in an alphabetical listing, like the telephone directory.[20] Such definitional concerns are more about the health of the business than the nature of the therapy.

However, the ethical dilemmas faced by counsellors and psychotherapists are identical. For this reason the generic term 'therapist' is used in this chapter to apply to both.

The ethics of therapy

The virtues of good professional conduct

Many of the ethical dilemmas associated with therapy are no different from those governing the provision of any public service. Indeed, to the layperson, *Codes of Ethics*[21] developed by various professional organisations might appear banal – and blindingly obvious.

For example, therapists should *always*:

- act in the person's best interests;
- respect confidentiality;
- maintain the highest standards of personal conduct;
- keep professional knowledge and skills up-to-date;
- communicate effectively; and
- keep appropriate records.

Alternatively, therapists should *not*:

- take any action without the consent of the person;
- claim to offer a service, which cannot be delivered;
- practise beyond the bounds of their training and qualifications;
- advertise services that are inaccurate or misleading; and
- abuse trust, for example, by exploiting the person emotionally, financially or sexually.

Such recommendations and prohibitions are no more relevant to therapists than to electricians or plumbers, working in someone's home. Here, I want to consider ethical dilemmas that appear particularly relevant to the practice of therapy.

Beginning therapy

Most dictionaries include psychoanalysis as one of the psychotherapies but this is misleading. Psychoanalysis involves a highly systematic, often lengthy, examination of unconscious conflicts. Many therapies do not accept the importance, or even, the existence, of such 'conflicts'. Psychoanalysis is an ambitious undertaking, requiring a major investment of personal commitment and time, from both the analyst and the person. By contrast, other therapies appear more practical: resolving discrete problems; even encouraging people to accept, or live with, problems as a way of dealing with their everyday lives. This does not mean that psychoanalysis occupies some higher ground, or is in any way 'better' than other therapies. That said, it will be more expensive, if only because of its length. However, because of its formal structure – and cost – stringent selection procedures usually operate.

Such stringency raises the next set of ethical dilemmas, for all forms of therapy. Analysts usually assess personality and motivational characteristics very carefully before enrolling someone in analysis. By contrast, the selection procedure for other therapies is much less stringent. However, if people are desperate, they might be willing to accept any offer of help, from anyone, to ease their difficulties. Such a person may be vulnerable and might accept either a grossly inappropriate offer of help, or something appropriate, but over a much longer time than is really necessary.

- How does the therapist decide whether someone is appropriate for a particular form of therapy?
- How do therapists determine what therapy might be appropriate for someone, given their various personal attributes, and the nature of their problems?
- What should therapists *do*, if they decide *not* to enrol a person in any form of therapy? Should they refer them to a colleague; offer a list of alternative therapists; or leave the person to decide his/her next move?

There are no clear, uncontested, answers to these questions. Many therapists now describe their approach as eclectic or integrative.[22] This implies that they have no preferences or prejudices, yet some therapists *never* give advice whereas others recognise 'advice giving' as, at least, a small part of their function.[23] Other therapists embrace a therapeutic philosophy, that is highly distinctive, and which forms the basis for all their work. For example, the *Institute of Transactional Analysis (ITA) Code of Ethics* notes that its fundamental philosophy is that:

- *everyone is OK;*
- *everyone has the capacity to think and influence his/her life by the decisions they make; and*
- *any decision can be changed.*

However, the ITA recognises that such principles had their origin in 1950s America and are individualistic rather than community focused. The organisation notes that any Code of Ethics needs to be 'considered within the context of benefit to the community as well as benefit to the individual'.[24]

This reminds us that, even before therapists sit down to begin the process of listening that exemplifies therapy, they bring certain personal values and beliefs, alongside their more clear-cut therapeutic philosophy. Therapists need to check, constantly, that they are listening to the person and not simply listening to the echo of their own prejudices.

The practice of therapy

Problems in living or illnesses?

As noted, therapy involves nothing more than two people talking; or in a group setting, several people taking turns to talk. Depending on their specific theoretical or philosophical orientation, therapists will spend varying amounts of time, listening, clarifying, interpreting and questioning. Other therapists might believe in the virtue of 'educating' the person about their 'illness', as a part of therapy.[25] For others, such obvious attempts to influence the person would be anathema, if not profoundly unethical.

Although the focus of psychotherapy can take various forms – addressing feelings, thoughts or disturbing patterns of behaviour – all such problems result in some kind of 'problem of living'. However, some therapists assume that they are helping people deal with aspects of their lives (or lived experience), whereas others assume that they are helping someone manage an 'illness' or 'psychiatric disorder'. Philosophically, these represent two very different approaches – one, akin to the pastoral 'soul work' of a hospital chaplain; and the other embedded in medical practice. However, even where people seek help to address their 'bipolar disorder' or 'schizophrenia', the resulting therapy will be obliged to address their experience: how they relate to their 'impulses' or the 'voices' in their head, as part of their whole, lived experience. There is nothing else.

Therapists face a major ethical dilemma around the extent to which they risk influencing the way people think about themselves or their lives. Some therapists do not so much take this risk, as rush to influence. However, if they intend to display a 'watchful practice' then all therapists might consider beginning by *asking* the person what kind of help they are seeking, in relation to what particular aspects of their lives or experience.

General or specific?

Some forms of therapy are highly problem-specific, aiming only to reduce the experience of distress or to promote a limited form of social adaptation. Others will be more concerned with the development of the personality: trying to free people from (apparently) limiting ways of thinking, feeling or behaving, which might restrict their 'full humanity'.

Of course, therapists need to embrace concepts like 'full humanity' or 'low self-esteem' before these can become part of the therapy process. Therapists might ask if they are shepherds, gently supporting people on their way home; or directing traffic, to maintain some social convention, with its own rules and regulations.

Who is the client?

Some people come to therapy because of their dissatisfaction with themselves or their lives. Others come because of someone else's dissatisfaction. Others seek therapy because they believe others want them to change, whether or not this is the case. Finally, some people are sent for therapy, and want nothing to do with it.

Where people make their own appointments, are prepared to pay and are prepared, at least, to discuss what *might* be the problem and what they *might* do, to resolve it, the therapist may feel very comfortable about proceeding.

Where people are less keen to make such a start, the therapist might wonder: do they really want to be here? or is someone obliging or coercing them? Where someone else has decided that 'change' is desirable, this particular ethical dilemma comes to a head. Therapists must decide if they are the person's agent; the family's agent; some other professional's agent; or agents of the state.

Does it work?

Most therapists promote the utility of their particular approach. Traditionally, it has proven difficult to evaluate most therapies – especially those which explore abstract concepts like 'conflicts' or 'personal growth'. However, with the emergence of highly problem-oriented therapies – like cognitive behavioural therapy (CBT) – which used rating scales and 'behavioural assignments', it appeared easier to judge whether someone's distress was reducing, or behaviour was changing. CBT is, presently, very popular – especially with the UK government. However, other therapists question whether this is merely a reflection of 'cost-effectiveness', rather than long-term usefulness.[26]

Therapy always needs to be tailored to suit the individual. This begs the question: what has something so personal in common with a research trial, involving carefully selected 'subjects', where the therapist's actions were governed by a 'therapy manual'?

In most public services the 'customer' is the final arbiter of quality and effectiveness. It is not clear why therapy should be judged differently. If someone returns after the first session and goes on to complete a lengthy course of therapy, does this not suggest a satisfied 'customer'. Unfortunately, therapy is still dogged, at least in some circles, by the idea that therapy is in the person's 'best interests', whether he/she agrees with this or not.

The focus of therapy

Although the number of therapies runs into the hundreds, the main functions of all therapy are to provide support and to enable re-education.[27]

Support: Most people who come for therapy experience distress, which they wish to be reduced, if not eliminated. They want to restore their emotional equilibrium, perhaps through developing some control over their circumstances.

Some therapies emphasise specific, even narrow, objectives: helping the persons to strengthen their existing defences, gaining some kind of security that will allow them to deal with their difficulties. To provide such support, the therapist may:

- *Offer guidance and reassurance*: encouraging people to accept some aspects of their experience, while 'normalising' others.
- *Facilitate emotional catharsis*: allow or encourage people to express their feelings.
- *Try to promote self-esteem*: help people identify and clarify personal assets or resources.
- *Enable coping*: helping them manage specific problems.

First of all, therapists should establish what kind of support the person is seeking, even before they begin to discuss any 'standard options'. This should be their primary ethical imperative.

Re-education: Others request help to make some change in their lives.

This may involve 'fulfilling their creative potential' or adjusting the way they approach their everyday lives. This may involve making changes within the person, their relationships with others, or both.

Here the therapy will emphasise making deliberate efforts to re-adjust. Reaching these goals may or may not require that people develop their understanding of what the problem was 'all about'. (I refrain from calling this 'insight'.) If re-education is to occur, the person must 'feel' some change within. This cannot occur without the full participation of the person. As Szasz noted:

> It is false to say that the psychotherapist *treats* or is a therapist. It would be more accurate to say that the 'patient' in psychotherapy treats or is a therapist, because he treats himself. But that would be using the term *treatment* metaphorically, inasmuch as such a person treats himself only in the sense in which any person too submits himself to and actively cooperates with athletic, educational, or religious influence or instruction treats himself.[28]

Ethics and the therapist

Authority

When people enter therapy they are likely to be demoralised, distraught or otherwise 'suffering'. The therapist must establish a relationship within which people feel sufficiently secure to begin to address whatever has brought them to therapy.

They are putting their destiny in the hands of someone they hope will be understanding, protective and helpful. This bestows an 'authority' on the therapist, which might appear lacking in everyone else, who so far has failed to help. However, authority and power go hand in hand, and raise several other ethical issues.

The more distressed someone is, the more likely that he/she will idealise the therapist, especially as a parent (authority) figure. Therapy often expresses a strong power dynamic. The therapist is very much in charge (control) and the person is dependent on support and approval. Even simple comments like 'would you like to come through?' or 'things seem to be going well' show how the therapist sits outside the person's field of distress, directing (however gently) the proceedings, making observations (from a safe distance).

During the 1930s, Harry Stack Sullivan,[29] was practising traditional psychoanalysis, sitting behind the person on the couch, silently making notes. One day, he decided to draw up his chair *beside* the person and began to converse with him.[30] This led to the development of his 'inter-personal theory', where he observed that problems did not exist *within* people, so much as *between* people. That spontaneous act probably marks the beginnings of what, today, is called the 'collaborative approach'.

Some therapists (especially psychoanalysts) use the power dynamic as part of therapy, while others try to reduce this, making the relationship more balanced. However, the power differential is central to all psychotherapy. By virtue of their expectation that the therapist will be helpful, patients project power (and authority) on to their therapist. However, the powerful nature of this union offers the therapist an opportunity to begin to restore the patient's morale, recognised as a core function of all therapies.[31]

However 'authoritative' the therapist might appear (or be viewed), the person is always the expert. Even where therapy runs several times a week, for years on end, therapists are still only sampling the person's experience. Sadly, some therapists still deceive themselves by falling for the idea, much beloved by early psychoanalysts that they might 'know the patient better than he knows himself'.

Communication

Therapy can be no more than a conversation, developed within an extraordinary relationship. Therapists use conversation to help people develop their understanding of the nature of some problem and, hopefully, what they might do to begin to address it, or live with it. This requires therapists to be able to communicate in a way that is not only intelligible to the person, using their language and vernacular, but also acceptable, given the stage of the relationship.

In addition to deciding what to say and how to say it, the therapist needs also to know when to stay silent. Although much more could be said about the conduct of this conversation, these few comments remind us that the *conduct* of the conversation always presents ethical challenges. Indeed, everything that the therapist says and does (or does *not* say or do) could represent an ethical problem.

Direction

Even when the therapist adopts a highly 'non-directive' stance, direction will be given (or at least interpreted by the person). People expect some direction if they are to alter the course of their lives. If they could do this alone, they would have no need of therapy. Deciding how much 'shepherding' or 'traffic direction' is appropriate can be demanding. If mechanics lie awake at night worrying about whether they have replaced the brake pads securely, therapists might be kept awake over their use of the 'wrong' phrase or the 'right' phrase at the 'wrong' moment.

Safe space

All conversations in therapy are about the person's life, attitudes, beliefs, thoughts, feelings and relationships. Therapists, in general, decline to talk about their lives. Not surprisingly, the resulting focus on the person's life can be intimidating. Therapy requires them to look at themselves (metaphorically) in a 'full-length mirror', perhaps even 'naked'. Each session's conversation places the person under the (metaphorical) spotlight. Care needs to be taken in deciding *when* would be the 'right' time to enable such close 'self-examination', or 'emotional undressing'. In all cases vital preparations need to be made, so that the person feels 'secure' in the relationship; confident that he/she will come to no harm; and aware of the point of taking such a potentially threatening step beyond their 'comfort zone'.

Creating these metaphorical 'safe spaces' is a critical aspect of the therapist's ongoing work with the person: a form of 'health and safety' checks. In therapy, such checks are not done at intervals, but run continuously in the background; sensitively monitoring the 'therapeutic atmosphere'.

Confidence

People like to believe that therapy is like confession, and that everything that they say will be treated in confidence. Indeed, most people need this kind of confidentiality to feel any degree of confidence in the therapist. Most professional Ethical Codes warn therapists that exceptional circumstances may arise where a breach of confidentiality may be indicated: for example, if it appears that the person may seriously harm someone else, or come to harm.[32] Clearly such a situation creates a major quandary for the therapist.

It *may* be possible to limit the potential damage that a breach of confidence would entail, by negotiating clearly, from the outset, the 'rules' of the therapeutic relationship. Before beginning, most therapists provide people with information about the conduct of the therapy: length of sessions, timekeeping, payment of fees and so on. There is no reason why they might not also discuss confidentiality, and the circumstances that might require them to breach a confidence. Many therapists are opposed to such gestures of 'transparency', on the grounds that it might encourage the person to conceal some 'dangerous' motives.

Conclusion

As an occupation, therapy is similar to other kinds of 'service industry'. To retain membership of a particular organisation, therapists must observe its particular Code of Ethics (or Standards), or risk being penalised or expelled. I have paid scant attention to such Codes, as they represent a moral 'bare minimum', which scarcely address the kind of dilemmas therapists encounter in practice.

The ethical dilemmas peculiar to therapy are at once simple and complex, revolving around a single dilemma: Is the therapist able (or willing) to *treat* the person as an autonomous agent? If they cannot, or will not, treat the person in this manner, for whatever reason, therapists risk becoming trapped in a protracted power game, where the person may nurture or reject their powerless role.

Notes

1 Hitchcock had a fascination with psychoanalysis. See: Gordon P *Dial 'M' for Mother: A Freudian Hitchcock*. Madison, NJ: Farleigh Dickenson University Press, 2006.
2 Gabbard G. *Psychology of the Sopranos: Love, Death, Desire and Betrayal in America's Favorite Gangster Family*. New York, NY: Basic Books, 2002.
3 See the essay written in 1932. Jung C. 'Psychotherapists or the Clergy'. Ch 11 in *Modern Man in Search of a Soul (Routledge Classics)*. London: Routledge, 2001.
4 Worthen V. Psychotherapy and Catholic confession. *Journal of Religion and Health* 2005: 13 (4) 275–84.
5 Spiegelman JM. Psychotherapists and the clergy: Fifty years later. *Journal of Religion and Health* 1984: 23 (1) 19–32.

6 Steere DA. *Rediscovering Confession: The Practice of Forgiveness and Where It Leads.* London: Routledge, 2009.

7 Ozawa-de Silva C. *Psychotherapy and Religion in Japan: The Japanese Introspection Practice of Naikan.* London: Routledge, 2006.

8 La Barre W. *Primitive Psychotherapy in Native American Cultures: Peyotism and Confession.* Indianapolis, IN: Bobbs-Merrill, 1947.

9 Norcross JC. 'A Primer on Psychotherapy Integration'. In JC Norcorss and MC Goldfried (Eds) *Handbook of Psychotherapy Integration.* Oxford: Oxford University Press, 2005.

10 See: Szasz TS. *The Myth of Psychotherapy.* Syracuse, NY: Syracuse University Press, 1988 (p 182).

11 Jung op. cit.

12 Cited by Szasz op. cit. (p 73).

13 From the Greek verb *therapeuo*.

14 Szasz op. cit. (p 208).

15 Szasz op. cit. (p 208).

16 *Rhetoric*: The art or study of using language effectively and persuasively. *Logic*: reasoned thought or argument, as distinguished from irrationality.

17 http://www.crusebereavementcare.org.uk/ (Accessed: 20/03/10).

18 http://www.relate.org.uk/home/index.html (Accessed: 20/03/10).

19 Client is the favoured term in most psychotherapy and counselling. However, in the rest of this chapter I shall call the 'client' the 'person', to emphasise the personal and inter-personal nature of the work of therapy.

20 See: Net Doctor for example: http://www.netdoctor.co.uk/diseases/depression/psychotherapy_ 000429.htm

21 For example, see: *United Kingdom Association for Psychotherapeutic Counselling*: http://www.ukapc.org.uk/ (Accessed: 26/03/10); *British Association for Counselling and Psychotherapy*: http://www.bacp.co.uk/ethical_framework/ (Accessed: 26/03/10); *UK Council for Psychotherapy*: http://www.psychotherapy.org.uk/code_of_ethics.html (Accessed: 26/03/10); *National Counselling Institute of Ireland*: http://www.ncii.ie/msa/Policy/Code%20of%20Ethics%20New.pdf (Accessed: 26/03/10).

22 Brooks-Harris JE. *Integrative Multitheoretical Psychotherapy.* Boston, MA: Houghton-Mifflin, 2008.

23 See: *AMHA Massachusetts and the Consortium for Psychotherapy.* http://www.oregoncounseling.org/ArticlesPapers/Documents/WhatIsPsychTx.htm (Accessed: 22/03/10).

24 http://www.ita.org.uk/modules/tinycontent/index.php?id=35 (Accessed: 22/03/10).

25 For example: Basco MR and Rush JA. *Cognitive-Behavioral Therapy for Bipolar Disorder.* New York, NY: Guilford Press, 1996.

26 See: Laurance J. 'The pursuit of Happiness: It's good to talk... or is it?' *The Independent* Tuesday, 8th July, 2008.

27 Barker P. *Talking Cures: A Guide to the Psychotherapies for Health Care Professionals.* London: NT Books, 1999.

28 Szasz op. cit. (p 190).

29 Evans FB. *Harry Stack Sullivan: Interpersonal Theory and Psychotherapy.* New York, NY: Routledge, 1996.

30 I was told this story by someone who had been a student of Sullivan towards the end of his life.

31 Frank JD and Frank JB. *Persuasion and Healing: A Comparative Study of Psychotherapy* (3rd ed.). Baltimore, MD: The Johns Hopkins University Press, 1994.

32 See: Section B. 4.4; *National Counselling Institute of Ireland*: http://www.ncii.ie/msa/Policy/Code%20of%20Ethics%20New.pdf (Accessed: 26/03/10).

9　The occupational therapist

Lesley Brady

Challenges to enablement

This chapter explores the dilemmas in practice experienced by occupational therapists within the context of Scottish mental health services. The dilemmas for occupational therapists in Scotland are, however, not considered to be significantly different from those of their colleagues in other parts of the United Kingdom and beyond. However, most of the practice examples provided are framed by the Scottish mental health legislation and relate to people resident in Scotland served by the devolved Scottish Government.

The chapter addresses issues highlighted in the literature and how this matches the reported quandaries experienced by a group of occupational therapists; the use of the occupational therapy Code of Ethics and professional conduct as a framework for reflecting the context of reported dilemmas on practice; and some discussion around the Millan principles as introduced within the Mental Health (Care and Treatment) (Scotland) Act 2003[1] (the Act).

The Act introduces new rights and safeguards for people with mental health problems. These include the opportunity to develop an Advance Statement and to choose a 'Named Person'. An Advance Statement outlines how he/she would like to be treated if they become unwell in the future. This might include specific treatments which are offered by occupational therapists (see Chapter 26).

The Named Person is someone nominated by the person to act as his/her supporter, protect his/her interests and be fully informed of progress and plans for changing any care arrangements.

The Advance Statement and the nomination of a Named Person must be witnessed by a relevant person as defined in the Act, but should be an assurance that the person has the capacity to understand what he/she is asking for. It is possible that occupational therapists may be asked by clients to witness these statements/nominations.

The Millan principles[2] are shown in Table 9.1 over page.

Table 9.1   The Millan principles

- *Non-discrimination* – People with mental disorder should, wherever possible, retain the same rights and entitlements as those with other health needs.

- *Equality* – All powers under the Act should be exercised without any direct or indirect discrimination on the grounds of physical disability, age, gender, sexual orientation, language, religion or national or ethnic or social origin.

- *Respect for diversity* – People should receive care, treatment and support in a manner that accords respect for their individual qualities, abilities and diverse backgrounds and properly takes into account their age, gender, sexual orientation, ethnic group and social, cultural and religious background.

- *Reciprocity* – Where society imposes an obligation on an individual to comply with a programme of treatment of care, it should impose a parallel obligation on the health and social care authorities to provide safe and appropriate services, including ongoing care following discharge from compulsion.

- *Informal care* – Wherever possible, care, treatment and support should be provided to people with mental disorder without the use of compulsory powers.

- *Participation* – People should be fully involved, so far as they are able to be, in all aspects of their assessment, care, treatment and support. Their past and present wishes should be taken into account. They should be provided with all the information and support necessary to enable them to participate fully. Information should be provided in a way that makes it most likely to be understood.

- *Respect for carers* – Those who provide care on an informal basis should receive respect for their role and experience, receive appropriate information and advice and have their views and needs taken into account.

- *Least restrictive alternative* – People should be provided with any necessary care, treatment and support both in the least invasive manner and in the least restrictive manner and environment compatible with the delivery of safe and effective care, taking account where appropriate of the safety of others.

- *Benefit* – Any intervention under the Act should be likely to produce for the person a benefit that cannot reasonably be achieved other than by the intervention.

- *Child welfare* – The welfare of a child with mental disorder should be paramount in any interventions imposed on the child under the Act.

Historical background

Occupational therapy is based on the theory that helping people to undertake a range of activities can help them to remain or become active, occupied and productive. In turn this helps keep people physically, emotionally and economically well. Purposeful activity has helped us survive through the ages.

Occupation as treatment for people with mental health problems has some roots in the eighteenth and nineteenth centuries, but became prominent in Scotland in the early twentieth century, when in 1922, instruction in occupational therapy – arts and crafts – was introduced in Gartnavel Royal Hospital in Glasgow.[3] Helping people to conduct their daily lives in a more hopeful and productive way appeared helpful to overall well-being.

Currently, connections can be made with occupational science in relation to understanding the meaning of occupation for an individual's potential and personal growth.[1] In terms of physical and mental well-being, this human potential leads us to the essence of occupational therapy in mental health: enablement and recovery.

In 2001 the *Core Skills and Conceptual Foundation for Practice*[5] as issued by the College of Occupational therapists in 1994 were:

> The occupational therapist assesses the physical, psychological and social functions of the individual, identifies areas of dysfunction and involves the individual in a structured programme of activity to overcome disability. The activities selected will relate to the consumer's personal, social, cultural and economic needs and will reflect the environmental factors which govern his life.

This definition emphasises dysfunction and disability, whereas today's language within mental health services is much more strengths driven and recovery focused. This change is evident in the description of core occupational therapy skills provided in a briefing note[6] from the College of Occupational Therapists in 2004:

- *Collaboration with the client* – to promote the client's autonomy and engagement in the therapeutic process.
- *Assessment* – a collaborative process aimed at identifying the client's functional potential.
- *Enablement* – the client identifying what's important to him or her.
- *Problem-solving* – cognitive strategies and experiential learning.
- *Using activity as a therapeutic tool*
- *Group work*
- *Environmental adaptation* – the modification of environments to increase function and social participation.

Occupational therapists aim to work within a person-centred approach which points to very real connections with the concept of recovery.[7] (See the Scottish Recovery Network website.[8]) An example from people who have experienced mental health problems helps reinforce this:

> Recovery is being able to live a meaningful and satisfying life, as defined by each person, in the presence or absence of symptoms. It is about having control over and input into your own life. Each individual's recovery, like his or her experience of mental health problems or illness, is a unique and deeply personal process.

Within the narrative research undertaken by the Scottish Recovery Network people identified the importance of having things to do that provide 'meaning and purpose, like working, volunteering and creativity'. The value of hope, self-belief and personal control were also stressed.

How does this relate to the ethical dilemmas facing occupational therapists in mental health today? To explore this topic, a literature review was undertaken, followed by focus groups, individual interviews and receipt of written testimonies from occupational therapists in inpatient, community, forensic and employment settings.

Background

Like other professions, occupational therapy has a Code of Ethics and professional conduct, which seeks to promote good practice and prevent malpractice. Sections of the Code provided by the College of Occupational Therapists[9] address:

- *Client autonomy and welfare* – autonomy, duty of care, confidentiality and protecting clients.
- *Services to clients* – referral, provision of services and record keeping.
- *Personal/professional integrity* – integrity, professional demeanour, fitness to practice, substance misuse, personal profit or gain, advertising, information and representation.
- *Professional competence and standards* – competence, delegation, collaborative working, lifelong learning, occupational therapy student education, research and service development.

The Code states: 'the College is strongly committed to client-centred practice and the involvement of the client as a partner in all stages of the therapeutic process'. There are, however, some challenges to the concept of true partnership where partners are equal, given the 'inherent imbalance of power between those seeking and those giving health care'.[10]

Working with people who are experiencing mental distress inevitably presents challenges for therapists who recognise the vulnerability of those who receive their services. Where there are conflicts regarding choice of interventions, ways of working or clarity about roles, there are potential dilemmas when fellow workers appear to have a different set of values and expectations.[11] For instance, greater value may be placed on medical solutions rather than on activity as a promoter of well-being. Similarly if several people are involved in care arrangements there is potential for discord and the autonomy of, and service to, the client can be compromised.[12]

The nature of mental distress/mental illness can often mean that occupational therapists are faced with addressing risks to themselves and others because of the level of emotional disturbance and behaviours exhibited by the person in their care.[13] The issues of risk assessment and management are complex and can, at times, present dilemmas regarding physical safety unless a comprehensive plan has been discussed with the client and his/her team in a coordinated way.[11] If the client is viewed as a true partner (as in the Code of Ethics), this can help the client explore and find solutions to the management of risk, which he/she and the team can agree upon.

The occupational therapist's role involves helping the person undertake activities to assist him/her to attain goals and strengthen his/her abilities to lead his/her chosen life. This can lead the therapist into situations where positive risk-taking is essential. Promoting safety and positive risk-taking form an integral part of the *Ten Essential Shared Capabilities* introduced by NHS Education Scotland as 'the foundation on which good mental health practice is set'.[15] Risk-taking often helps people find creative ways of solving lifestyle problems. When this work leads to a requirement to share information regarding the client, there are moral and ethical issues that need to be considered before this sharing can be undertaken, as this can be a worrying and confusing process for the occupational therapist and the client. The potential for damage regarding sharing information without due process and discussion is significant.[16]

Focus groups, interviews and written testimonies

Through focus groups, interviews and written testimonies, I gained an understanding of some of the issues faced by occupational therapists in contemporary practice. These included the following:

- Discrete ethical challenges inherent in the occupational therapist–patient relationship.
- Potential ethical challenges faced by occupational therapists in inter-disciplinary working.
- How changes in practice have (or have not) brought new ethical dilemmas.

Occupational therapists are expected to work within the ethical framework described earlier in this chapter. In Scotland, this involves taking account of the Millan principles (see Table 9.1). These ten principles are also found within the spirit of the Code of Ethics.

Table 9.2 summarises the themes occupational therapists reported during focus groups, individual interviews and in written testimonies. These are linked to the headings within the Code of Ethics and are followed by some discussion of these themes in more depth.

There are clear connections between issues raised in the literature and apparent consistency within the staff group, including issues relating to people who use forensic services.

Using the four main sections of the Code of Ethics I explore these issues more closely, clarifying the perspective of the staff group and the issues which challenge their thinking and practice.

Client autonomy and welfare

Several comments were made regarding the challenges of inter-agency working where there can be 'culture clashes' that often are not addressed. Occupational therapists reported unease when transferring people's care to other agencies who do not necessarily demonstrate similar beliefs and values. This was reported with particular emphasis on 'retraction processes', where people can be discharged to other care providers before the occupational therapists think they are ready, or to agencies that may be able to provide only basic care, thus restricting the client's day to day living. This raised the issue of whether clients really have the opportunity to be autonomous and make choices as these choices might be divergent with people providing services. The outcome of this issue may result in potential conflict with the principles of participation and least restrictive alternative as defined by Millan. The occupational therapist may seek to address this potential conflict through care management/case review process and through robust clinical supervision.

Another concern related to 'risk behaviour', whether actual or threatened: for example, harm to self or others. Occupational therapists described the challenges when clients' behaviour posed the risk of possible harm to themselves or the public, and how best to manage this; particularly in the situation of lone working. Often the risk involved self-harm where the client embarks on a course of action that inevitably would have a negative health outcome. In contrast, deliberate self-harm can often be viewed by the client as helping achieve relief: for example, intense emotional pressure. In these circumstances the duty of care can become a challenge in terms of the client's autonomy, welfare and decision-making abilities, along with the principle of benefit and protecting the client. Involving the client in the care planning process is paramount, linking this with case review and supervision.

Where clients are subject to compulsory measures under legislation (see Chapters 23–25) and experience restrictions of their liberty, occupational therapists can play a key role in helping them towards their recovery. There are challenges where risk assessment and management processes are not robust and the client has been excluded from the discussion. The overall care provided by the occupational therapist can be compromised if the care plan is viewed as restrictive, thus challenging the duty of care and client's autonomy as far as this can be exercised, and challenges the principle of reciprocity (see Table 9.1). The potential for

Table 9.2   Ethical issues and sections of the Code of Ethics

Code of Ethics section heading	Reported issues
Client autonomy and welfare – autonomy, duty of care, confidentiality, protecting clients	Inter-agency working and transferring care on to agencies with different standards
	Confidentiality, protection of the public/society versus the freedoms of the individual. Specific issues within forensic care
	Risk behaviour/risk-taking – whose risk is it?
	Occupation involves risk
Services to clients – referral, provision of services, record keeping	Raising expectations/practice versus time constraints
	Discharge too early versus recovery focus
	Government/organisational targets versus person-centred care services
	Forensic issues in relation to recall to hospital – losing liberty, safety to self, public, staff
Personal/professional integrity – integrity, professional demeanour, fitness to practice, substance misuse, personal profit or gain, advertising, information and representation	Inter-agency working, clashes of culture
	Living and working in a target-driven world
	Inpatient services – joint decision making.
	Standing up for professional role and other people's expectations of role. Many masters. Team players, challenges to practice. Role clarity – differences of opinion regarding role – able to say 'no'
Personal competence and standards – professional competence, delegation, collaborative working, lifelong learning, occupational therapy student education, research and service development	Confidence, robust supervision and support systems, reflection
	Lone working and professional isolation
	Supervision, thinking time
	Strong leadership/team/shared vision

disruption to or restriction of purposeful activity in terms of the individual's recovery requires careful consideration with the client and the clinical team.

Services to clients

The Code of Ethics states that services to clients 'shall be client-centred and needs-led'. The occupational therapists reported significant challenges to this. Time pressures and workloads often dictated the amount of time therapists could engage with clients. There were some worries that these issues, along with the 'target-driven' culture, compromised quality of care, which could become service/therapist driven, rather than client-centred and needs-led. Coupled with this were the pressures of different models of care and complex methods of recording outcomes, which usually excluded the client's input, and took much time to complete. The principles of participation and benefit were challenged and could be resolved through robust clinical and managerial supervision structures and through open discussion with the client, their families and other members of the team.

In forensic care, clients could be recalled to hospital on the instruction of Scottish Government ministers; for example, following an incident that caused concern. The consequent loss of liberty required sensitive management. Clients needed to continue, as far as possible, with a therapeutic regime that promoted recovery and addressed the issues that precipitated the hospital recall. Occupational therapists reported that this was challenging in terms of how their interventions were delivered, as part of the role might be to assess suitability for leaving hospital and resuming life in the community whilst the client was in a low secure setting and his/her liberty restricted. A shared approach within the team is paramount and there needs to be scope for risk-assessing clients' strengths as well as the topics that needed some intervention, so that they could anticipate and prepare for possible discharge. There are therefore challenges to ensure that the principles of reciprocity, participation and least restrictive alternative are adhered to. The occupational therapist needs to explore creative ways to ensure that the focus remains on the client's recovery whilst being mindful of the reasons for the hospital recall.

Personal and professional integrity

Occupational therapists need to be clear about their 'core business' and how they execute it. An occupational therapist in a large multi-disciplinary/agency team felt that the role was compromised by the need to be a 'team player' and therefore part of all team processes. There are concerns about 'standing up for your professional role' rather than merely fitting in with others' expectations of the occupational therapist. Moreover, there was a strong emphasis on retaining core skills.

Other issues arose where clients were aiming to alter their lifestyle and activities of daily living by exploring employment or volunteering opportunities. Here the occupational therapist's role became one of broker. Dilemmas occurred when other agencies and employers expected levels of information regarding the client's history that the therapist and client felt need not be revealed. This posed challenges to the principle of non-discrimination. The occupational therapist has a key role in identifying these dilemmas so that a compromise can be reached within the limits of policy and procedure. Additionally there may be advantages in carefully designing a strategy to ensure that the client's strengths continue to be emphasised.

Therapists often reported a growing unease when working in situations that did not sit well with their professional ideology concerning recovery and person-centred care. The expectations of the organisation may conflict with the assessed strengths, needs and length of time the client requires to reach his/her goals.

Professional competence and standards

Occupational therapists may be members of many teams and as such are pulled in many directions. Teams develop and grow differently and this can be challenging if the therapists are not viewed as contributing significantly to the overall teams' approaches. A balance needs to be struck where the occupational therapist and the team need to clarify how the occupational therapist's role will complement the overall role of the team in which they work.

Occupational therapists recognise the importance of strong professional leadership in an ever-changing world. Regular clinical supervision is vital to professional competence and standards, where the therapist has opportunities to explore and reflect on issues of professional contribution, personal learning and confidence.

Robust partnerships within clinical supervision are by no means universal, and occupational therapists described some dilemmas, especially if the supervisor was not the person perceived as best placed to offer a supervisory role in the clinical setting.

Back to the future

- Are there discrete ethical challenges inherent in the occupational therapist–patient relationship?

The answer to this question appeared to be yes *and* no.

Challenges often occur when enabling people to carry out their daily living tasks. Risk-taking is required to assist an individual to reach his or her aspirational level of ability. Sometimes the aspirations of the client conflict with the opinion and assessment of the occupational therapist or other team members. This has the potential for an ethical dilemma, and may affect the relationship if compromise and agreement cannot be reached. It is important to be mindful of the clients' autonomy, their expertise in their own lives, how they view themselves in terms of the mental health problems they are experiencing and how to assist progress in their quest for recovery.[17] Co-creating a structured programme of activity with the individual has some challenges for negotiation but has the potential for a more helpful outcome in the spirit of true partnership.

- Potential ethical challenges faced by occupational therapists in inter-disciplinary working

Working within a recovery-focused, person-centred framework can cause some conflict within the multi-disciplinary setting. Often 'occupation', and the creative use of activities as interventions, is not valued highly by some other practitioners. These practitioners may give emphasis to other therapies or medication, and consider activity as diversionary rather than therapeutic. The occupational therapists can, as a result, be undervalued.

The integrity of the professional role can be challenged where there is no strong professional leadership and confidence in the role. There are risks that the occupational therapist may be cast in the role of 'generic worker' rather than *specialist* contributor.

Additionally, there are potential challenges in the previously discussed circumstances surrounding the issue of transfer of care when the occupational therapists are not confident about the values and recovery focus of the new service providers.

- How changes in practice have (or have not) brought new ethical dilemmas

Occupational therapists have opportunities to work in a wide range of settings – statutory, non-statutory, third sector and private settings. Expectations of the role can vary greatly. The structures within which an occupational therapy service operates can influence how the role expectations are addressed.

Financial constraints, targets, raising standards, working within the Code of Ethics and the Millan principles all present challenges. Some of these are new and some not so new.

Conclusion

Are the issues and dilemmas described throughout this chapter unique to occupational therapists? Probably not! The Scottish Government continues to emphasise *a values based, recovery-focused* health service and a *mentally flourishing* Scotland.[18] These ambitious Government goals fit comfortably with the integrity of the role of the twenty-first century occupational therapist, both in the context of working with people recovering from mental health issues and in the context of promoting well-being and illness prevention.

Acknowledgements

The author offers grateful thanks to the staff of Occupational Therapy service in NHS Ayrshire and Arran, for their information and support, and to Derek Barron, Associate Nurse Director, NHS Ayrshire and Arran for his encouragement and mentoring.

Notes

 1 Scottish Executive, 'Mental Health (Care and Treatment) (Scotland) (Act) 2003', 2003, Edinburgh.
 2 Scottish Executive, 'The new mental health act – What's it all about? A short introduction', 2004, Edinburgh.
 3 C.F. Paterson, 'A short history of occupational therapy in psychiatry' in J. Creek, L. Lougher (Eds.) *Occupational Therapy and Mental Health* (4th ed.), Elsevier, 2008, pp. 3–14.
 4 S.E.E. Blair, C.A. Hume, and J. Creek, 'Occupational perspectives on mental health and well-being' in J. Creek and L. Lougher (Eds.) *Occupational Therapy and Mental Health* (4th ed.), Elsevier, 2008, pp. 17–28.
 5 R. Hagedorn, 'An introduction to philosophy, principles and practice' in *Foundations for Practice in Occupational Therapy* (3rd ed.), 2001, p. 4.
 6 College of Occupational Therapists, 'Briefing 23 – definitions and core skills for occupational therapy', 2004, London, COT.
 7 College of Occupational Therapists, 'Recovering ordinary lives: The strategy for occupational therapy in mental health services 2007–2017, a vision for the next 10 years', 2006, London, COT.
 8 Scottish Recovery Network website, 2009, online, available at: www.scottishrecovery.net
 9 College of Occupational Therapists, 'Code of ethics and professional conduct', 2005, London, COT.
10 J. Butler, J. Creek, 'Ethics' in J. Creek and L. Lougher (Eds.) *Occupational Therapy and Mental Health* (4th ed.), Elsevier, 2008, pp. 199–210.
11 K.W. Hamell, 'Client centred practice: Ethical obligation or professional obfuscation?' *British Journal of Occupational Therapy*, June 2007, 70, pp 264–6.
12 A. Kassberg and L Skar, 'Experiences of ethical dilemmas in rehabilitation: Swedish Occupational Therapists' perspectives' *Scandinavian Journal of Occupational Therapy*, 2008, 15, pp. 204–11.
13 R. Barnitt, 'Ethical dilemmas in occupational therapy and physical therapy' *Journal of Medical Ethics*, June 1998, 24, pp. 193–9.
14 Scottish Office, 'Community Care: Care Programme Approach for people with severe and enduring mental illness, including dementia', Social Work Service Group Circular 16/96, 1996, Edinburgh.
15 NHS Education Scotland, 'The Ten Essential Shared Capabilities for mental health practice: Learning materials (Scotland)', 2007, Edinburgh.
16 J. Sim, 'Client confidentiality: Ethical issues in occupational therapy' *British Journal of Occupational Therapy*, February 1996, 59, pp. 56–61.
17 J. Howard, 'Expecting and accepting: The temporal ambiguity of recovery identities' *Social Psychology Quarterly*, December 2006, 69, pp. 307–24.
18 Scottish Government, 'Towards a mentally flourishing Scotland: The future of mental health improvement in Scotland', 2007, Edinburgh, online, available at: http://www.scotland.gov.uk/Publications/2007/10/26112853/0

10 The chaplain

Kevin Franz

Introduction

The history of chaplaincy to the sick predates not only the National Health Service (NHS) but modern health care. For most of that time chaplaincy has been linked to the Christian church, and chaplains drawn from its priests and ministers. To understand a chaplain's perspective on ethical dilemmas, it is important to be alert both to the history and to contemporary practice. Some aspects of this chapter emerge from a Scottish context but its broad outline should be recognisable elsewhere.

The superficial cause of change for chaplaincy lies in the context of the altered religious map of society. As with most Western cultures, Christian dominance in Britain has come to an end through a process of secularisation and the development of a multi-faith society. For chaplaincy these changes prompted the move from a ministry offered by the church to an instrument of spiritual care offered within the NHS.

Chaplaincy has also been affected by new understandings of the relationship between spirituality and institutional religion: 'believing without belonging'.[1] As the perceived importance of the church and of church-going has ebbed, the significance of 'the spiritual' in people's lives has grown. In the response of the healthcare system to the needs of individuals, chaplaincy has been able to point to a distinctive set of skills and knowledge-base which are integral to modern understandings of person-centred care.

Responding to the *World Health Organisation (WHO)* description of health as requiring a spiritual and compassionate element alongside the physical, psychological and social, the Scottish Government Health Department developed a policy for spiritual care in NHS Scotland.[2] In requiring each Health Board to draw up a spiritual care policy it envisaged a spiritual care service which was equitable and accessible to people of any faith and of none. All staff have a responsibility to deliver spiritual care in a broad sense, with the result that the specialist role of chaplains took on a new character. While conscious of being heirs to a long tradition many chaplains perceive themselves as part of a new and emerging profession. This gives rise to some discrete ethical dilemmas.

At the heart of contemporary practice lies a judgement about where the chaplain 'belongs,' setting the context for the ethical questions which he/she faces. The working context can be described as if chaplaincy were simply analogous to other allied healthcare professions, something many chaplains aspire to. Yet the 'place' of the chaplain is one which takes its character not from the institution but from the task: the spiritual care offered both to individuals and to the institution, from a place which may be described as 'marginal' or 'counter-cultural'. The ambiguity in the chaplain's role sets the context for the ethical dilemmas he/she faces. Perhaps it is implicit in the nature of religious and spiritual care. I consider briefly these two modes of care, and then offer a model of the chaplain's role: one of *accompaniment*.

'The glory of God is a human being fully alive'

These words of St Ireneaus, written in the second century CE, may act as a bridge between two apparently different ways of conceiving the chaplain's task: one religious, the other spiritual, by recalling the well-being of the individual who is at the heart of each.

On the surface it is easier to illustrate what *religious care* is: a response to a person's religious personality, itself a mix of culture, language, ritual and identity. What distinguishes religious care is that it commonly involves some measure of belonging: being part of a community where the experience is shared. In many cases a person will look to that community to meet a felt religious need. The chaplain's understood role is to act simply as the contact with that community. Yet there can be challenges here.

Historic religions such as Christianity, Islam and Buddhism are not simple monolithic structures. The Catholic–Protestant polarity in the west of Scotland is only the most obvious example. Most religions are multiple in their expression, with differing traditions, not all at ease with one another. The tensions within religious traditions can be as tenacious as those between them. At the simplest level the chaplain needs to be at ease with this diversity. If someone describes himself as a Quaker and asks for baptism the chaplain has to know enough about Quakerism to realise that it is a non-sacramental church and that baptism is not practised. But that does not resolve the question. How best to respond? There are two diverging understandings implicit in the request. Which religious language is the one to follow? What 'religious' care is required, if any? Does the chaplain himself act as a filter for such a request or hand it over to the faith community to resolve?

More challenging are the instances where a person's religious identity offers a negative perspective on his/her current situation. If a woman is rescued from the river after an attempted suicide and speaks afterwards of her membership of a local protestant church, religious care might at first sight suggest enlisting its support as a source of care. What if she is reluctant, even resistant, when the offer to make contact is made, and it emerges that the church is strongly and theologically opposed to suicide, so that an attempt on one's life poses a risk to the immortality of the soul? What does a commitment to religious care require? If that conviction is at odds with what is known about that church the chaplain faces a task of gentle clarification. If, however, there are good grounds for believing that this is the authoritative teaching how is the chaplain to respond?

Religious care in the context of spiritual emergence is even less straightforward. A man with a long history of living with a severe personality disorder describes himself as a new adherent of the spiritualist church, speaks freely and often of the spirit world, and of the active presence of good and bad spirits. Further, he sees in the chaplain a spirit guide or higher soul with access to a greater wisdom than the spiritualist church community itself. He then speaks of how his response to what he learns from the spirits is drawing him to decide whether he should give up his life to be of more 'use to them'. At this point spiritual care better describes the chaplain's response as he moves from active listening to a more proactive role.

The attempt to describe *spiritual care* is more elusive because spirituality itself can be a slippery concept. One helpful understanding is that it can refer to the 'essence of human beings as unique individuals: "what makes me, *me*, and you, *you*". It is the power, energy and hopefulness in a person: life at its best; growth and creativity, freedom and love. It is what is deep set in us – what gives us direction, motivation. It is what enables a person to survive bad times, to overcome difficulties, to become themselves'.[3]

This is a good description of a healthy spirituality, one that enriches and sustains. This has little to do with what can be described as 'shallow' spirituality which, like a shallow religiosity, will have little to offer at a time of crisis.

Those we accompany also help us recognise a more difficult truth: the spiritual identity some feel themselves given by God, fate or genetic inheritance is lived in pain. It can be a source of torment, even a matter of life and death. In a bleak description of this spiritual journey Vicky Nichols wrote:

> the dark night of the soul, experienced as a stage on a spiritual journey that then moves on for many, is a landscape that can remain home, or non-home, for people whose access to internal and external sources of hope and renewal is blocked or just not enough to pull them out of the abyss.[1]

We shall return to this linking of spiritual experience to Christian mysticism later.

The chaplain needs to recognise that if spiritual insights, language and practice can be benign they can also appear to be malignant or pathological. Yet there should be no lazy assumption that what is to the outsider a confusing spiritual language is damaging. Just as our mental state influences our spirituality, so the spirituality (if authentic to us) will be shadowed by our mental distress. A critical point of exploration for an accompanier is to help sift through what may seem unconnected, random, even chaotic, spiritual language to find the core, which may hold part of the key to recovery. To dismiss apparently distorted expressions of spirituality as 'nothing more' than the illness runs the risk of failing to nurture the place where a person's fragile meaning is preserved.

Perhaps the best way to conceive of the religious/spiritual dynamic is to picture a continuum on which at every point the chaplain, through conversation and listening, must discern how best to accompany the other in the search for well-being.

Of all the representations of the inner experience of mental distress, Edvard Munch's image of '*The Scream*' is the most famous. Munch's painting shows a lonely figure on a wooden bridge, with eyes wide open in distress, hands clasped to the head, while in the background two well-dressed figures walk on unconcernedly. Munch was concerned here to push to the limit the power of a work of art to reproduce what he called 'das Geschrei', the scream. Munch helps us see not only the inner experience of mental distress, but also the outer experience of loneliness and isolation.

It is in response to these twin aspects of the experience of others that the chaplain develops a way of being and working. This takes shape for me primarily in the model of friendship: a way of relating on the basis of trust and exchange.[5] Of course, there are limits to the mutuality of the relationship, dangers of dependence, and the need constantly to negotiate boundaries. Yet it is well-grounded in many religious traditions. It helps model what human beings need to flourish, and helps determine the chaplain's role of accompaniment: a willingness to travel with the other wherever the journey leads. Eva Hoffman suggested that we are 'keepers of one another's stories', and out of such friendship may come new maps of a shared reality.[6]

A complementary model arises not so much from the relationship with the individual as with the institution. Society invests a great deal of power in the mental health system (see Chapters 23–27). Mental health professionals must be willing to meet the challenge that power – even when benignly exercised – is inextricably part of their practice and of how they are perceived. Chaplains may be caught in a tension here. As they seek to be regarded as fellow professionals by others, and as they are properly accountable within the structures of the health service, do they become 'insiders', part of the establishment, distinct from the person they seek to accompany? This is not easy territory to explore. My own conviction is that the art of chaplaincy is to be both insider *and* outsider: moving with integrity from the edge to the centre, both within *and* at a distance from the structures of power. There are two spheres where this is particularly necessary: confession and what is currently described as spiritual emergence.

Confession and confidentiality

The contemporary chaplain's task is rooted in a long-established practice which can loosely be described as 'priestly'. The increasing professionalisation of chaplains means that such a description of the role might now appear counter-cultural or even alien. Yet, one specific dimension of the chaplain's task does have a priestly character, which illustrates the inter-weaving of religious and spiritual care, and presents discrete ethical dilemmas: *confession*.

We need to confront and then set aside the images conjured up by the word 'confession'. Embedded in all Christian culture, confession commonly finds liturgical expression in worship, and is related to a cluster of ways of understanding the world, its social structures and the relationship between individuals as marked by failure and fracture. It is a way of responding to the human experience of disappointment and our desire for change. It is not accidental that in Catholicism individual confession is part of the sacrament of reconciliation. This shows that the focus is not on sin or failure but on making things good: on restoration of well-being within the person and in the person's relationships with others. The gift of individual confession, whereby an individual 'makes' his confession to God in the presence of a priest, has been a key element in enabling that change. Here it is important to note what the role of the priest is and is not. The confession is not made 'to' the priest but rather 'in the presence of' a priest, who acts as the representative of the wider community of the church, or of God. Through presence, listening, advising and reassuring, the priest helps the individual work towards the desired change.

Even if this is a legitimate religious activity, what makes this other than a 'religious' act, appropriate only to those from a particular Christian tradition? Is there anything here other than a residuum of an older pattern, a redundant way of conceiving chaplaincy? I would argue that the four modes in which a priest operates in sacramental confession – being present, listening, advising and reassuring – can unlock some of the dynamics in the relationship, even when the person has no religious belonging.

One distinctive aspect of the relationship is free choice. There is no obligation for the person to relate to a chaplain, as there may be to other professional staff. Whether a person seeks the chaplain out through self-referral, or is referred at the suggestion of a carer or staff member, the initiative lies wholly with the person. This is especially important in an in-patient setting where there are elements of compulsion or expectations of compliance at the heart of most of the other relationships someone contracts. It may be worth recalling what we explored earlier about the 'friendship' model of chaplaincy. It is for the person to decide the level and degree, the content and the pace of the conversation. The chaplain may or may not have access to the person's history and current treatment plan. Information may or may not be offered by staff or by carers. Yet the discipline within which the chaplain operates is to trust what is shared by the person, to offer respect for him and most importantly, to be wholly present. This implies being wholly focused on the person's good. Here the parallel with sacramental confession may be instructive. In the chaplain's presence the person explores, seeks truth, expresses feelings of regret, speaks of fear and hope, and in doing so moves from an inner monologue into something heard and responded to.

It is in seeking to respond that the chaplain (in 'priestly' mode) faces discrete ethical challenges.

Most centre on the issue of confidentiality. It is self-evident that in the context of sacramental confession there is an overriding obligation to respect the confidential nature of what
is 'overheard', what is often referred to as the 'seal of the confessional'. Even here, in practice, that is not an absolute, but there is a strong presumption that what is shared remains
sealed within the penitent/confessor relationship.

Yet it is important to distinguish between 'confidential' and 'secret'. If someone shares
with the chaplain in the course of an exchange that he made a violent knife attack on
another within his family, and that this is the basis for his detention, this is hardly a secret. It
is a public fact. If he then speaks of his sense of shame, of deep regret both for the physical
hurt caused and for the effect it has had on his relationship with his whole family we move
into a place in the conversation where the use of moral language has been initiated and to
which the chaplain may respond. If the person then asks for a copy of the bible the chaplain
may want to suggest certain passages or narratives which from knowledge may deal with
violence and forgiveness. When the conversation is over he may ask the person's permission
to alert nursing staff that this is one of the actions he proposes to take.

If the person speaks further about the weight of the knowledge of the consequences of his
action the chaplain may respond by asking him to identify practical steps he might take to
repair the harm, and elicit what might stand in the way. If the person then asks if he can ever
be forgiven, the chaplain may respond to the implicitly religious nature of the question.
Throughout this exploration the chaplain must judge what is 'confessional' or 'confidential',
and having made that judgement suggest that there are things here which it would be helpful
for other staff to be aware of. It is always more creative for the person to undertake that sharing but it can be the chaplain's role to seek permission to share key issues with staff.

If the person speaks of his fear that, given the opportunity, he would carry out another
attack, or if the level of shame and hopelessness is so deep that he might commit suicide,
then the chaplain's responsibility is to alert other staff. Too narrow a commitment to confidentiality would produce negative results for the person's good or the good of others. This
is not a breach of confidentiality. It is part of what being wholly present implies: being atten-
tive to and focused on the good of the other; being alert to moments of collusion in a 'secret'
conversation; and holding in balance friendship with the person and the responsibilities of
belonging within a professional multi-disciplinary team.

It recalls what we characterised earlier as the insider/outsider nature of the chaplain's
role. There is value in what people perceive as the marginality of the chaplain, someone on
the edge. Yet the chaplain is also a privileged member of a multi-disciplinary team. The
craft requires finding the right balance. For example, a service user concerned about drug
treatment or mounting anxieties about an imminent tribunal may make negative comments about staff. It may be helpful for the chaplain to act as a 'lightning conductor' for
frustration, knowing that there will be no negative consequences. If, however, the grievance seems well-founded the chaplain should be ready either to clarify the grievance and
help identify some strategies, or to offer to act as an advocate. All of this is implicit in the
friendship model.

What can be more troubling for the chaplain is when someone speaks of an intention to
'play the game': to be outwardly compliant with a treatment regime he/she has no confidence
in. A chaplain has to discern when he is simply offering space for the discharge of emotions of
fear or frustration, when he is in danger of colluding with someone over unproven criticism of
colleagues and therefore damaging trust, and when the sense of grievance is so deep-seated as
to have a potentially negative impact on recovery. The guide in this is likely to be a fairly
straightforward: 'what works for this person's greatest good?' (see Chapter 30).

If the dilemmas which emerge from the confessional/confidential aspect of the chaplain's relationship with a person relate to a tradition of religious care and to some extent are familiar, those which arise in the context of spiritual emergence require a different set of skills.

Spiritual emergence and spiritual emergency

'What I was experiencing was a spiritual emergency and not a mental illness'.[7]

It has long been a complaint that mental health service providers either ignore or pathologise the spiritual dimension of people's lives, proof of what has been described as a peculiar cultural insensitivity, a 'religiosity gap'[8] between clinicians and patients. This is eloquently expressed in the following:

> . . . it is, to my mind, little short of miraculous that in the lives of so many people, the heart and soul are awakened by what appears to be the direct intervention of spiritual reality. The difficulty . . . is to recognise such an intervention when it comes and to be able to hold on to its authenticity in the face of scepticism or outright ridicule. Most difficult of all . . . is to hold on to it when others deem it to be madness or the unmistakable evidence of psychosis.[9]

This makes the development, from the 1980s onwards, of clinical interest in 'spiritual emergence' all the more significant, even if the research base remains small. Much of the experience which is described under this term could be found in the traditions of many historic religions. Thus heightened perhaps even ecstatic experiences, the inner assault on established ways of being, a sense of the thinning of the veil between the inner world and the outer world, the visionary and the ordinary, are familiar spiritual territory, albeit uncommon. What makes such experiences significant in terms of mental health is that they may be accompanied by distress, by unusual or bizarre references such as near death experience, close encounters with extra-terrestrial beings or communication with spirit guides. Some factors peculiar to our time may make this phenomenon potentially volatile for the person experiencing them.

The person living through such a time of awakening may be unconnected with any formal religious tradition. Perhaps significantly, web-based support networks refer to the hazards of practising spiritual techniques which in the past were either restricted to an inner elite or were always taught by 'masters' who accompanied the learner. Similarly, they may warn against 'a do it yourself' approach to spirituality. At the most basic level each religious system has a language to help give shape to such deep inner experience which might be called loosely the 'mystical'. Without a commonly agreed vocabulary how is the person living through such a time to trust it, to discern what is authentic and to find ways of communicating it meaningfully to others? This takes us back to the picture which Munch gave, of the mirroring of internal distress by outer isolation.

In a very helpful approach a model was developed which distinguished three different kinds or levels of such experience.[10] Prefaced by criticism of 'spiritual illiteracy' not only among professionals but also in the wider culture it suggested that it is helpful to discriminate between spiritual development, seen as a gradual and untroubled process, spiritual emergence which is connected to enhanced emotional and psychological health and a deeper connectedness, and spiritual emergency which can appear to be identical to psychosis. In this last, spiritual emergency, while not doubting that there may be a serious psychotic condition in which the psyche fragments, the model offers the possibility of healthful emergence.

Thus, in the face of a deep-seated and recurrent depression someone in a gradual process of spiritual development may reconnect with a Catholic childhood faith, finding in its rituals a response to the depression which is being lived through. That reconnection is not to be dismissed as simply reversion or flight, although those elements may be present. The dilemma to the one accompanying here may be that reconnecting with a conservative faith perspective brings in its wake negative perceptions of, say, a sexual identity which is too sinful to be acknowledged. However, the reconnection, the breakthrough from loneliness into community is benign.

Less benign may be the experience of someone who sees his life as a re-enactment of Christ's life and who points to marks on his body which echo the marks of the crucifixion. How best to counter the delusion while responding to the evident search to 'make sense' of current experience? Although there is an older tradition of piety which would have affirmed this as a sign of spiritual growth, the dangers here are all too evident. It is crucial to discern if there is a potential link between a conventional (and therefore healthy?) Christian under-standing of Christ's death and suicidal ideation. Is such an experience one which will lead to spiritual growth, is it psychotic or a mix of the two?

To illustrate some of these dynamics it may be helpful to look at the insight of the nineteenth century poet Gerard Manley Hopkins who knew what it was to stand on the edge of the men-tal abyss. In his poems he helps those who seek to be accompaniers catch sight of the inner experience not only of mental distress but also of spiritual emergence. A Jesuit priest, Hopkins was alert to the complex interplay between the life of the mind and the life of the spirit, between the life of a mind assailed and a spirit tested to the point of destruction. Through his poems he helps us approach the difficult questions which surround that relationship:

> No worst there is none. Pitched past pitch of grief, more pangs will . . . wilder wring. Comforter, where, where is your comforting? Mary, mother of us, where is your relief? . . . O the mind, mind has mountains; cliffs of fall Frightful, sheer, no-man-fathomed. Hold them cheap May who ne'er hung there.[11]

His image of mental illness as the experience of being suspended over the abyss is echoed by many. As he wrestles with what the spiritual significance of his mental illness might be, or worse might not be, he helps us see that the first need is to find a language. It is striking that many of the discussions of the connections between 'breakdown' and 'breakthrough' begin with a consideration of what growth may occur in the midst of, or even in despite of, mental illness. Yet the religious heritage has a prior part to play in spiritual emergence. It can help find words for the present distress, providing stories and narratives which move on a different plane from the objectivity of diagnostic language. It can provide analogies for the person's experience which may help break through the sense of isolation and loneliness.

If the religious and spiritual heritage have the potential to be helpful in setting an indi-vidual's experience in a wider frame, offering words, images and stories which resonate with their present experience, there is an important caveat which the chaplain has to be alert to. Indeed it is the dilemma which confronts chaplains in the whole of their craft, the danger that professionals 'colonise' this most intimate part of a person's identity. The following observation is instructive:

> My spirituality is intensely personal and one of the few things I can really call my own. I fear professionals invading my personal space. It is important that those who are meant to care for me do not take over aspects of my identity.[12]

In sum, the chaplain, rooted in a craft which has a long reflective tradition, is to act as a friend to the other, to complement what all those involved in a person's care may bring to the search for recovery, and above all to be ever alert to the mystery and dignity of each person's inner world.

Notes

1 The concept was first developed by G. Davie (1994) *Religion in Britain since 1945: Believing without Belonging*. London: Wiley Blackwell.
2 NHS Education for Scotland, *Spiritual Care Matters: An Introductory Resource for all NHS Scotland Staff*. 2009, pp. 7–9. Online. Available. http://www.nes.scot.nhs.uk/documents/publications/classa/030 309SpiritualCareMatters.pdf Other key documents are collected in Scottish Government Department of Health and Wellbeing *Spiritual Care and Chaplaincy in NHS Scotland*. Online. Available. http://www.sehd.scot.nhs.uk/mels/CEL2008_ 49.pdf
3 Quoted in P Gilbert (2007) The Spiritual Foundation: Awareness and context for people's lives today. In: ME Coyte, P Gilbert, and V Nicholls (eds.) *Spirituality, Values and Mental Health: Jewels for the Journey*. London: Jessica Kingsley Publishers, p. 23.
4 V Nicholls (2007) Connecting Past and Present: A survivor reflects on spirituality and mental health. In: Coyte, Gilbert, and Nicholls, op. cit. p. 106.
5 For a full exploration of the model see J. Swinton (2000) *Resurrecting the Person*. Nashville, TN: Abingdon Press.
6 Quoted in P Gilbert The Spiritual Foundation op. cit. p. 31.
7 W Brown and N Kandirikirira (2007) *Recovering Mental Health in Scotland: Report on Narrative Investigation of Mental Health Recovery*. Scottish Recovery Network: Glasgow, p. 36.
8 N Crowley, *Psychosis or Spiritual Emergence? – The Transpersonal Perspective within Psychiatry*. p. 4. Online. Available. http://www.rcpsych.ac.uk/members/specialinterestgroups/spirituality/publications.aspx
9 B Thorne (2007) Awakening the Heart and Soul: Reflections from therapy. In: ME Coyte, P Gilbert, and V Nicholls op. cit. p. 273.
10 Ibid.
11 Gerard Manley Hopkins (1970) *Collected Poems*. London: OUP, p. 100.
12 W Edwards and P Gilbert (2007) Spiritual Assessment – Narratives and responses. In: ME Coyte, P Gilbert, and V Edwards, op. cit. p. 149.

Section 2 – Ethical dilemmas

Phil Barker

A deeply personal common thread runs through the seven contributions in Section 2. Each acknowledges that there is good reason to doubt his/her professional integrity: history often provides only the cruellest of mirrors. However, if there is any criticism – of professional role or function – it comes from the professionals themselves. They are only too aware of their limitations and the imperatives necessary to fulfil their professional obligations.

There are also clear tensions between these 'team members'. All seem to be asking, in different ways: to whom do I owe my allegiance?

What is my professional duty?

All professionals are expected to ensure that people do not come to any foreseeable harm as a direct (or indirect) result of their fulfilment of any aspect of their professional practice. This applies as much to an engineer involved in the building of a bridge, as a nurse involved in caring for a vulnerable person. The 'duty of care' is, as a result, enshrined in law. All mental health professionals are expected to adhere to some reasonable standard of care in the fulfilment of their practice. While specific examples may be given, especially by governing professional bodies, the range of possible situations is infinite.

However, aside from the legal concept of 'duty of care', all professionals might consider their 'moral responsibility' in any given situation. This might be similar to a duty of care but might, conceivably, be quite different.

How do my personal and cultural beliefs affect the care I offer?

All professional disciplines develop a discrete professional philosophy, which guides their practice, at least in principle. The Hippocratic Oath, which involves upholding a specific set of ethical standards, is the oldest example of such a belief system. However, individual practitioners also hold particular beliefs, which may conflict with the general guidance offered, for example, by a professional Code of Ethics.

All professionals might reflect on their 'personal' belief system. What do they understand by concepts such as: 'health' and 'illness'; 'care' and 'treatment'; and 'right' and 'wrong'? To what extent do such 'personal beliefs' fit or conflict with professional Codes of Conduct, or other ethical frameworks in common use?

Who am I working for?

In principle, all professionals are working for the person who is the 'patient' or 'client'. In practice, professionals are likely to feel pulled in several directions at once: by their responsibilities towards families, managers, society and healthcare funders among others.

All professionals might reflect on the inherent tensions in their work related, specifically, to this notion of *allegiance*. How might they begin to address the ethical problems that might emerge from such a conflict of loyalties?

What is my role and function?

Although the specific roles of different professionals appear, in principle, to be clear-cut, in practice there can be considerable overlap. The demands of teamwork often blur the distinction between one professional and another.

All professionals might consider what, exactly, is their professional responsibility, in any given situation: as a psychiatrist, nurse, chaplain and so on. In particular, professionals might consider to what extent 'teamwork' conflicts with the fulfilment of their role as a discrete professional. How do they address the possible tensions between being a 'team member' and an autonomous individual professional?

How 'good' is my practice – or that of the service in general?

Many professionals cultivate – or are encouraged to cultivate – a sense of emotional distance between themselves and the person in their care. This defines the 'boundaries' of the professional relationship; distinguishing it from 'casual' relationships or friendship. However, this can result in a view of the person as the 'object' of care and treatment, rather than the 'subject'.

All professionals might consider how appropriate the service on offer – by themselves or the team – would be if the person receiving it was a member of their family, a friend or some other 'significant other'. How would they *judge* the quality as well as the appropriateness of the service? How would they address any shortfall in the standard of care or treatment they would expect would be necessary for some 'loved one'?

Section 3

Care and treatment

Section preface

Phil Barker

'Mental health' implies many different things – from vague ideas about 'well-being' to strict, but equally vague, rulings in law. The key focus of all mental health services is *care* and *treatment*, definitions of which can also be vague, if not contradictory.

Although relatively young, the institution of 'modern psychiatry' has changed direction several times: assuming new identities; of necessity, shedding the skin of its last incarnation. What has remained constant is the assumption that psychiatry – and its contemporary incarnation, mental health – provides 'care' and 'treatment' for those who need it; even if they do not actually *want* it. Long seen as something soft and supportive, *care* is usually delivered by nurses or other relatively low-ranking carers. By contrast, *treatment* is assumed to be more sophisticated and scientific, if not daring and heroic, offered by doctors and other expert 'therapists'.

Section 3 profiles five aspects of contemporary mental health care and treatment. There are many other areas that could have been considered but, arguably, these represent the most important aspects of contemporary practice, if not also those most fraught with ethical problems. Perhaps, not surprisingly, the 'high profile', technical or sophisticated aspects of care and treatment are most often delivered by the medical specialist – the psychiatrist. The grittier, awkward, troublesome aspects – I hesitate to call it 'dirty work' – tend to be done by anyone *but* the psychiatrist.

A **psychiatric diagnosis** is necessary, in most countries, before anyone can be offered any kind of care and treatment. It is widely assumed that mental health (or more accurately, *psychiatry*) is a medical speciality, so it is unsurprising that *diagnosis* should be considered so important. Even the layperson knows that a proper diagnosis is necessary before the appropriate treatment (or therapy) can be determined. Here, however, the parallels with medical diagnosis begin to collapse, if not also the blind faith in psychiatry as a branch of medicine. It has become clearer, over the past 30 years, that psychiatric diagnosis is merely a powerful form of name-calling: describing, in lofty terms what people *do*; or giving a name to what other people *think* of the actor. Psychiatric diagnosis is, primarily, the preserve of the psychiatrist.

Professional relationships form the basis of all care and treatment. Even the effectiveness of a physiotherapy session for a pulled muscle will be judged, in part, on how we *felt* about the therapist. In mental health, unlike physiotherapy, there is little 'laying on of hands'. Almost everything done in the name of care and treatment is expressed through professional relationships – most often through conversation. Even when professionals are not intending to 'make' a relationship, this becomes the key focus of almost everything that they do. Although all disciplines are required to engage in such 'relating', some groups – like nurses – do much more of this than anyone else. Indeed, *relationships* and *mental health nursing* have become almost indistinguishable concepts.

One could be excused for thinking that **restraint** belonged to the past: an unsavoury image from a Hogarth engraving: pointing backwards to the asylum era. This appears to be no more than wishful thinking. Various forms of restraint, and other coercive practices, remain firmly embedded in contemporary services. There may no longer be 'rubber rooms' or 'shackles' but 'creative' ways of holding people in check still exist, albeit disguised by 'politically correct' language. Do we lack the ingenuity to develop alternatives, or do we simply lack the motivation?

Electroconvulsive therapy (ECT) is another psychiatric 'treatment' with a poor track record in the public imagination; inspired partly by its depiction in many Hollywood films over the decades. Shock therapy was always seen as a drastic intervention; one of the 'necessary evils' of psychiatry. However, discharging an electric current through the brain might be necessary, providing it was not *your* brain. In principle **consent** is necessary for any form of care and treatment, but where the treatment is potentially dangerous – as in ECT – very specific conditions need to be put in place, before treatment can proceed.

Finally, **medication** is part of the staple fare of all medical treatment. People who visit the doctor and are *not* given a prescription for some drug are often sorely disappointed. However, most drugs prescribed by physicians are highly specific in their intended action: like *anti*convulsants, or *anti*biotics, seeking to control or eliminate a very specific medical problem. Psychiatric drugs are, by contrast, fairly blunt instruments. For a long time we have developed hopes of a pill for every ill, something like Aldous Huxley's *soma*, which could keep the world at bay. The history of psychiatric medication was full of such expectation, but ultimately the price for the boasting and mendacity had to be paid. That said, for many people medication is still the 'best option': a much easier route to relief than actually dealing with one's life problems.

11 Psychiatric diagnosis

Phil Barker

Introduction

Judgement – not *diagnosis*

However much psychiatric diagnosis may *share* the language of medicine, it is a completely different, if not alien, form of classification. All medical diagnoses begin with a hypothesis, based on the physician's observations of *signs* of possible illness, displayed by the body, and *symptoms* reported by the person. The formal diagnosis – especially where the condition is severe or life-threatening – is dependent on pathological corroboration. After examining me, the physician may *believe* that I have swine flu (H1N1) but would need the results of a laboratory test of a viral culture to confirm this. If my condition appears related to a more complex, or rare disorder, the physician might need to call on the support of radiographers, toxicologists, pathologists or other medical scientists, to confirm the diagnosis.

By contrast, if I go (or am sent) to a psychiatrist complaining of *troubling* thoughts, feelings or patterns of behaviour – or indeed if a member of my family views any of these as troublesome – a psychiatrist may decide, on the basis of an interview, that I have a psychiatric disorder. None of the blood tests, urine tests, X-rays, biopsies or computerised body scans, commonly used to confirm a medical diagnosis, will be used to help confirm the presence of my 'illness'. Although I may be interviewed several times, in principle a *single conversation* with a *single psychiatrist* is all that is necessary to judge whether or not I am 'mentally ill'.

However odious the comparison might seem to psychiatrists – if not other mental health professionals – all psychiatric diagnosis is mere *opinion*, based on the professional's 'powers of observation'. These are the same 'tools' used by the art or theatre critic, or the judges in boxing or gymnastics. Of course, these critics and judges might be described as experts, having witnessed hundreds if not thousands of 'performances', and their judgement might carry considerable authority. However, the audience, the general public and the performers are free to disagree. Indeed, time will tell whether these opinions were flawed if not actually 'fixed'.

However, because a psychiatric diagnosis is made by a doctor it is assumed to relate to an *actual* illness.[1] In that sense, it is nothing like judging the results of a boxing match. If those judges make errors of judgement, or even 'fix the fight', the loser can still fight again later for another title. By contrast, if I am judged to have a psychiatric disorder, this may (indeed likely *will*) affect, among other things: my freedom to travel internationally; my career opportunities; my chances of adopting or fostering a child; or even my right to cast my vote in an election. Unlike sports, making a comeback from a psychiatric diagnosis is fraught with many more complications.

Distress or disturbance – not *illness*

Fifty years ago, Thomas Szasz described the concept of 'mental illness' as a myth: something people believed in, which had great symbolic power, but which was literally impossible.[2] The *mind* is a concept. An abstract idea cannot become *ill* in the sense that a bodily organ becomes diseased. 'Mental illness' merely refers to particular kinds of human behaviour, which either the person (who becomes a 'patient') or others – friends, family or society at large – find *troubling*, in one way or another. A woman who complains that she is afraid to leave the house might be diagnosed with 'agoraphobia'; a man believed to have a compulsion for abusing young children, might be diagnosed with 'paedophilia'. However, if offered 'psychotherapy' for their respective 'disorders', the woman's anxiety might be reduced and the man's compulsion might be 'minimised'. No amount of talking will affect a genuine illness, characterised by a low blood count, malignant tumour or a systemic infection.

The ethics of 'mental illness'

Clearly, some people, or their families, friends and others, may be *troubled* by the way they behave; the ideas they embrace; or the emotions they experience (or do not appear to experience). Some of these people may appear distressed to such an extent that they are unable to work, relate to others, or otherwise get on with their everyday lives. Something – or several things – might be going on in the person's life, which might require attention. However, it would be wrong – in an ethical sense – to refer to these 'happenings' – or 'problems in living' – as manifestations of a 'mental illness'.

The metaphor of mental illness

First of all, however *distressed* someone might feel or however *disturbing* the person might be to others, the person is 'sick' *only* in the same sense that a joke or a building might be considered 'sick': disturbing to *some* people in *some* way. Any 'mental illness' exists only as a metaphor.

The psychiatric cliché states that: '*mental illness is just like any other illness*'. However well-intentioned this remark, it is based, at the very least, on a complete misunderstanding of medical diagnosis. At worst, it is a *lie*: used by the disingenuous, to promote particular social or political ends. Politicians, and psychiatric professionals, have *argued* repeatedly that:

- 'mental illnesses are diagnosable disorders of the brain';
- (which) 'can be accurately diagnosed, successfully treated, just as a physical illness'; and
- that 'one of the most widely believed and most damaging myths is that mental illness is not a physical disease; nothing could be further from the truth'.[3]

It is unlikely that advocates of the '*like any other illness*' view, believe that each one of the hundreds of psychiatric disorders defined in the *Diagnostic and Statistical Manual of Mental Disorders* (DSM) is a 'brain disorder' or 'physical disease'. Despite all the rhetoric there is no evidence that even the most intensively researched forms of 'mental illness' – 'schizophrenia' and 'bipolar disorder' – are 'disorders of the brain', far less 'physical diseases'. Moreover, if they were, then people with such 'diseases' should be in the care of neurologists, the medical experts in brain pathology, not psychiatrists.[4]

Ideas have consequences

Throughout most of its history, psychiatry promoted the fiction that 'mental illness' was a life-long condition. People might experience some 'remission' but recurrence (relapses) was likely. Psychiatry also promoted vigorously the idea that people could *only* get better (recover) with the help of psychiatric professionals. Where this was not wishful thinking it was mendacity writ large.[5] Evidence has accumulated over the past 50 years regarding the damage done by psychiatry in the name of 'care' or 'treatment'. Over the past 20 years it has, however, become clearer that people can and do 'recover' from the states called 'mental illness'; including the so-called 'serious' states called 'schizophrenia' or 'bipolar disorder'. Most of these recoveries owed nothing to psychiatric treatment by drugs or other physical methods. Instead, the *social support* of professional staff,[6] friends or peers,[7] or even self-belief,[8] held the key. Increasingly, research by psychiatrists and psychologists also challenges the assumption that drugs, far less other more drastic forms of psychiatric 'treatment', are necessary.[9] Sadly, many people continue to be misled into thinking that their 'diagnosis' means that they have an 'illness'; and that their recovery depends on a life-long regime of psychiatric drugs. The UK charity *Rethink* offers fairly typical advice:

> Accepting your diagnosis can be the first step to recovery. Acceptance can lead to an understanding of the value of ongoing treatment, which in turn improves the chances of recovery. Such beliefs can help you to stick to taking your medication.[10]

The history of psychiatry tells a sobering story of the consequences of the idea of 'mental illness', which fostered the development of bogus psychiatric diagnoses, which in turn consigned many people to a career of damaging psychiatric 'interventions', and a lifetime of dependency and social exclusion. As noted earlier, the key consequence of a psychiatric diagnosis is that people given such diagnoses risk losing many of the rights most of us take for granted.

Power and coercion

Unlike other forms of 'serious' illness – cardiovascular disease, cancer, AIDS – people with 'mental illness' may be *obliged* to accept a diagnosis and be *compelled* to accept 'treatment'. Professionals may argue that such 'treatments' – by psychiatric drugs, ECT or some 'talking cure' – are 'effective'. In any democracy, this should be irrelevant. The person should be *free* to reject it. People with serious medical conditions can, and often do, reject offers of life-saving treatment (see Chapter 2). People with a psychiatric diagnosis remain the only people who can lose their liberty *and* be forced to accept some 'treatment', against their wishes. This state of affairs is merely the latest chapter in the long history of psychiatric containment and control (see Chapter 3).

Illness or disorder?

Today, psychiatrist talk less about 'mental illness' and more about 'psychiatric disorder; however the implication of some 'underlying illness', 'genetic influence' or 'biological basis' remains.[11] Arguably, the general public – including politicians and medical journalists – represent the greatest believers in 'mental illness'. They may talk about 'mental health problems' but this is only a synonym for 'mental illness'. Without doubt, the new 'politically correct' language can be traced to Szasz's influence. No satisfactory genetic or biological evidence has ever been produced to account for any of the hundreds of forms of psychiatric disorder in the *DSM*. Everyone knows that talk of 'mental health problems' carries little *authority*. If people are to obtain any help, such 'problems' must be translated into one form of 'mental illness' or another; and codified as a particular 'mental disorder'.

The classification of psychiatric disorders

The two main forms of classification in psychiatry are: the *International Statistical Classification of Disease and Related Health Problems*[12] (ICD-10) published by the *World Health Organisation* (WHO); and the *DSM-IV*,[13] published by the *American Psychiatric Association* (APA). Both aim to distinguish groups of 'patients' with identical or similar 'clinical symptoms'. This serves as the first step towards care or treatment. A *formal* psychiatric diagnosis is necessary before people can be treated in state-funded hospitals, or private insurance companies will pay the bills.

Following a *medical* diagnosis most physicians would be able to make a prediction of the prospects of recovery for any patient (prognosis). This is *not* the case in psychiatry, as most psychiatrists readily admit: 'Diagnosis in psychiatry increasingly struggles to fulfil its key purposes, namely, to guide treatment and to predict outcome'.[14]

The ICD-10

The statistical classification of diseases dates from the nineteenth century and until the early twentieth century focused on causes of death.[15] The *WHO* took over the classification in 1948 and the system was renamed the *International Classification of Diseases and Related Health Problems*. The ICD is used to classify diseases and other health problems on health and vital records, such as death certificates and hospital records. The latest version – *ICD-10* – has 22 chapters, ranging from 'Infectious and parasitic diseases' to 'External causes of morbidity and mortality'. Chapter 5 addresses: '*Mental and behavioural disorders*'. Although this WHO system is focused on the classification of *diseases*, it carries the following cautionary note:

> The term 'disorder' is used throughout the classification, so as to avoid even greater problems inherent in the use of terms such as 'disease' and 'illness'. 'Disorder' is not an exact term, but it is used here to imply the existence of a clinically recognizable set of symptoms or behaviour associated in most cases with distress and with interference with personal functions.[16]

Even the compilers of the ICD were uncomfortable with the notion that 'mental disorders' might be mistaken for *actual* diseases or illnesses. Szasz's 50-year-old critique of the metaphor of 'mental illness' appears, finally, to have been accepted, however grudgingly. That said, the terms 'clinical' and 'symptoms' are commonly understood to refer (only) to medical phenomena. By cunningly conjuring with medical language, the authors of the ICD continue to give the reader the impression that mental 'disorders' are 'medical disorders'.

The DSM-IV

Not surprisingly, given its origins in the USA, the *DSM* has become the most influential psychiatric classification system.[17] Like the ICD, its origins lie in the mid-nineteenth century, when the US Census department began to count the number of people detained in asylums. The idea of developing a uniform system for classifying 'madness' was first proposed in 1849 by an association of Medical Superintendents, which evolved into the APA in 1921, when formal data began to be collected.[18] By 1950 these statistics had become the responsibility of the *National Institute of Mental Health* and the first version of the DSM was published in 1952.

DSM-I (1952): Adolf Meyer's 'psychobiological' approach was a major influence on this first manual.[19] Meyer understood 'mental illness' as a reaction of the personality to psychological, social and biological factors. Meyer's concept of 'reactions'[20] was used to define most of the 'mental disorders' included in this first edition.

DSM-II (1968): The second version had no dominant theoretical framework. Although it emphasised Kraepelin's approach to diagnosis – focusing on symptoms rather than underlying 'pathology' – the 'symptoms' were not defined in any great detail. Instead, disorders were seen as reflecting broad underlying *conflicts* or *maladaptive reactions* to life problems: evidence of the continued influence of psychoanalysis.

DSM-III (1980): Work began on the third revision in 1973 and introduced detailed descriptions of symptoms, removing all reference to possible aetiology. In abandoning the notion of 'cause' DSM-III became firmly phenomenological. This version also abandoned the concept of 'neurosis', much to the disgust of psychoanalysts.

Two significant developments occurred within DSM-III.

1   The diagnosis of homosexuality had been withdrawn from DSM-II in 1973, mainly because of the negative publicity generated by Gay Rights activists.[21] In DSM-III, homosexuality, once integral to the psychoanalytic construction of 'mental illness', was formally 'declassified' and became 'normal' behaviour.

2   Biological psychiatrists were keen to dismiss all terms and theories associated with hypothetical or explanatory concepts. As a result, the DSM shifted from *explaining* 'mental illness' – for example by reference to 'conflicts' – to a wholly *descriptive* (phenomenological) approach, which continues to the present day: the 'neo-Kraepelinian revolution'.[22] The term *empirical* also began to be used, emphasising the reliance on experience or experiment, without the need for theories or hypotheses.[23] This move towards a more detailed diagnostic process was influenced by the scandal that followed the publication of the Rosenhahn's study[24]; psychiatrists appeared unable to discriminate between 'real' patients, and people 'pretending' to be 'patients'.[25]

DSM-IV (1994): Further revisions were made in 1987 (DSM-III-R), but by the early 1990s the APA had developed DSM-IV, which displayed much closer co-operation with the WHO and the designers of ICD-10.

The most recent version – DSM-IV (the 'text revision') was published in 2000. This continued the emphasis on gaining approval for diagnoses. The APA noted that: 'more than 1000 people (and numerous professional organisations) have helped in preparation of this document'.[26]

DSM-V

Work on a further revision has been ongoing for several years and *DSM-V* is expected to be published in 2010. The APA continued to develop its emphasis on consultation, and established a website at which people could comment on the proposed revisions. Doubtless such 'polling' of opinion might appear bizarre to other physicians. Genuine diseases or illnesses are *discovered* by medical science, not *constructed* by committee. For almost 40 years, the APA has brought together various groups of psychiatric 'experts' who have voted for the inclusion or exclusion of disorders. This method began with Robert Spitzer, architect of DSM-III and DSM-III-R.[27]

During the development of DSM-V the APA were lobbied by gay/lesbian/transgendered people, who were opposed to classifying 'Gender Identity Disorder' as a 'disorder'. This echo of the removal of 'homosexuality' in 1973 reminds us that if sufficient pressure can be brought to bear, 'mental disorders' can be created or made to disappear. This begs the question: are psychiatric diagnoses *medical*, *social* or *political* phenomena?

The ethics of psychiatric diagnosis

All systems of diagnostic classification in psychiatry have been widely criticised.[28–32]

- Psychiatric diagnosis reduces people to one-dimensional sources of 'data', obstructing any attempt to consider the 'whole person'.
- Psychiatric diagnosis 'medicalises' problems in human living,[33] perpetuating the social stigma associated with 'insanity'; avoiding addressing the complex personal, interpersonal and social issues at play.
- The use of 'symptom-based criteria', in the absence of any classic 'signs' of disease or bodily disorder, has resulted in a seemingly endless multiplication of the original number of 'mental disorders'. Within 30 years the DSM grew from 134 to 943 pages.
- The politics, and inherent values, of the criteria for inclusion and/or exclusion of disorders are self-evident. 'Post-traumatic-stress disorder' was included following *positive* lobbying from trauma victims and homosexuality was dropped following *negative* lobbying from Gay Rights groups. A similar scenario would never have happened in relation to the diagnosis of genuine illnesses or disorders – such as cancer or hypertension.
- Diagnostic criteria within both DSM and ICD imply, but do not state directly, the notion of psychological 'well being'. In principle, almost any experience, or behaviour, could be classed as a disorder, if it is considered 'odd' (i.e. pathological) by enough people.
- The current classification systems are heavily biased towards states for which people want 'treatment'. Despite the socially disruptive and 'unhealthy' nature of anger, hostility and aggression, only one DSM-IV disorder explicitly addresses this area (intermittent explosive disorder). By contrast, entire categories are devoted to 'depression' and 'anxiety'. Few film or television 'heroes' are depressed and anxious; many are 'intermittently explosive'. The classification systems appear to reinforce popular stereotypes of failure and success.
- The diagnosis of 'mental disorders' implies some underpinning biological disorder. This is expressed by the widespread borrowing of terminology from general medicine: 'symptoms', 'relapses', 'prodromes' and so on. This contributes greatly to the popular belief that problems of human life are disorders, which can be solved by taking medication or some other kind of 'therapy'.[34] This is the 'medicalisation of everyday life'.[35] However, many members of society appear more than willing to support attempts to 'medicalise' the myriad moral problems they encounter in their lives. Slavery, apartheid and anti-semitism, all have been *popular* at some time in some society. This did not make them 'right'.

Conclusion

People have developed systems of classification for all manner of things, for thousands of years. The classification of 'mental disorders', in one form or another, has been around for a long time, and today the medical language of psychiatric diagnosis, however false, is firmly established within everyday conversation. To impress the laity, physicians adapted Greek or Latin words to describe the body and its various diseases. Psychiatrists followed suit. As Szasz noted:

> They called inflammation of the lung 'pneumonia' and kidney failure 'uraemia'. The result is that people now think that any Greco-Roman word ending in *ia* – or with the suffix *philia* or *phobia* – is a bona fide disease. This credulity would be humorous if it were not tragic.[36]

A century ago there were only a handful of forms of 'insanity'. Today, there are literally hundreds of forms of 'mental disorder', many carrying Greco-Roman suffixes: kleptomania, anorexia nervosa, hypomania, paraphilia, and so on. Ironically, despite the alleged 'advances' in psychiatric research and treatment, there are many more people now with some 'mental disorder' than was the case, even 20 years ago. Moreover, so-called epidemics of 'bipolar disorder',[37] 'borderline personality disorder',[38] 'multiple personality disorder'[39] and 'narcissistic personality disorder'[40] are frequently said to be sweeping the Western world. However, unlike influenza, such psychiatric 'epidemics' either signal changes either in the psychosocial milieu, or the influence of the drug industry. Whitaker argues that the massive increase in the diagnosis of 'bipolar disorder' is due, largely, to marketing pressures from drug companies.[41]

In general medicine, diagnosis provides an economical means of communicating clearly and precisely about the presence of *actual* bodily disease, or the presence of actual organic or functional disorder. Medical diagnosis gives a name to a process that is already evident *within* the body itself. By contrast, psychiatric diagnoses are names for complex patterns of *behaviour* and/or *subjective experiences*, which are *exhibited* by people, interpersonally or socially. The very same behaviour, occurring or exhibited in private or alone, is excluded from diagnostic consideration. *Homosexuality*, along with various other 'sexual perversions', was long considered not simply a vice, but a serious form of 'mental illness'. Now, people are 'gay' and their identity merely reflects a 'sexual preference'. Most forms of sexual behaviour were heavily controlled by the Christian church, and others, throughout history: the translation of such taboos into forms of 'mental illness' was a reflection of late nineteenth century morality. Today, many societies appear to have a 'positive obsession' with sexuality, with the result that forms of behaviour that once were taboo – such as 'fetishes' or 'cross dressing' – are now lauded as liberating.

These are examples of cultural 'shifts' that also reflect the *politics* of diagnosis. Szasz commented:

> Psychiatrists diagnose the person who eats too much as suffering from 'bulimia' and the person who eats too little as suffering from 'anorexia nervosa'. Similarly the person who has too much sex suffers from a 'sex addiction', while the person who shows too little interest in sex suffers from 'sexual aversion disorder'. Yet psychiatrists do not consider celibacy a form of mental illness; celibate persons are not said to suffer from 'anerotica nervosa'.[42]

Celibacy, especially as practised by Catholic priests, is valued as a sign of religious commitment: a 'good' thing. Within conventional medicine, a condition that may be classed as an illness is never considered to be a 'good' thing.

Recently, a campaign has emerged focused on the 'abolition of the schizophrenia label' (CASL).[13] The campaign's argument is that 'schizophrenia' as a diagnosis is 'unscientific' and 'has outlived its usefulness'. Moreover, the campaign argues that the label is damaging to people so labelled. This is all too obvious, and clearly is the case for many other psychiatric 'disorders'. It is not clear if the supporters of this campaign wish to get rid of all psychiatric diagnoses or just 'schizophrenia'. CASL supporters appear enthusiastic about the Japanese decision to re-label *Seishin Bunretsu Byo* ('mind-split-disease') as 'integration disorder' (this Japanese term is the closest thing to 'schizophrenia' in the West). This appears to be a rather modest kind of campaigning: the replacement of an anachronistic, fake medical term with psychobabble. However incensed the CASL group appear to be about the immorality of 'labelling', they appear disinclined to call for its full-scale abandonment.

On one level, DSM and ICD are *benign* – merely bureaucratic systems for classifying the states people find themselves to be in, or are viewed by others as occupying. Such classification systems can be seen to 'open the door' to offers of help, care or treatment for the said 'mental disorder'. The situation becomes *malignant* when the person does not seek such a classification; or wishes to avoid such care or treatment. Classically, people who deny that they have a 'mental disorder' are either 'in denial' or 'lack insight'. The more they protest, the more 'seriously' their 'mental disorder' is viewed.

Given that most health and social care is dependent on funding by central government or insurance companies, most mental health professionals are uncomfortable with any critique of psychiatric diagnosis. Many professionals argue that without diagnosis people could avail themselves of care and treatment. It is worth asking why this is the case. What is this all about? Others will, mistakenly, assume that any criticism of psychiatric diagnosis – especially of the concept of 'mental illness' – implies a denial that people might be experiencing some distress or difficulty; or represent a 'risk' to themselves or others. It is self-evident that some, perhaps many, people experience distress and difficulty in their lives, or endanger the welfare of others. Attributing this to some abstract process called 'mental illness' merely perpetuates the kind of mythology that once blamed demons or bad spirits for some human misadventure. More importantly, it maintains the helplessness of the individual person, who is encouraged to put all his or her faith in psychiatric professionals, in seeking a solution for the problem. Clearly, many mental health professionals are driven by self-interest; fearing for their professional livelihood should their opposition to the use of psychiatric diagnosis become widely known.

Any attempt to deal, constructively, with the ethical dilemmas raised by psychiatric diagnosis will be difficult and probably lengthy. Both psychiatric professionals (of all disciplines) and the general public have invested heavily in this mythology, which helps absolve individuals from the need to take responsibility for their lives, and helps others make a living by acting as a 'good Samaritan'. However, it is self-evident that the provision of necessary support to people experiencing any kind of distress or difficulty must begin by asking them: What is distressing you? What has happened to bring you here, looking for help? What do you think needs to be done, to begin to help you deal with this?[14,15]

In what way does a diagnostic interview, using some classification system, represent a better alternative?

In ethical terms, how is the application of a diagnosis – of whatever kind – the 'right' thing to do as a *first* step, if one is genuinely seeking to help the person?

Notes

1 In some countries, like the USA, some specialist nurses apply psychiatric diagnoses, to enable the funding of mental health care by insurance companies.
2 Szasz TS *The Myth of Mental Illness: Foundations of a Theory of Personal Conduct* (50th Anniversary Edition). New York, NY: Harper Perennial, 2010.
3 These quotes are from the White House Fact Sheet on Myths and Facts about Mental Illness, President William Jefferson Clinton and Tipper Gore, the President's mental health adviser. For the original sources, see: Szasz TS *Psychiatry: The Science of Lies*. Syracuse, NY: Syracuse University Press, 2008, p. 89.
4 People with epilepsy and Huntington's chorea were once institutionalised in 'mental hospitals'. As soon as the neurological basis of their condition was identified, the care of such people was transferred to neurology.
5 See: Whitaker R *Mad in America: Bad Science, Bad Medicine and the Enduring Mistreatment of the Mentally Ill*. New York, NY: Basic Books, 2001.
6 Read J, Mosher L and Bentall R *Models of Madness*. London: Brunner Routledge, 2004.
7 Chamberlin J *On Our Own: Patient-Controlled Alternatives to the Mental Health System*. New York, NY: McGraw-Hill, 1979.
8 Deegan P 'Recovery as a journey of the heart' *Psychiatric Rehabilitation Journal*, 1996: 19 (3), 91–8.
9 See: Read, Mosher and Bentall op. cit.
10 http://www.rethink.org/about_mental_illness/how_is_mental_illness_diagnosed/accepting_your_diagn.html (Accessed: 28/03/10).
11 Joseph J *The Gene Illusion – Genetic Research in Psychiatry and Psychology under the Microscope*. New York, NY: Algora Publishing, 2004.
12 World Health Organisation *The International Classification of Disease and Related Health Problems* (10th Revision). Geneva: WHO, 1992.
13 American Psychiatric Association *Diagnostic and Statistical Manual of Mental Disorders*, Fourth Edition, Text revision (*DSM-IV-TR*). Washington, DC: APA, 2004.
14 McGorry PD, Hickie IB, Yung AR, Pantellis C and Jackson HJ 'Clinical staging of psychiatric disorders: A heuristic framework for choosing earlier, safer and more effective interventions' *Australian and New Zealand Journal of Psychiatry*, 2006: 40 (8), 616–22.
15 History of the development of the ICD. In: World Health Organization. *International Statistical Classification of Diseases and Related Health Problems*, 10th revision (Vol. 2, Ch. 6), Geneva: WHO, 1993.
16 http://www.who.int/classifications/icd/en/bluebook.pdf (Accessed: 28/03/10) p. 11.
17 Currently DSM-IV-TR. See: http://www.psych.org/mainmenu/research/dsmiv/dsmivtr.aspx (Accessed: 26/03/10).
18 Grob GN 'Origins of DSM-I: A study in appearance and reality' *American Journal of Psychiatry*, 1991: 148, 421–31.
19 Meyer A *Collected Papers* (Four Volumes) E Winters (Ed.). Baltimore, MD: John Hopkins University Press, 1952.
20 Mazure CM and Druss BG A historical perspective on stress and psychiatric illness. In CM Mazure (Ed.) *Does Stress Cause Psychiatric Illness?* Arlington, VA: American Psychiatric Publishing Inc., 1995.
21 Boorse C 'Homosexuality reclassified' *The Hastings Center Report*, June, 1982: p. 42.
22 Compton WM and Guze SB 'The neo-Kraepelinian revolution in psychiatric diagnosis' *European Archives of Psychiatry and Clinical Neuroscience*, 2005: 245 Special Issue (4/5), 196–201.
23 Kirk SA and Kutchins H *The Selling of DSM: The Rhetoric of Science in Psychiatry*. Hawthorne, NY: Aldine de Gruyter, 1992.
24 Rosenhahn T 'On being sane in insane places' *Science*, 1973: 179, 250–8.
25 See: Barker P *Assessment in Psychiatric and Mental Health Nursing: In Search of the Whole Person* (2nd ed.). Cheltenham: Nelson Thornes, pp. 290–1.
26 APA 2004 op. cit. p. xix.

27 See: Speigl A 'The dictionary of disorder: How one man revolutionized psychiatry' *The New Yorker* http://www.newyorker.com/archive/2005/01/03/050103fa_fact?currentPage=1 (Accessed: 29/03/10).

28 Pilgrim D 'Psychiatric diagnosis: More questions than answers' *The Psychologist*, 2000: 13, 302–5.

29 Boyle M *Schizophrenia: A Scientific Delusion?* (2nd ed.). London: Routledge, 2002.

30 Kutchins H and Kirk SA *Making Us Crazy: DSM – The Psychiatric Bible and the Creation of Mental Disorders.* New York, NY: The Free Press, 1997.

31 Bentall RP *Madness Explained: Psychosis and Human Nature.* London: Penguin, 2003.

32 Caplan PJ and Cosgrove L *Bias in Psychiatric Diagnosis.* New York, NY: Rowman and Littlefield, 2004.

33 Robert Spitzer acknowledged the 'medicalization' of such problems as integral to the DSM. See: Speigl op. cit.

34 See: Furedi F *Therapy Culture: Cultivating Vulnerability in an Uncertain Age.* London: Routledge, 2004.

35 Szasz 2007 op. cit.

36 Szasz 2007 op. cit. p. 101

37 Whitaker R *Anatomy of an Epidemic: Magic Bullets, Psychiatric Drugs and the Astonishing Rise of Mental Illness.* New York, NY: Crown, 2010.

38 Millon T The borderline personality: A psychosocial epidemic (Ch. 10) In J Paris (Ed.) *Borderline Personality Disorder: Etiology and Treatment.* Washington, DC: American Psychiatric Press, 1993.

39 Furedi 2004 op. cit.

40 Twenge JM and Campbell KW *The Narcissism Epidemic: Living in an Age of Entitlement.* New York, NY: Free Press, 2009.

41 Whitaker 2010 op. cit.

42 Szasz 2007 op. cit. p. 96

43 http://www.caslcampaign.com/news.php (Accessed: 29/03/10).

44 See: Barker P and Buchanan-Barker P *The Tidal Model: A Guide for Mental Health Professionals.* London: Brunner Routledge, 2005.

45 See also: Mosher LR, Hendrix V and Fort DF *Soteria: Through Madness to Deliverance.* Philadelphia, PA: Xlibris Corporation, 2004, p. 298.

12 Professional relationships

Vince Mitchell

Introduction

Offering people professional help for their problems involves forming a relationship with them. As with all relationships, this has an ethical dimension. People may be, in varying degrees, *caring* or *indifferent*; *contrived* or *genuine*; *coercive* or *collaborative*; *honest* or *deceptive*. Furthermore, the notion of the relationship being professional and helpful gives it *purpose* and *boundaries*. Therefore, we have different considerations than we have with other relationships, even though many of the principles that underlie our conduct will be shared.

The nature of these boundaries will depend on the profession to which we belong. As a nurse, my perspective may differ from other helping professionals or people who are cast in the role of needing help. However, we should not run away with the idea that the relationships we form in professional helping and health care are different in any absolute sense. The relationship is still one between two (or more) people and most of our conduct can be shaped by our understanding that the relationship is a *human* one. We can also relate to our work colleagues in this way and avoid what has been referred to as professional tribalism.[1] Furthermore, should we find ourselves in the position of being the person receiving help, we relate then to our professional helpers in a way that recognises our common humanity, rather than just the 'professional–patient' labels.

The purpose of the professional helping relationship is to improve how people *experience their lives*, referred to by some as their 'mental health'. Having such a professional purpose can be challenging, due to problems pertaining to subjective and conflicting definitions of mental health. These problems cannot be allowed to detain us here. Nevertheless, the relationship ought to fulfil the purpose of improving people's experience by addressing their problems of living, however conceived. I am not advancing here the view that the relationship *must* promote the value of therapeutic outcomes *at any cost*. Instead, I hope to show that how we relate to each other is a *moral pursuit*. In promoting the desired outcome, constraints exist on our conduct. I will outline the importance of developing relationships in our professional life that, as well as being helpful, are genuine and respectful. I will suggest how we might think about the concept of autonomy regarding these professional relationships and explore some tensions that exist.

Professionalism and the interpersonal

Early origins

The notion that the sort of relationships we form with each other can affect our mental health is not new. In 1813, Samuel Tuke[2] argued that relating with 'patients' in a respectful manner, by valuing their interests and expertise, promoted an improvement in their mental condition. A century later, the psychodynamic approach that evolved from Freud's work enhanced understanding of human relationships.[3] However, Freud's work did not seem to emphasise the qualities in the therapeutic relationship *itself* that could be of help to the client. Along with this, Freud appeared to hold a rather pessimistic view of humanity: having a non-moral destructive id at its core that could only be restrained by an equally powerful but cruel super-ego.[4] By the 1950s, Carl Rogers was arguing for a more optimistic view of human nature and motivation.[5] From this, Rogers developed the idea of the therapeutic importance of having a genuine, trusting and positively regarding relationship with the person you are helping. Interestingly here, Rogers[6] argued that professionalisation could act as a barrier in the helping relationship.

> We are afraid that if we let ourselves freely experience these positive feelings towards another we may be trapped by them . . .. So as a reaction we tend to build up distance between ourselves and others – aloofness, a 'professional' attitude, an impersonal relationship.

Rogers advocated that our relations *should* be personal. We should free ourselves to care. This leaves some difficult questions for the notion of professionalism. Would we be better helpers if we were not professionals at all? I think that professionalism, when correctly conceived, *can* bring strength of purpose. It also enables us to decide what is not acceptable in practice – such as sexual relations and sharing alcohol. What professionalism should *not* be is a reason to avoid engagement or objectify the other. It provides us with *opportunity* to form relationships with people who may benefit from our help and *special reasons to care* beyond everyday human concern.

The importance of being human

An understanding of the importance of forming personal relationships was also a cornerstone of Hildegard Peplau's work on nursing practice in the early 1950s. Among professional groups, nurses spend more time with the person in distress than any other. For better or for worse, nurses share with people many intimate moments. For Peplau, nursing is a journey where both start as strangers, but develop through mutual respect and shared experience. Or as Peplau puts it[7]

> It is likely that the nursing process is educative and therapeutic when nurse and patient can come to know and to respect each other, as persons who are alike, and yet, different, as persons who share in the solution of problems.

Although these words are part of a definition of *nursing*, I think that it can apply to the many and various professional relationships that are formed.

The importance of engaging on human terms was brought to light for me in practical terms early on in my nursing practice, when I was assigned as the primary nurse to a woman newly admitted to the ward. By coincidence, I happened to know some words in her native language. Although there were no communication difficulties as she spoke English perfectly, I found that saying good morning and a few other words in her own language brought a certain connection between us. It enabled us to talk a bit about her country and her broader interests. By sharing her language, I acknowledged her existence as a *person beyond the role of patient*. As time went on, I was able to assist with her recovery or 'healing' as she referred to it. I believe these foundations were built on this initial connection. However, we don't need to have a shared interest by coincidence, as in this example. There are likely to be many things that we share with the people in our care, if we take the time to find them.

Helm[8] speaks of the importance of *realness* and authenticity in relationships. From her own experience, the relationships that were healing were those where the other person acted kindly or when they were able to share some of their own lives with her. The picture is not always straightforward, though. Jackson and Stevenson[9] found that as well as people valuing closeness, ordinariness and friendship in their relationships with nurses, there is also the perceived need for nurses to be able to move into a more distant professional stance at certain times.

A further complication lies in the possibility of a mixed intention in the development of a more friendly relationship. There is the danger of professional boundary violations but there is also the more subtle concern that a friendly association becomes a mere means to a *non-collaborative end*. Professionals may believe that by being friendly with the person in their care they will then be more able to *persuade* them into doing something that they otherwise would not have wanted to do. An example of this (to be explored later) is in a community mental health team where the client accepts medication, wishing not to damage his relationship with the mental health worker, despite not agreeing with the medication. Concerns such as these are all grist for the ethical mill. Relationships have often been so undermined by paternalistic practices that many see the promotion of *individual autonomy* as the only way that they can have their rights respected in healthcare environments (see Chapter 1).

From individual to principled autonomy

Individual autonomy and paternalism

According to Beauchamp and Childress,[10] the question of whether individual autonomy or professional beneficence should take precedence in decision making has reached the point where it has become 'a central problem in bioethics'. The sharp end of professional beneficence is *paternalism*, and it is understandable in this context that people strive to emphasise the importance of making autonomous choices about their lives and treatment. However, this move to individual autonomy has been criticised in recent years for reducing trust in professional relationships[11] and for its overemphasis on the exclusion of all other principles.[12]

Despite the seemingly obvious applications to mental health, this central question is often conspicuous by its absence. There is some discussion relating the question to mental capacity and competence (see Chapter 26). The upshot of this is that if competence to give consent to treatment is deemed insufficient, then paternalism is back on the agenda. For example, Manson and O'Neill[13] state that where the level of understanding is insufficient '. . .paternalism is not always avoidable in medical practice'. Although, I am in agreement with the thesis that the promotion of individual autonomy can undermine the formation of trusting relationships, I will argue here that it does not follow that the paternalism is inevitable in situations where competence is considered insufficient.

I am not equating 'mental health' and 'competence'. The relationship is a complex and contentious one. I will assume that in some situations mental distress affects the decisions that people make in a way that prevents them from following their broader life-plan or 'critical interests'.[14] Psychiatric advance directives are a promising way of allowing people to make choices that cohere with these critical interests but I am not elaborating on this here (see Chapter 26).

Principled autonomy, trust and moral distress

I wish to focus on the possibility of understanding autonomy in a way that promotes trusting and respectful relationships. This autonomy, though, is not the right to absolute independence that appears to follow from the arguments of some. A more ethically robust alternative is advanced by O'Neill.[15,16] To act with *principled autonomy* is to choose *within the constraint* that the principle on which the decision is based is one which everyone could consistently understand and choose to act on. For example, this means that acting on a principle of deception or indifference would be *disallowed*, as this is not a principle that could be consistently chosen by all. By acting in this way, trust can be more *reliably* placed in relationships based on principled autonomy, making it possible for others to protect and guide us. To call this 'paternalism' is misleading as it is not a wilful overriding of an individual's preferences. Instead, we can learn to recognise the wisdom of the other and develop a *shared understanding*. If strong enough relationships can be developed, then the person will trust the judgement of the other sufficiently to make a decision, when it cannot be made by the person on his/her own. These decisions could include critical matters such as the person accepting another's recommendation for how their current distress may best be resolved.

It is essential to point out here that this process is reciprocal. We can learn from each other's expertise. As a professional, some of the choices of people that we have previously considered *pathological* may well be understood now as a proper response to their problem. Some of our new understandings could be in tension or even conflict with local constraints or national policies. *Moral distress* is a real possibility when the professional is conscious of a required moral action but cannot act because of 'institutionalized obstacles'.[17] How we choose to reconcile this is one of the most important concerns facing professionals working in this area.

How we can respect people in relationships

Principles and respectful dialogue

I return to the example of a client (Tom) who feels compelled to take his medication in order to maintain his relationship with his community worker (Bob). My concern highlighted above was that that the relationship was being used as a means to gain the *non-collaborative* end of compliance. How could this be different? First, respectful relationships cannot be based on deception. Both Bob and Tom need to be open and honest about their views and intentions. Bob may believe that medication would be of assistance and Tom may disagree. Despite this initial difference of opinion, Bob and Tom may still develop their relationship by Bob assisting Tom with projects which are of interest to him. The *purpose* of developing the relationship should be a *collaborative end* – a genuine intention to help Tom by a creative process. In this process, Bob can learn from Tom what needs to be done for the situation to improve and Tom can develop a deeper personal wisdom.[18] It may be that over time Tom begins to place more trust in Bob as he has always been respectful in his transactions with him. As a result, Tom may decide that he can trust Bob's judgement and, after entering a *dialogue* regarding medication, agrees to give it a try. The *way* in which information is communicated is important.[19] The communication should be relevant to Tom, understandable and honest. For example, if a side effect such as sexual dysfunction is important to him, it should be discussed in an open and considerate manner, not 'veiled over'.[20]

Importantly, there needs to be the possibility of the opposite result. Bob must also trust Tom's judgement when entering into the dialogue. It may be that, as a result of the dialogue, Bob now understands that medication would *not* be an appropriate response to

Tom's problems. This second result would *not* be possible if the essential purpose of the relationship was one to ensure *compliance*. To be a respectful relationship, the purpose must be to reach a solution that could be mutually agreed and any means employed must be respectful to the capabilities of others to act.

I will concede that this is an ideal picture and that in practice situations can be a lot more messy or urgent than this. However, it is worth considering some of the practices that are *ruled out as principles* by this perspective.

> **Deception**: Bob enters into what Tom believes to be a 'genuine relationship' when Bob's purpose is to ensure 'compliance' to medication.
> **Indifference**: Bob makes no effort to assist Tom in any of his projects.
> **Manipulation**: Bob says he will assist Tom with his projects *only* if he has his medication.
> **Coercion**: Bob uses a *threat* of force to coerce Tom to take his medication.

There may be some overlap. For example, an action could have some elements of deception and manipulation if Tom is unaware that Bob is shaping his behaviour towards a certain end using manipulative means. It is argued here that in our relationships with others, the four practices outlined above, if made principles, would be incompatible with living the sort of life that respects our *dignity* as human beings. In other words, living in a world where everyone deceives, coerces or is indifferent, if such a world is possible, would be intolerable. It could be argued that there are some situations where we can make exceptions *in particular* such as using restraint in order that a principle of rejecting violence is upheld *in general*. However, it seems reasonable to state that we cannot build our professional helping relationships on practices such as coercion and deception. Therefore, at the very least, the above practices should be prohibited except in the most extreme of circumstances (see Chapter 13).

Dignity as the origin of respect

The above example outlines how we can relate to one another with *respect*. The theory that underlies this conceives of respect in a particular way. The respect outlined here is *recognition respect*.[21,22] This recognises a dignity or authority in the entity respected. This is either present or not depending on the nature of the entity. In the case of human beings, we can recognise an *equal standing as persons* on the basis of our shared dignity and this understanding regulates our conduct to each other. According to Kant,[23] the origin of this dignity lies in our rational nature. It is necessary to point out that rational nature is not intended to be equated with competence or sanity. Rational nature is defined here, in similar terms to Korsgaard,[24] as being the special ability we *all* have to choose to act based on our desired ends, rather than having these actions determined merely by instinct. With principled autonomy,[25] we respect the dignity of persons by acting on principles that could be chosen coherently by *all* producing a morality that is grounded in this equal status. It follows from this that we ought to engage with others in a way that recognises their inherent dignity as people to be reasoned with and not compelled.

Relational autonomy

Traditional notions of autonomy and the ideas that underpin them have received a substantial feminist critique. It is of particular interest here as feminist writers argue that relationships are neglected in many ethical accounts and that a broader conception is required.

Gilligan[26] argued that when it comes to ethical reasoning women speak in a *different voice*, which has been downplayed by traditional theories. The female voice speaks in terms of emotions, caring and relationships, rather than rules, rights and justice (see Chapter 1). In making decisions, it tends to focus more on relationships in the particular situation than on universal principles. This approach emphasises the importance of context, both personal and social; on how decisions are made. As has been pointed out by Tong and Williams,[27] feminist ethics seeks to reflect the everyday life of 'differentially empowered people' not the relations between business people during a 'contract negotiation'.

As a result, some feminist writers have developed a new conception of autonomy that develops this 'richer account of agency'.[28] Relational autonomy allows for the fact that people are socially embedded and our views are shaped by these forces. It is sensitive to the view that for some people the socialisation and the relationships that result are oppressive and that, as a result, some people have few *real* options. Relational autonomy refers to a number of different approaches, which cannot be fully expanded on here. Yet, all accounts argue for *interdependence* against individualistic notions of autonomy that promote values of atomistic self-sufficiency.[29]

Principled autonomy shares many of these criticisms of individualistic approaches to autonomy. As it has been outlined above, it is more concordant with feminist voices by emphasising the importance of *human* relationships that promote dialogue and a *shared understanding*. However, it could still be argued that the universal nature of Kantian ethics with its emphasis on rationality relegates the importance of emotions in caring, and fails to fully reflect the influence of social factors on decision making.

Interprofessional considerations

Many professionals work in teams with other professionals. The individual, as a member of a profession, has conferred on them a professional *identity* and arguably a status and power within the team. Along with this, there is the professional *culture* that is developed from a process of socialisation into that profession and the separate education experience.[30] As a result, individuals within the team can have greatly varying perspectives and roles.

Professional autonomy is the notion that a profession can govern itself. This is different from the descriptions of autonomy above that have considered how *individuals* relate to each other. However, MacDonald[31] argues that the concept of professional autonomy has both an individual and collective nature, as it is individuals who work to honour and protect the standards of their particular profession from outside pressures. He adds that due to the nature of social structures and uneven power between the separate professions (and the public) these forms of professional autonomy are best understood by the relational view already described. The relational view captures the richer context in which professionals make decisions. However, it is argued here that principles outlining our obligations are still needed in order to actually *make* a respectful decision. Furthermore, these principles are aligned with the ones outlined above in developing the therapeutic relationship. Decisions need to be conducted in an atmosphere of mutually respectful dialogue fostering the development of trust and shared understanding. It should go without saying that the person who is the *subject* of the discussion is equally (not tokenistically) part of the conversation. However, it is worth noting again that equal status also brings equal obligations to be considerate and responsible for the decisions made.[32]

The confrontational nature of some interprofessional encounters has proved a serious barrier to this form of relating. I was involved in such a drama some years ago. I mistakenly promised a client that I would be able to argue successfully for some leave off the ward in the multi-disciplinary team meeting. I went in confident of this. However, we came up against a cautious junior doctor who did not wish to take the risk. A heated discussion ensued but I could not *persuade* the doctor (with the power invested in her) to change her mind. There is very little that is right about this. I entered into a false promise; there was little or no dialogue; trust was absent; and relationships were damaged. If we had been able to enter into a dialogue then it may well have been possible for us all to understand each other's needs, obligations and vulnerabilities.

Although this encounter took place with each of us cast in our separate roles, we must (in Peplau's words above) see ourselves '... *as persons who are alike, and yet, different, as persons who share in the solution of problems*'.[33] The interprofessional angle is still the interpersonal angle. The professionals would be more likely to understand the point of view of other professionals if more trusting relationships (accompanied by an equalising of power structures) were accomplished. On a brighter note, there is evidence to suggest that professional autonomy can be in synergy rather than conflict with team working.[34] We need to understand autonomy in a way that promotes this collaborative approach. The democratic structure of therapeutic communities may well provide a useful example for this.[35]

Boundaries and professional purpose

There are, however, important distinctions between helping relationships and other relationships that we form. The *purpose* of helping relationships is to assist another person in solving particular problems. *This is the reason that the relationship exists.* Being professional gives special reasons to care, helping more than a usual member of the public. Yet, unlike other close relationships with friends and family there is not the expectation of the professional being helped in return. Furthermore, these special reasons give professionals further obligations to the person in their care. Part of developing a shared understanding is that the person is able to appreciate that the professional has these obligations. Although the nature of these obligations varies, all helping professions share some form of commitment to respect dignity. Social workers are committed to enabling people develop their potential;[36] counsellors pledge to alleviate suffering;[37] occupational therapists to promote well-being through occupation.[38] In the case of nursing and medicine, professionals are told to make 'the *care* of people your first concern'.[39,40]

There is a need for professional boundaries to uphold the intention of the relationship. Some of the common areas for boundary dilemmas include the following:[41]

Gifts
Self-disclosure
Sexual misconduct
Role, time and place.

Working in a helping profession can be a hugely rewarding experience – we learn a great deal and will share many positive experiences with people. However, that reward must always be secondary to the reward for the person we seek to help. There is, of course, a salary, but any reward outside of this needs to be carefully handled. I once encountered a community nurse who always ensured that boxes of chocolates given to her by her clients were shared with the team, in an effort to be clear that no preferential treatment would result. Should she have refused the chocolates? Probably not, but she certainly shouldn't have visited the client because of the chocolates!

Another potentially difficult area is self-disclosure. It can form a valuable part of the help-ing process.[42] Much of this chapter has emphasised the importance of sharing our experi-ences on human terms. However, despite this closeness, we need to remain in some sense separate from the other.[43] We need to be able to distinguish our own feelings from the person in care.[44] Again, the purpose must be clear. Professionals should not use the *opportunity* of a therapeutic encounter to burden people they hope to help with their own problems. Neither should they burden them with their own successes. A person once described to me how his community nurse on a home visit spoke with him at some length about her forthcoming holiday to Greece. As someone who is unlikely to have such a holiday, the person found this self-disclosure rather insensitive.

Professional organisations are categorical in their forbidding of sexual relations between professionals and people in their care. In some cases the behaviour is morally wrong because of an intentional and manipulative use of *power* by a 'predatory therapist'.[45] However, a consciously malicious intention may not be present. Appeals may be made to the existence of consent by both parties to the sexual behaviour. However, these appeals are weakened by the possibility of transference and counter-transference in the relationship,[46] or other vul-nerabilities.[47] Transference is where the individual unconsciously transfers thoughts and feelings from an experience in the past to his/her current relationships. Counter-transference is the therapist's response, which may also be unconscious, to a client's transference.[48] If these unconscious elements are outside of the person's rational agency, then, arguably, any consent that *relies* on these hidden motivations is invalid. This is a vexed issue. However, even if considerations of consent are taken out of the picture, the robust point can still be made that there is an abuse of the *purpose* of the professional relationship by entering into sexual rather than a helping relationship.

Finally, unlike other relationships, the goal of a therapeutic relationship will often result in its own extinction. The importance of working towards the end of the relationship has been referred to as its resolution phase.[49] At the relationship's end, the person who was once in need of help can now find his/her way without professional support or guidance. It is important that the relationship has met a need rather than fostered dependency. This brings another boundary. People must be able to withdraw when the purpose of the relationship is no longer therapeutic. Similarly, people may wish to meet outside of the working relation-ship for other reasons. This is probably unwise considering the strength of the roles that the helping relationships cast us in. Unfortunately, it is a reality that some roles in life have boundaries defined by power imbalances and this is often the case in mental health.[50] As a result we may never fully lose our role as a 'powerful' professional, even after the purpose of the professional relationship has been extinguished. Therefore any non-professional relation-ship we try to form with the same person is likely to have a 'dual' character.[51]

Conclusion

Professional relationships share much with other interpersonal relationships. As profession-als, we need to form relationships where we can engage with people in a way that is per-sonal, respectful and real. I have advanced the view that the most coherent way to respect each other is to understand autonomy as a principled rather than an individualistic notion, following the work of O'Neill.[52] To act with autonomy in this sense is to make decisions based on principles on which all of us could consistently act and understand. It seems to follow that seeing autonomy in this way meets some of the criticisms of (individualistic) autonomy by emphasising the importance of human relationships that promote dialogue and a shared understanding. I have considered how this could be applied in scenarios that may be encountered by mental health professionals. I have argued that the key to collaborative working is the development of a relationship that, if strong enough, will allow recognition of the wisdom of the other. The professional can develop a new understanding of the person's experience that allows the professional to trust the person's judgement in matters where previously he/she believed the person to be incompetent. Reciprocally, the person can trust the judgement of the professional sufficiently for that professional to make decisions at times when they cannot be made by the person on his/her own.

This approach to trusting relationships was also applied to interprofessional relations. It was concluded that in these relationships professionals take different roles but we must also be aware of what we share, which is our humanity and shared purpose to help solve a particular problem. Finally, professional purpose brings professional boundaries. Professional relationships bring special considerations above standard human relationships. Professionals must act in a way that preserves this purpose, which means that certain actions are forbidden. However, all these constraints exist only so that they allows us to have genuinely respectful professional relationships with each other.

Notes

1 A. Beattie, 'War and peace among the health tribes', in K. Soothill, L. Mackay and C. Webb (eds.) *Interprofessional Relations in Health Care*, London: Edward Arnold, 1995, pp. 11–26.

2 S. Tuke, *Description of the Retreat [1813]*, London: Process Press, 1996.

3 S. Freud, *An Outline of Psychoanalysis*. J. Strachey (ed.), London: The Hogarth Press, 1969.

4 S. Freud, *The Ego and the Id*. J. Strachey (ed.), London: The Hogarth Press, 1962.

5 C. Rogers, 'A note on the 'nature of man'', *Journal of Counseling Psychology*, 1957, vol. 4(3), pp. 199–203, reprinted in H. Kirschenbaum and V.L. Henderson (eds.) *The Carl Rogers Reader*, London: Constable, 1989.

6 C. Rogers, 'The characteristics of a helping relationship', *Personnel and Guidance Journal*, 1958, vol. 37, pp. 6–16, reprinted in H. Kirschenbaum and V.L. Henderson, op. cit., p. 120.

7 H. Peplau, *Interpersonal Relations in Nursing: A Conceptual Frame of Reference for Psychodynamic Nursing*. New York, NY: Springer, 1991, p. 9.

8 A. Helm, 'Recovery and reclamation: A pilgrimage in understanding who and what we are', in P. Barker (ed.), *Psychiatric and Mental Health Nursing: The Craft of Caring*, London: Arnold, 2003, pp. 50–5.

9 S. Jackson and C. Stevenson, 'What do people need psychiatric and mental health nurses for?' *Journal of Advanced Nursing*, 2000, vol. 31(2), pp. 378–88.

10 T.L. Beauchamp and J.F. Childress, *Principles of Biomedical Ethics*, New York, NY: Oxford University Press, 2009, p. 207.

11 O. O'Neill, *Autonomy and Trust in Bioethics*, Cambridge: Cambridge University Press, 2002.

12 C. Foster, *Choosing Life, Choosing Death: The Tyranny of Autonomy in Medical Ethics and Law*, Oxford: Hart Publishing, 2009.

13 N.C. Manson and O. O'Neill, *Rethinking Consent in Bioethics*, Cambridge: Cambridge University Press, 2007, p. 156.

14 R. Dworkin, *Life's Dominion. An Argument about Abortion, Euthanasia and Individual Freedom*. New York, NY: Albert A. Knopf, 1993.

15 O. O'Neill, op. cit.

16 G.M. Stirrat and R. Gill, 'Autonomy in medical ethics after O'Neill', *Journal of Medical Ethics*, 2005, 31, 127–30.

17 M.C. Corely, P. Minick, R.K. Elswick and M. Jacobs, 'Nurse moral distress and ethical work environment', *Nursing Ethics*, 2005, 12, 381–90.

18 P. Buchanan-Barker and P.J. Barker, 'The tidal commitments: Extending the value base of mental health recovery', *Journal of Psychiatric and Mental Health Nursing*, 2008, vol. 15, pp. 93–100.

19 Manson and O'Neill, op. cit.

20 A. Higgins, P. Barker and C.M. Begley, 'Iatrogenic sexual dysfunction and the protective withholding of information: In whose best interest?', *Journal of Psychiatric and Mental Health Nursing*, 2006, vol. 13, pp. 437–46.

21 S.L. Darwall, 'Two kinds of respect', *Ethics*, 1977, vol. 88(1), 36–49.

22 S.L. Darwall, *Second-Person Standpoint*, Cambridge, MA: Harvard University Press, 2006, pp. 122–6.

23 I. Kant, *Grounding for the Metaphysics of Morals [1785]* J.W. Ellington (trans., 3rd ed.), Indianapolis, IN: Hackett, 1993.

24 C. Korsgaard, *Creating the Kingdom of Ends*, Cambridge: Cambridge University Press, 1996, pp. 110–11.

25 O. O'Neill, op. cit.

26 C. Gilligan, *In a Different Voice: Psychological Theory and Women's Development*, Cambridge, MA: Harvard University Press, 1993.

27 R. Tong and N. Williams, 'Feminist ethics', in E.N. Zalta (ed.) *The Stanford Encyclopedia of Philosophy*, 2009, Available online: http://plato.stanford.edu/entries/feminism-ethics/

28 C. Mackenzie and N. Stoljar, 'Introduction: Autonomy refigured', in C. Mackenzie and N. Stoljar (eds.) *Relational Autonomy*, New York, NY: Oxford University Press, 2000, p. 21.

29 Ibid.

30 P. Hall, 'Interprofessional teamwork: Professional cultures as barriers', *Journal of Interprofessional Care*, 2005, vol. 19, supplement 1, pp. 188–96.

31 C. MacDonald, 'Nurse autonomy as relational', *Nursing Ethics*, 2002, vol. 9(2), pp. 194–201.

32 Stirrat and Gill, op. cit.

33 H. Peplau, op. cit.

34 A.M. Rafferty, J. Ball and L.H. Aiken, 'Are teamwork and professional autonomy compatible, and do they result in improved hospital care?' *Quality in Health Care*, 2001, vol. 10, supplement 2, pp. ii32–7.

35 P. Campling, 'Therapeutic communities', *Advances in Psychiatric Treatment*, 2001, vol. 7, pp. 365–72.

36 British Association of Social Workers, *Code of Ethics for Social Work*, 2007, Birmingham: BASW, Available online: http://www.basw.co.uk/Default.aspx?tabid=64

37 British Association for Counselling and Psychotherapy, *The Ethical Framework for Good Practice in Counselling and Psychotherapy*, Lutterworth: BACP, 2009.

38 College of Occupational Therapists, *The College of Occupational Therapists' Code of Ethics and Professional Conduct*, London: COT, 2005.

39 Nursing and Midwifery Council, *The Code: Standards of Conduct, Performance and Ethics for Nurses and Midwifes*, London: NMC, 2008.

40 General Medical Council, *Good Medical Practice*, London: GMC, 2006.

41 T.G. Gutheil and A. Brodsky, *Preventing Boundary Violations in Clinical Practice*, New York, NY: Guilford Press, 2008.

42 G. Egan, *The Skilled Helper* (6th ed.), Pacific Grove, CA: Brooks/Cole, 1998.

43 Rogers, 1958, op. cit.

44 P. Barker, 'Person-centred care: The need for diversity', in Barker op. cit., pp. 3–9.

45 W.R. Procci, 'A cautionary tale about boundary violations in psychodynamic psychotherapy and psychoanalysis', *Focus*, 2007, vol. 5, pp. 407–11.

46 A. Celenza and G.O. Gabbard, 'Analysts who commit sexual boundary violations: A lost cause?', *Journal of the American Psychoanalytic Association*, 2007, vol. 51, pp. 617–36.

47 C.A. Galletly, 'Psychiatrist-patient sexual relationships: The ethical dilemmas', *Australian and New Zealand Journal of Psychiatry*, 1993, vol. 27, pp. 133–9.

48 A.C. Jones, 'Transference and countertransference', *Perspectives in Psychiatric Care*, 2004, vol. 40(1), pp. 13–19.

49 H. Peplau, op. cit.

50 J. Henderson, 'The challenge of relationship boundaries in mental health', *Nursing Management*, 2004, vol. 11(6), pp. 28–32.

51 Gutheil and Brodsky, op. cit.

52 O. O'Neill, op. cit.

13 Restraint

Brodie Paterson

Introduction

> Our science enables us to call your madness illness and diagnose a madness in you that prevents you being a patient like other patients: hence you will be a mental patient.[1]

Unlike most other medical specialists, psychiatrists have the legal power to coerce patients into accepting treatment.

In a UK post-asylum era, it is tempting to suggest that the complex ethical questions about coercion in treatment are somehow less relevant or less important than they once were. Nothing could be further from the truth. Coercion in its various forms continues to play a central role in mental health practice both in the United Kingdom and across the world. This chapter briefly explores the history of coercion, and discusses its use in contemporary practice. The primary focus will be on an evaluation of whether (and if so how) restraint, seclusion and compulsory medication can be justified ethically. For the purpose of this chapter, however, *both* seclusion and compulsory medication will be considered sub-types of restraint: seclusion, because substituting a locked door for a restraining hand or belt, merely replaces one means of restricting movement with another; compulsory medication – particularly rapid tranquilisation – because *'a medication used to control behaviour or to restrict a patient's freedom of movement'*, is in reality *'not treatment but restraint'*.[2] The focus of the discussion will be on their use in services for working age adults but it is acknowledged that such interventions are used in other services.

As Thomas Szasz[3] observed, state legitimised coercive interventions whilst *'always morally problematic'* are also always *'inherently political in nature'*. This chapter eschews therefore the use of a more conventional ethical framework in favour of two post-modernist constructions of validity: the 'pragmatic' and the 'psychopolitical'. The decision to do so requires, however, some justification for those unfamiliar with this approach. Validity as a concept has several well-known dimensions central to the positivist tradition in research in the behavioural sciences, particularly 'content', 'construct' and 'predictive' validity.[1] This 'traditional' construction of validity reflects a modernist worldview, whereby knowledge provides a map of a reality, which is assumed to be objective. If instead an alternative post-modern worldview is taken the search for certainty in knowledge is replaced by that of identifying defensible 'claims' regarding all knowledge. Validation then becomes the process of choosing among competing interpretations each framed as potentially falsifiable and thus open to exploration.[5] Truth in this context is not defined with reference to an objective reality but retains significant value as a concept, albeit interpreted now, in terms not of accuracy, but of utility, in the sense of *'whatever assists us to take actions that produce the desired results'*.[6] The process however, whereby *'the results desired'* are agreed upon, involves consideration of both values and ethics. The consequence is that validity itself becomes an ethical question and it is this perspective, which will inform the exercise undertaken.[7]

The coercion continuum

It is necessary to clarify exactly what coercion involves and to describe contemporary practice in this area. Coercion is defined here as: '*any action or threat of actions, which compels the patient to behave in a manner inconsistent with his own wishes*'.[8] It exists on a continuum and can be overt and explicit – such as the *use of restraint* (whether accomplished by means of physical holding or mechanical device), *seclusion* (whether accomplished through locked doors or threats to enforce isolation) or '*as required medication*' administered in the absence of consent. It can also be implicit. The suggestion that if medication is not taken orally 'other options will have to be explored' is readily understood as a barely veiled threat by the service user in many mental health in-patient services.

Notably, 48 per cent of service users who responded to an audit of English in-patient services agreed that '*they felt that the threat of medication or seclusion was used to control behavior*'.[9] Such threats are not idle. In the first national audit 8 per cent of in-patients in England and Wales were reported to have been restrained at least once during their current stay in hospital; with 1.5 per cent having been restrained more than five times and 0.7 per cent restrained on more than ten occasions. Seclusion was less common with 3 per cent of patients reported as having been secluded at least once.[9]

Similar if not higher figures for the use of coercive interventions are reported across Europe and the rest of the world[10] although remarkable variation in the specific type of coercion used exists.[11] The use of mechanical restraint is almost unknown now in the United Kingdom but remains common practice in much of Europe, with less common variations such as the use of net beds (large cot type structures) in widespread use in Austria. Seclusion, used in much of Europe, is banned in Italy. Compulsory medication in the form of rapid tranquilisation is however, it appears, used almost everywhere.[11] Such variation in an era of evidence-based practice and common European guidance[12] requiring that services adopt and implement the principles of least restrictive environment and least intrusive treatment may seem surprising. The pattern and frequency of use of such interventions reflect however the gradual emergence over time of consensus on what represents acceptable practice, which has eventually become enshrined in local and sometimes national guidance.[13] These are not evidence-based interventions but forms of 'custom and practice' reflecting local culture, and hence the variation.[13] Ultimately, these practices represent value judgements. This is best illustrated perhaps with reference to an example in British Colonial India. When the non-restraint movement swept the United Kingdom in the 1800s many British psychiatrists came to view mechanical restraint as archaic and sought to eliminate it. Interestingly however, British psychiatrists practising in India during the colonial period dissented vehemently. This was not because they saw mechanical restraint as necessary to control the 'native' population. Rather, it was because the public institutions for the insane, which catered for European colonials, employed only Indian orderlies and nurses. In practice such direct care staff (as today) were largely responsible for managing aggressive and violent patients. The discourse then prevalent made mechanical restraint essential for British patients because it avoided what, for a British patient, would have been profoundly shaming in that culture, at that time: that is, physical domination by 'native' orderlies.[14] What practitioners judged 'reasonable' and thus acceptable reflected the local cultural imperatives. Whilst the nature of these imperatives will vary over time and place, the process by which it is decided which coercive interventions are used remains the same, explaining the wide variations in practice observed.

Coercion: a brief history

The use of coercion to manage acute mental distress is not new, predating both the development of the asylum and psychiatry itself. The origins of organised care in mental health stem in part from desires to protect those vulnerable to abuse and exploitation from the public and also to protect the public from those whose behaviours were perceived as representing a threat to themselves or others, or to the broader social order. Legal provisions in England dating back to at least the fourteenth century have provided for the '*imprisonment of a lunatic*'.[15] Such legislation permitted not only detention but also that they might '*bind him and beat him with rods*' not as punishment but in an attempt to restore sanity.[16] The use of coercion in the form of mechanical restraint to protect staff from dangerous behaviour was, however, also commonplace. Michael Foucault[17] records that a variety of '*marvelous instruments*', including the '*fixed chair*', '*handcuffs, muffs straitjacket*' the '*fingerglove garment*' and '*wicker caskets in which individuals were enclosed*' were in widespread use in French hospitals before the actions of Pinel at the Bicetre called them into question. It has been suggested that Pinel, while widely credited with freeing lunatics from their chains, remained comfortable with threatening patients with the *camisole* or *gilet de force* (the straightjacket) and considered the effects achieved by such intimidation justified to gain compliance.[18]

The practice of coercion also came to be questioned in the United Kingdom. Inspired initially by the treatment of a fellow Quaker admitted to York asylum in England and his horror at the conditions he subsequently found there William Tuke went on to establish 'The Retreat', a service based on the principles of 'moral treatment' (see Chapters 2 and 3). A critical element of moral treatment was '*A system which, by limiting the power of the attendant*' made '*it his interest to obtain the good opinion of those under his care*'. This approach, Tuke argued, provided more '*effectually for the safety of the keeper, as well as of the patient*' than any '*chains, darkness, and anodynes*'.[19]

In a bizarre irony, because Tuke rejected the medical treatment of insanity as ineffective, 'moral treatment' came to be adopted by medical campaigners in favour of the asylums. They were eventually successful in entwining the notion of cure with the concept of the '*benign institution*'.[20] Later advocates of what eventually became known as '*non restraint*' in the new system of asylums, which developed in the United Kingdom during the nineteenth century, including James Connolly,[21] were however subject to considerable criticism. Concerns were expressed about '*serious physical effects (such as broken ribs,)*' sustained by staff in struggles with service users in at least one asylum.[22] Non-restraint was therefore never universally popular or adopted everywhere despite the somewhat mythical status it has since come to enjoy.[23] Although mechanical restraint did fall out of favour in the United Kingdom, at least for adults of working age, physical restraint, strong clothing and 'strong rooms' (later renamed *seclusion)* remained part of common practice in many British institutions and elsewhere throughout the nineteenth and twentieth centuries.[24]

The debate over the use of compulsion in services for people with mental health needs is therefore far from new. The dominant conceptualisation of validity adopted by those who support the need for seclusion, restraint and compulsory medication even if only implicitly, can be described as 'pragmatic'. Kvale[25] asserts that, in a pragmatic construction of validity, the need for theoretical '*justification is effectively superseded by application*'. In the context of the use of coercion in-patient mental health in-patient services interventions that 'worked' in terms of their effectiveness in producing the desired results (e.g. improving service user's mental health; reducing injuries to staff; or even increasing the likelihood of future compliance with 'treatment' for fear of repetition) might therefore be considered to enjoy *pragmatic* validity. Unfortunately, whilst we may know which combinations of 'as required medication' can achieve rapid tranquilisation most effectively, and with fewer adverse effects,[26] evidence of the effectiveness of restraint and seclusion, as systematic review indicates, is at best ambiguous.[27]

Justifying coercion

The legal justification for the use of restraint, seclusion or compulsory medication is that such forms of coercion represent forms of necessary 'treatment' so that staff can fulfil their 'duty of care' and *'ensure that control is exercised over the patients'*.[28] It has been suggested that coercive interventions might be more usefully understood not as part of 'treatment' but instead as indicative of *'treatment failures'*, suggesting a need to urgently review the care delivered.[11] In English law however, a treatment need not be effective to be considered 'lawful' and can even be harmful.[29]

An in-patient unit in which service users were free to refuse all medication and to refuse to have their persons or their rooms searched for contraband items, such as illegal drugs, might in certain circumstances spiral out of control, leading to an unsafe environment for both staff and service users. Mental health in-patient settings consistently emerge from research as potentially violence-prone.[30,31] Such a situation calls for staff to be trained in restraint and rapid tranquilisation, and the case for the use of seclusion, once in decline, to be revisited, as an option can seem compelling. Coercion in this framing of the problem is represented as undesirable but 'progress in treatment can only be expected if safety has been established',[32] According to this justification, restraint, seclusion and 'as required medication' are therefore 'regrettable necessities', used only with extreme reluctance, as an absolute last resort to manage dangerous behaviour arising from the service users' 'mental illness', which poses a serious risk to the safety of the service user or others.

Suggestions that restraint, seclusion or as required compulsory medication actually 'work' in terms of improving safety are however scant. Evidence for the necessity of restraint must be considered, therefore, in the light of evidence garnered largely from studies on the effects of training.[33]

There are potentially strong arguments in favour of training in restraint as part of wider training in the prevention of violence.

Fisher[34] argued that restraint can prevent: imminent harm to self or others; substantial damage to the physical environment; and the serious disruption of treatment programmes. It can also decrease stimulation. He has also raised the issue that it may be valuable when implemented in response to service user requests.

Lee *et al.*'s[35] review found that the literature indicates several potential benefits arising from the introduction of structured training in physical restraint, including an increase in staff confidence, a decrease in the seriousness of assaults and assault-related injuries and a decrease in the levels of fear expressed by staff when interacting with patients. Reductions in the use of restraint following training have also been reported.[36]

Unfortunately, as Allen[37] observes, negative outcomes have also been found with all these measures. In the United Kingdom one explanation offered for the negative results associated with training has been that the 'importing' of training models from non-health service (prison) led to a widespread and persistent overemphasis on physical intervention during training in the prevention and management of violence in some programmes.[38] Unfortunately, this led to the neglect of training in interpersonal skills and the wider aspects of violence prevention. Such training was it appears misconstrued as a 'stand-alone' intervention: that is, it was interpreted as capable by itself of resolving the problems of workplace violence rather than as a necessary, but discrete, component of a total organisational commitment to a public health model.[39] This led, at least in some settings, to the development of service cultures in which nurses were *'trained to expect violence and how to react it but not how to stop it happening'*.[40] Such approaches it is suggested contributed to the emergence of a *'culture of violence in mental health care in the UK'*.[40]

Framing the problem of safety in mental health services as one that can be solved by increased control, whether by restraint, seclusion or compulsory medication, is at best simplistic if not profoundly misleading. An emerging body of research into the perceptions of service users around coercion suggests that many consider it is being used to *punish* rather than enable treatment, or manage high-risk behaviours.[11] Given the history of mental health services this is unsurprising. The use of systematic punishment to induce compliance was once orthodox practice, and threats of such 'punishment' as service users perceive it are clearly commonplace. The belief that *'fear (is) the most effectual principle to reduce the insane to orderly conduct'* may have appalled Daniel Tuke[12] in the nineteenth century. However, to assume that such long-established discourses no longer exert any influence on practice would be naive. As Shapiro[13] observed it is precisely because such discourses are so familiar that they are able to 'operate transparently'. Those affected are effectively blinded to such influences on both their thinking and behaviour.

In settings where the needs of service users have become superseded by the needs of the culture for order, routine, predictability and deference to power, the misuse of such interventions to enforce compliance can easily become commonplace. Wardhaugh and Wilding[14] have described this process as *'An active betrayal of the values upon which the organisation is supposedly based'*. In such services *'the primary aims of care have become subordinate to what are essentially secondary aims such as the preservation of order, quiet and cleanliness'*.[15] The problem is that giving permission to staff to use such interventions, whose subtle (or not so subtle) misuse under the guise of treatment has long been identified as a key factor in the development of corrupted cultures, can then become self-perpetuating.[16] Over time a range of explanations have been offered as to the origins of what we presently choose to describe as 'mental health needs' or 'problems'. Amongst the lesser known is the phenomenon of the 'insane ear'. A characteristic swelling of the ear lobe was once thought by some asylum physicians in the early nineteenth century to be a symptom of the long-sought physiological basis of insanity.[17] It took William Tuke[19] to suggest a somewhat more prosaic explanation. In what might be described as an early epidemiological study he noted the phenomenon now described as 'haematoma auris' occurred much more frequently in the left ear of 'disruptive' male patients than their right. This led him to suggest that this was more to do with the majority of asylum attendants being right handed than any underlying propensity in the population to the condition known more colloquially in the United Kingdom as 'cauliflower ear'.

Considering alternatives

If the problem of violence or other disturbed behaviour is framed as something to be controlled, needing restraint, seclusion and rapid tranquilisation, what are the alternatives? Prilleltensky[48] asserts that a focus on causation is of critical importance. He has criticised approaches to defining and/or assessing validity, which focus merely on 'what works', arguing that implicit to such approaches is a reductionist perspective on pathology, which neglects the social dimensions of causation. This he observes neglects the potential for the transformation of the conditions that may have given rise to the phenomena in question, typically in this case violence in in-patient mental health settings. Instead, he argues in favour of a model of validity which he terms 'psychopolitical', arguing that interventions must be judged on the extent to which they seek to transform the conditions that give rise to the problem.[48] To qualify as 'psychopolitically valid' an intervention must:

- recognize and challenge inequalities of power and their negative effects on both service users and staff;
- help to prevent the acting out of one's own oppression on others;
- build awareness of internalised oppression;
- illustrate and challenge dominant discourses that promote victim blaming;
- challenge collusion with exploitative systems, the causative role of these inequalities in terms of their impact on communities and individuals and the need for interventions to address such inequalities; and
- contribute towards the struggle to establish and sustain a positive individual identity.

This perspective on validity prompts a focus on primary prevention and consideration of the structural determinants of violence that might otherwise be neglected. Irrespective of the setting, common reactions in staff exposed to aggression and violence include fear, frustration and anger. Unless recognised and constructively managed, such feelings can influence their future interactions with patients and other staff. Counter transference, in the form of the adoption of aggressive coping styles by staff, can then embed a cycle of retaliation and revenge in the culture.[49] Counter transference by staff can, however, have roots other than in violence by service users. Bowie[50] proposes an extension to the violence typology proposed by the California Division of Occupational Safety and Health, that is:

Type 1 *intrusive violence*: Criminal intent by strangers; terrorist acts; mental illness or drug-related aggression; and protest violence.
Type 2 *consumer-related violence*: Consumer, clients, patients (and family) violence against staff; vicarious trauma to staff; staff violence to clients and consumers.
Type 3 *relationship violence*: Staff-on-staff violence and bullying; domestic violence at work.

Bowie proposes a further '*Type 4*' category, which he suggests, comprises '*organisational violence*', that is, that which 'the organisation' perpetrates against consumers, clients and patients.[50] Direct care staff in many services are invariably at the lowest point in organisational hierarchies, often marked by rigid boundaries.[51] These hierarchies can however all too readily foster the development of abusive, bullying or 'toxic' cultures. The central dynamic of such toxic organisations is a culture of shame and humiliation, which can be pursued actively or allowed to happen by default.[52] Workers (and even whole professional groups) at the bottom of hierarchies can become acutely sensitised to any perceived threat to their limited degree of status and self-esteem. One consequence is that, low-level verbal abuse, or even non-compliance by a service user, can evoke a disproportionate emotional response because of the implicit threat to the staff member's vulnerable self-esteem. Restraint, seclusion and/or 'as required medication' provide an all too ready means for staff to exorcise such feelings by controlling, punishing and humiliating the service user.[53]

Actual or threatened violence is the most commonly reported reason for the use of seclusion, restraint or rapid tranquilisation in mental health in-patient services. However, such violence appears much more often to escalate from low-level conflict related to rules, rather than stemming directly from the individual's pathology.[51] The use of restraint, seclusion or 'as required medication' in services for people with mental health needs must therefore be understood as arising not simply from the pathology of the individual, however construed, but as stemming from the pathology of a society whose individualising and victim-blaming processes the service cultures may simply replicate.

To reduce the use of coercive measures transformative interventions are required.[48] These focus on the primary prevention of violence, recognising and addressing the central role the culture of individual mental health services should play in preventing violence. The underlying reasons for violence in in-patient settings often lie in structural inequalities of power, the unrecognised effects of trauma on both service users and staff, and the failure to develop supportive and therapeutic cultures. The potential effectiveness of system-wide meta-interventions, complemented by targeted training in crisis management to reduce restraint and seclusion, has now been convincingly demonstrated.[55-58] David Colton has produced a checklist for services contemplating pursuing restraint and seclusion reduction, to assess their readiness to implement such initiatives.[59]

Key ethical dilemmas

Even where the root causes of violence have been identified and addressed there may still be situations where coercion occurs. Whether or not to restrain, seclude or medicate patients can present with a decision dilemma for nursing staff, where they attempt to manage the risks to all involved including themselves. In such circumstances, nurses may regard the conflicting choices of intervention/non-intervention as equally unwelcome options.[60] However, there remain scenarios where restraint, seclusion or rapid tranquilisation may be warranted in exceptional circumstances.

- A service user diagnosed with bipolar disorder, who is experiencing an acute crisis, has repeatedly refused oral medication. She is manifestly psychotic, delusional and evidently pyrexic, appears acutely dehydrated and repeatedly refuses fluids. She is reported as not having slept for 72 hours. Her physical health will rapidly deteriorate in such circumstances. Should staff decline to enforce medication?
- A service user detained under mental health legislation refuses access to his/her room by standing in front of the door obstructing the planned search of a room carried out as part of a 'random search' strategy in a medium or high secure service. The service user has a previous history of constructing and using weapons. Should staff physically restrain him to permit the search?
- A service user with a diagnosis of anorexia refuses to accept oral supplements or oral sedation to permit intravenous feeding. Medical opinion is that without rapid intervention she will die within days or weeks. Should staff restrain her to administer treatment?
- An acutely psychotic young service user, also diagnosed with autistic spectrum disorder, struggles badly to manage his symptoms in an acute in-patient unit which can be noisy and sometime chaotic. When acutely distressed he aggressively confronts other service users and will repeatedly attempt assault. If physically restrained he reacts badly continuing to struggle for long periods, causing staff serious anxiety that he may experience acidosis and suffer cardiac arrest. If secluded the low stimulus environment appears to help him calm. Should staff seclude him?

Conclusion

Recent years have seen the emergence of a new restraint reduction movement whose aims include the reduction of all forms of coercion. This movement has explicitly sought to reframe the problem of violence towards staff and to challenge what it has described as the almost exclusive focus on the pathology of the individual resulting from the dominance of biological psychiatry and the near demise of social psychiatry. In seeking to reduce recourse to coercion it has argued that the root causes of the behaviours leading to such interventions can often be found in what services do to both service users and staff. The role of the organisation is thus increasingly recognised as of critical importance.

There is now persuasive evidence that multi-dimensional meta-interventions are capable of significantly reducing the use of seclusion, restraint and as required compulsory medication. As the examples above illustrate, it may be impossible to eliminate the use of such interventions in all settings. However, it may be possible to reduce them significantly in most. It is also clear that such reduction strategies offer the most effective route to making mental health in-patient settings safer for both service users and staff. Given such clear evidence, and the legal requirement now imposed on many European countries to provide services in the 'least restrictive manner', any service that fails to attempt to reduce the use of such interventions, must offer good reason.

It may be apt to end with the words of a service user, once a mental health nurse, who may be uniquely qualified to comment. Discussing his experience of restraint he observed:

> For me the real issue is not so much about restraint per se, but about restraint carried out by people who think restraining a patient is not a violent act. There may be times when it is a necessary violent act. A person who knows this, and believes violence to be basically wrong, will strive to minimise the violence. A person who thinks restraining a patient is not a violent act will not. They will also not understand why someone would be upset by being restrained and will not be in a position to deal with that upset in a positive way.[61]

Coercive interventions remain commonplace in mental health but can be open to abuse in the corrupted cultures that continue to exist in some in-patient settings.

Coercive interventions can be significantly reduced in most in-patient settings via meta-interventions that start by reframing the problem of violence toward staff.

All services should be required to publish their rates of restraint, seclusion and compulsory medication. Such transparency would do much to encourage services to reduce their use.

Notes

1 La Grange, J. (Ed.). (2006). *Michel Foucault Psychiatric Power: Lectures at the collège de France 1973–1974*. Basingstoke: Palgrave Macmillan, p. 35.
2 Health Care Finance Administration. (1999). *Medicare and Medicaid Programs: Hospital Conditions of Participation: Patients Rights; Interim Final Rule*. Department of Health and Human Services, Health Care Financing Organisation; Federal Register; part II. 465.
3 Szasz, T. (2007). *Coercion as Cure: A Critical History of Psychiatry*. New Brunswick, NJ: Transaction Publishers.
4 Kerlinger, N. (1973). *Foundations of Behavioral Research*. New York, NY: Holt, Rinehart & Winston.
5 Polkinghorne, D. (1992). Postmodern epistemology of practice. In S. Kvale (Ed.), *Psychology and Postmodernism*. London: Sage, pp. 146–66.
6 Kvale, S. (1995). The social construction of validity. *Qualitative Inquiry*, 1(1), 19–40.

7 Lather, P. (1993). Fertile obsession: Validity after post-structuralism. *The Sociological Quarterly*, 34, 673–93.

8 Breggin, P. (1982). Coercion of voluntary patients in an open hospital. In R. Edward (Ed.), *Psychiatry and Ethics*. New York, NY: Prometheus.

9 Health Care Commission. (2005). *Count Me In: Results of a National Census of Inpatients in Mental Health Hospitals and Facilities in England and Wales*. London: Health Care Commission.

10 Bowers, L., Douzenis, A., *et al.* (2005). Disruptive and dangerous behaviour by patients on acute psychiatric wards in three European centres. *Social Psychiatry and Psychiatric Epidemiology*, 40(10), 822–8.

11 Whittington, R., Baskind, E., and Paterson, B. (2006). Coercive measures in the management of imminent violence: Restraint, seclusion and enhanced observation. In D. Richter and R. Whittington (Eds.), *Violence in Psychiatry; Causes Consequences and Control*. New York, NY: Springhouse.

12 Paterson, B. and Duxbury, J. (2006). Developing a perspective on restraint and the least intrusive intervention. *British Journal of Nursing*, 14(22), 1235–41.

13 Council of Europe. (C.oE.). *Recommendation (2004)10 to Member States, Concerning the Protection of the Human Rights and Dignity of Persons with Mental Disorder*. Strasbourg. Council of Europe.

14 Waltraud, E. (1991). *Mad Tales from the Raj: The European Insane in British India, 1800–1858*. New York, NY: Routledge.

15 Alldridge, P. (1990). Hospitals, madhouses and asylums: Cycles in the care of the insane. In R. M. Murray and T. H. Turner (Eds.), *Lectures in the History of Psychiatry*. London: Gaskell.

16 Alldridge ibid.

17 Lambard 1581:138 cited by Alldridge ibid. p. 35.

18 La Grange op. cit. p. 105.

19 Tuke, S. (1813). *Description of the Retreat, an Institution near York for Insane Persons of the Society of Friends*. York: W. Alexander, p. 5.4

20 Thompson, C. (Ed.). (1987). *The Origins of Modern Psychiatry*. Chichester: John Wiley and Sons, p. 13.

21 Connolly, J. (1856). *The Treatment of the Insane Without Mechanical Restraints*. London: Dawsons of Pall Mall.

22 Tuke, D. H. (1847). Amelioration of the condition of the insane. In D. H. Tuke and J. C. Buckness (Eds.), *Manual of Psychological Medicine*. London: J. Churchill, p. 78.

23 Yellowlees, D. (1872, June 22). Mechanical restraint in cases of insanity. *The Lancet*, 1872, 880–1.

24 Soloff, P. H. (1984). Historical notes on seclusion and restraint. In K. Tardiff (Ed.), *The Psychiatric Uses of Seclusion and Restraint* (1st ed.). Washington, DC: American Psychiatric Press.

25 Kvale op. cit. p. 31.

26 National Institute of Clinical Excellence. (2005). *Violence: The Short-Term Management of Disturbed/ Violent Behaviour in Psychiatric In-Patient Settings and Emergency Departments*. National Institute of Clinical Excellence.

27 Sailas, E. and Fenton, M. (1999). *Seclusion and Restraint as a Method of Treatment for People with Serious Mental Illness*. The Cochrane Library, Issue 3. Oxford: Update Software. Cochrane Library number CD001163.

28 Lord Widgery (R v. Bracknell J.J, ex parte Griffiths p. 318 E-G).

29 Keywood, K. (2005). Psychiatric injustice? The therapeutic presumption of behaviour management in mental health law. *The Journal of Adult Protection*, 7(4), 25–30.

30 Estryn-Behar, M., Duville, N., Menini, M. L., Camerino, D., and Le Foll S and le Nezet O. (2007). Factors associated with violence against healthcare workers: Results of the European Presst-Next study. *Presse Medicale*, 36(1), 21–36.

31 Health Care Commission. (2007). *A Mental Health and Learning Disability Trusts: Key Findings from the 2006 Survey of Staff*. London: Health Care Commission.

32 Bloom, S. (1997). *Creating Sanctuary: Toward an Evolution of Sane Societies*. New York, NY: Routledge, p. 11.

33 Wright, S. (1999). Physical restraint in the management of violence and aggression in in-patient settings: A review of issues. *Journal of Mental Health*, 8(5), 459–72.

34 Fisher, W. (1994). Restraint and seclusion: A review of the literature. *American Journal of Psychiatry*, 151(11), 1584–91.

35 Lee, S. Wright, S., and Sayer, J. (2001). Physical restraint for nurses in English and Welsh psychiatric intensive care and regional secure units. *Journal of Mental Health*, 10(2), 151–62.

36 Parkes, J. (1996). Control and restraint training: A study of its effectiveness in a medium secure psychiatric unit. *Journal of Forensic Psychiatry,* 7, 525–34.

37 Allen D. (2000). *Training Carers in Physical Interventions: Towards Evidence Based Practice*. Kidderminster: British Institute of Learning Disabilities.

38 Leadbetter D. and Paterson, B. (2004). Exploring safe physical interventions. *Nursing & Residential Care*, 6(5), 232–4.

39 Paterson, B., Miller, G., and Leadbetter, D. (2005). Beyond zero tolerance: A varied approach to workplace violence. *British Journal of Nursing*, 14(15), 811–15.

40 Tucker, R. (2004). *NMC National Conference on Violence: Some Nurses Too Quick to Restrain Patients*, Press Statement 27-2004, 21 April 2004.

41 Duxbury, J. (2002). An evaluation of staff and patient views of and strategies employed to manage inpatient aggression and violence on one mental health unit: A pluralistic design. *Journal of Psychiatric and Mental Health Nursing*, 9(3), 325–37.

42 Tuke, D. H. (1882). *Chapters in the History of the Insane in the British Isles*. London: Kegan Paul, p. 90.

43 Shapiro, M. J. (1988). *The Politics of Representation: Writing Practices in Biography, Photography and Policy Analysis*. Wisconsin: University of Wisconsin Press, p. xi.

44 Wardhaugh, J. and Wilding, P. (1993). Towards an explanation of the corruption of care. *Critical Social Care*, 37(13), 4–31, 5.

45 Martin, J. P. (1984). *Hospitals in Trouble*. London: Blackwell, p. 108.

46 Page, C. W. (1904). Mechanical restraint and seclusion of insane persons. *Boston Medical and Surgical Journal*, December, 590–5.

47 Mills, C. K. and Yawger, N. S. (Eds.) (1915). *Lippincott's Nursing Manuals Nursing and Care of the Nervous and the Insane*. Philadelphia, PA: J. B. Lippincott Company.

48 Prilleltensky, I. and Nelson, G. (2002). *Doing Psychology Critically: Making a Difference in Diverse Settings*. London: Palgrave.

49 Maier, G. J. (1999). Psychological issues in treatment: Transference and counter transference. In K. Tardiff (Ed.), *Medical Management of the Violent Patient: Clinical Assessment and Therapy*. New York, NY: Dekker, pp. 277–309.

50 Bowie, V. (2002). Defining violence at work a new typology. In M. Gill, B. Fisher, and V. Bowie (Eds.), *Violence at Work Causes Patterns and Prevention*. Uffculme, Devon: Willan Publishing.

51 Frost, J. (2003). *Toxic Emotions at Work: How Compassionate Managers Handle Pain and Conflict*. Boston, MA: Harvard Business School Press.

52 Wyatt, J. and Hare, C. (1997). *Work Abuse: How to Recognize and Survive It*. Rochester, VT: Schenkman Books.

53 Paterson, B. and Duxbury, J. (2007). Restraint. A question of validity? *Nursing Ethics*, 14(4), 535–45.

54 Whittington R. and Wykes, T. (1996). Aversive stimulation by staff and violence by psychiatric patients. *British Journal of Clinical Psychology*, 35(1), 11–20.

55 Jonikas, J., Cook, J., Rosen, C., Laris, A., and Kim, J. (2004). A program to reduce use of physical restraint in psychiatric inpatient facilities. *Psychiatric Services*, 55(7), 818–20.

56 Schreiner, G. M., Crafton, C. G., and Sevin, J. A. (2004). Decreasing the use of mechanical restraints and locked seclusion. *Administration Policy Mental Health*, 31, 449–63.

57 Murphy, T. and Bennington-Davis, M. (2005). *Restraint and Seclusion: The Model for Eliminating Their Use in Healthcare*. Marblehead, MA: Hcpro.

58 Sullivan, A. M. and Bezmen, J. (2005). Reducing restraints: Alternatives to restraints on an inpatient psychiatric service – utilizing safe and effective methods to evaluate and treat the violent patient. *Psychiatric Quarterly*, 76(1): 51–65.

59 Colton, D. (2004). *Checklist for Assessing Your Organization's Readiness for Reducing Seclusion and Restraint*. Staunton, VA: Commonwealth Center for Children and Adolescence.

60 Marangos-Frost, S. and Wells, D. (2000). Psychiatric nurses' thoughts and feelings about restraint use: A decision dilemma. *Journal of Advanced Nursing*, 31(2), 362–9.

61 Davis, P. (2004). Critical thoughts on restraint in hospital. *Mental Health Nursing*, May 2004.

14 ECT and informed consent

Phil Barker

Caveat

Electroconvulsive therapy (ECT) and informed consent are, potentially, highly complex issues but, ethically, there is not a lot that *needs* to be said:

- If people *want* to receive ECT (or any service, treatment, therapy), they *should*, at least in principle, be free to *ask* for and *receive* it.
- If people are to receive *any* professional service, they are entitled to know: what it will involve; how it is likely to affect them; what it will cost; and whether or not the 'professionals' are qualified to deliver this service.

What could be simpler?

Introduction

Origins of ECT

Apart from psychosurgery, which is rarely undertaken today, ECT[1] is the most controversial form of psychiatric 'treatment'.[2] ECT is defined as:

> . . . involving the passage of an electric current across the brain. The treatment is only administered to an anaesthetized patient who has also been administered a muscle relaxant. The electric current induces seizure activity in the brain which is necessary for the therapeutic effect of treatment.[3]

Today, the emphasis is very much on the potential 'therapeutic value' of the electrical current. How the 'seizure activity' becomes 'therapeutic' remains, to a large extent, a mystery and much contemporary theorizing even doubts the need for electricity as a means of inducing seizures.

ECT is a left over from the dark age of psychiatry, where the 'Great and Desperate Cures'[4] of insulin coma, and lobotomy were developed. In 1933, the fertile imagination of the Hungarian psychiatrist *Laszlo Meduna* led him to believe that epilepsy and schizophrenia were antagonistic.[5] This reversed the established view that epilepsy and schizophrenia were actually related. However, for Meduna: 'No longer did epilepsy cause insanity; instead it cured it'.[6] This was all part of the misguided fashion for iatrogenic epilepsy.[7] *Insulin shock therapy*[8] enjoyed a brief reign, but proved, medically, too demanding and was overtaken by the use of *camphor oil* and then *metrazol*:[9] all were used to induce convulsions in people – something which people with epilepsy were very keen to avoid.

The 'therapeutic value' of shock methods was taken for granted by the 1940s when the Italian psychiatrists, *Ugo Cerletti* and *Lucio Bini*, began to experiment with *electrically* induced seizures. After witnessing the use of electricity to stun pigs at a slaughterhouse, Cerletti experimented on a vagrant picked up at Milan railway station. As Cerletti noted, the experiment was: 'carried out in an atmosphere of fearful silence bordering on disapproval in the presence of various assistants belonging to the clinic and some outside doctors'.[10]

The unfortunate vagrant was shocked repeatedly, despite his explicit protests. Cerletti, however, was clearly pleased with the results, if not also pleased with himself: 'That is how the first epileptic fit experimentally induced in man through the electrical stimulus took place. So electroshock was born: for such was the name I forthwith gave it'.[11]

Notably, the 'subject' of Cerletti's 'experiment' had not asked for any psychiatric help. Instead, he had been arrested for vagrancy and sent to Cerletti by the police 'for observation'. Cerletti disobeyed the Police Commissioner's instructions, and experimented on the man; without any consent, or authority. After the first shock, the man protested: 'Not another one! It's deadly!' That the man could speak at all appeared only to encourage Cerletti to press on with his 'shocking' experiment.[12]

Sixty years later, all this seems barbaric. Today, we run the risk of public censure, if not criminal proceedings, for merely using 'politically incorrect' language. Cerletti's arrogance is writ large on the pages of psychiatric history. However, everyone involved in the organization and delivery of ECT today, treads in Cerletti's footsteps. They may not appreciate the historical link, but it is entirely apposite.

ECT and the brain

As soon as it became apparent that epileptic seizures signalled a sudden burst of electrical activity in the brain, rather than demonic possession, every effort was made to reduce the likelihood of the person having such 'fits'. Once the neurophysiology became clearer, it was apparent that the seizures were accompanied by cerebral anoxia,[13] which caused brain damage. The more seizures a person experienced, the more brain damage would occur.

Despite his neurological background, this fact appeared to escape Cerletti. Ever since, psychiatrists have denied that ECT causes any brain damage, although neurologists continue to issue counter-claims. Indeed, advocates make grandiose claims for ECT[14] including the idea that it: 'has proved to be one of the safest procedures in medicine'; and that there is a 'myth, largely promoted by anti-psychiatrists, that ECT damages . . . brain functioning'.[15] It is ironic that the complaints of 'anti-psychiatrists' need to be trotted out, as if neurologists – the actual authorities on brain anatomy and function – were not sufficiently savage in their criticisms.

Dr Peter Sterling, a professor of neurobiology, offered a well-considered critique of ECT, to the Standing Committee on Mental Health of the Assembly of the State of New York, in 1978.[16] Thirty years later, his testimony is still relevant. Moreover, Sterling has not changed his views over the years, especially concerning ECT advocates' denial of ECT-induced brain damage:

> One can be sympathetic to psychiatry (as I am) and still imagine that passing 150 V between the temples to evoke a grand mal seizure might cause brain damage, especially when you realize that this 'cure' for depression requires this procedure to be repeated 10–20 times over a week or so. And when you talk to a friend who has been so treated and discover that a year later she is still experiencing huge gaps in recall of major life

events, you begin to worry. Finally you discover that ECT's benefit is only temporary, so that many psychiatrists administer it chronically.[17]

As a neuroscientist, Sterling understood only too well brain physiology, and how ECT causes neuronal death. It comes as no surprise to him that observers: 'describe people who have had many ECT treatments as "punch drunk" – resembling boxers who have sustained chronic brain damage'.[18]

This is a powerful echo of another neurologist, from almost 30 years ago, who commented on the brain-damaging effects of ECT.

> As a neurologist and electroencephalographer, I have seen many patients after ECT, and I have no doubt that ECT produces effects identical to those of a head injury. After multiple sessions of ECT, a patient has symptoms identical to those of a retired, punch-drunk boxer . . ... After a few sessions of ECT the symptoms are those of moderate cerebral contusion, and further enthusiastic use of ECT may result in the patient functioning at a subhuman level. Electroconvulsive therapy in effect may be defined as a controlled type of brain damage produced by electrical means.[19]

A recent review offered a sobering summary of its brain-damaging effects:

> . . . One of its adverse secondary effects is neurocognitive dysfunction . . ... Declarative memory is clearly impaired after ECT. Immediate memory, however, is broadly preserved. Few studies have addressed procedural and incidental memory. Selective memory is impaired, probably due to the disruption of specific brain regions.[20]

Moreover, such cognitive dysfunction is increased where the dose of electricity is higher or it is administered more often.[21]

As Read noted,[22] none of this is surprising. When *Walter Freeman* (see Chapter 2) 'imported' ECT from Europe to the USA in the 1940s, it was accepted that ECT 'worked' because it *caused brain damage*. Freeman commented: 'The greater the damage, the more likely the remission of psychotic symptoms. . . . Maybe it will be shown that a mentally ill patient can think more clearly and more constructively with less brain in actual operation'.[23]

The ethics of ECT

As discussed in Chapter 1, ethics can be a very complex business. At least in a democratic society, people are free to do almost anything, provided that it does not harm anyone else. That said, in paternalistic societies,[24] laws or policies are often established to 'look after' sections of the community; or to prevent almost everyone from coming to grief – whether literally or metaphorically. Psychiatry offers a fine example of just such paternalistic influence.

My personal view is that if people wish to experience electrically induced, grand mal seizures, on a repeat basis, as part of some 'course of treatment,' in an effort to remedy some 'emotional ills', or otherwise 'fix' their lives, they *should be free* to ask for, receive, and pay for such a 'service'. However, whether or not any mental health professional should feel *obliged* to deliver such a service, is another matter. Whether or not such a service should be paid for by a National Health Service is also questionable.

Regrettably, however, within the psychiatric community some take the view that people are not *able* (i.e. competent) to make such a decision; and someone else should decide on their behalf (see Chapters 23–26). Often the view is also taken that any psychiatric/mental health professional worthy of the name should aid and abet the delivery of ECT, if it is deemed necessary.[25]

The situation becomes more complicated when we consider the situation of people, like Cerletti's famous 'subject', who do not ask for such 'shock treatment'; and may actually protest against being given such unwelcome 'treatment'.[26] In most Western societies, the public invest such a degree of faith in medicine and physicians that if ECT is prescribed, then friends and family will assume, automatically, that the person must need such 'treatment'.

Most of the ethical dilemmas associated with ECT hinge on consent, which is addressed briefly later. However, such ethical issues also are influenced by popular (and professional) beliefs regarding the effectiveness of ECT as a 'treatment' balanced against its potential for causing harm (brain damage). We should not forget also the risk of psychological harm, although this has rarely been addressed by researchers.

General efficacy: The ethical case against ECT has been presented, in great detail, by several authors: including psychiatrists, neurologists and 'survivors' of ECT[27–30] Most of their criticisms relate to the brain-damaging effects of ECT, but they also challenge the repeated assertions of efficacy that have been proposed over the past 60 years, many of which have little serious scientific basis.

Suicide: Psychiatrists who favour the use of ECT[31] often claim the 'need' to use it as a 'life-saving intervention' and this idea has now become a popular fiction.[32] However, the evidence supporting the use of ECT to 'prevent suicide' is weak, where it is not actually contradictory.[33] Many studies show *no* difference between the rate of suicide in people given ECT and a similar cohort of 'patients'.[34,35] A major study of over 1,000 patients with 'major affective disorders' showed that:

> mortality did not differ between patients having a lifetime history of ECT and patients never having had ECT. We conclude from a short-term follow-up of depressives that mode of therapy received in the hospital has minimal influence on subsequent mortality, including suicide.[36]

Schizophrenia: Although commonly used with people with an affective disorder (forms of depression) it was also used widely, as noted already, with people with a diagnosis of schizophrenia. This practice was largely displaced by the introduction of 'anti-psychotic' drugs in the 1950s. However, many 'patient support groups' like the National Alliance for the Mentally Ill (NAMI) continue to enthuse about the usefulness of ECT.[37] However, the Royal College of Psychiatrists (United Kingdom) now acknowledges that ECT has no role in the general treatment of schizophrenia, and also acknowledges that ECT might 'work', at least in part, because of the extra attention, support and the general anaesthetic.[38]

Women and older persons: Women received ECT more frequently than men and the rates of administration for both genders increased with age.[39–41] For many older people, especially older women, the use of ECT appears to further confirm their weakness and vulnerability. Orr and O'Connor interviewed women in depth and concluded: 'the central theme underpinning all of these women's stories was the shifting of power from themselves to others'.[42]

The Cochrane review concluded that: 'it is not possible to draw firm conclusions on whether ECT is more effective than anti-depressants, or on the safety or side effects of ECT in elderly people with depression'.[43] Given that many older persons are already experiencing a degree of cognitive decline, due to the ageing brain, the induction of even more cognitive impairment in the name of 'treatment' seems suspect, to say the least.

Young persons: Although ECT has been used with young people for over 50 years, there are signs that its use is increasing in some countries, at the same time as it goes into decline (or is banned) in others.[14] It seems all too apparent that any procedure that risks injuring the brain is ill-advised in the case of young people, where the brain is still developing.[15,16] In the State of Victoria, Australia, for example, there has been a significant outcry over the use of ECT with children as young as four.[17]

Psychological effects: Although some people choose ECT, perhaps on the basis of past experience, considerable evidence supports the view that as many as *one-third* of people receiving ECT found the experience deeply traumatic, in both the short and longer terms. Lucy Johnstone's research describes how the experience of ECT can worsen feelings of shame and failure. Not surprisingly, many wish to avoid ECT if offered again but others may comply out of a sense of powerlessness, fearful of confiding their true feelings to professional staff.[18]

Most ECT research has concentrated on the procedure, its 'outcome', in terms of reported 'improvement' in 'symptomatic presentation', and the extent to which memory is impaired. Little attention has been paid to the psychological effects of ECT. Johnstone's study focused on individuals who had some kind of negative experience of ECT.[19] The participants in Johnstone's study had many criticisms of the process itself:

- the lack of proper discussion of the procedure beforehand;
- the sight of trolleys and medical equipment as they waited their turn;
- being able to overhear people being given ECT; and
- the 'distant or offhand staff attitudes'.

As Johnstone noted, all this could easily be remedied but, arguably, at the cost of being seen as 'window-dressing' or 'hypocrisy'. The main concern of the participants in this study related to 'having electricity passed through your head'. As Johnstone noted, not only did this carry powerful symbolic meanings, it was also seen as 'irrelevant and damaging'.[50]

Perhaps unsurprisingly, most of the participants in Johnstone's study believed that their 'breakdowns' were meaningful: involving factors that could not be addressed by some physical procedure. However, the evidence for the 'effectiveness' of ECT is so poor that one needs to ask whether or not it is worth all the emotional trouble. As Johnstone concluded:

> If up to a third of people will suffer psychological trauma after ECT, and if there is no way of identifying these individuals in advance, the ratio of costs to benefits may begin to seem unacceptably high. As always, more research is needed. However, this should not be an excuse for complacency about the experiences of those for whom the description of ECT as 'a helpful treatment and not particularly frightening' is profoundly untrue.[51]

Informed consent

The concept of informed consent applies to all aspects of psychiatric, psychotherapeutic or other 'mental health' care and treatment, but it is especially relevant to ECT, which is on a par with surgery. Apart from the induction of the seizure the 'patient' will need to be anaesthetized, which carries obvious risks.

[*Note*: Although even ECT advocates acknowledge that deaths do occur, the statistics are often minimized by suggesting that it is no greater in ECT than with general anaesthesia for minor surgery.[52] However, this ignores the obvious fact that, even if this comparison is true for an individual treatment, a course of ECT usually involves at least *eight* treatments in close succession. Statistics on the death rate where someone has similar repeat doses of anaesthetic for minor surgery are, of course, not available].

Informed consent is a complex legal/ethical concept, with several different meanings, referring to:

- A set of legal rules, which prescribe certain patterns of behaviour for all health care staff, in their interactions with patients. Informed consent rules also provide certain penalties, should the practitioner deviate from the recommended course of action.
- An ethical doctrine, which seeks to promote an individual's right of self-determination regarding any medical treatment.
- A specific interpersonal process, within which health staff and the 'patient' interact, in an effort to select the most appropriate course of medical care or treatment.[53]

Indeed, informed consent involves all three of these definitions. All medical treatment involves some degree of risk. In principle, patients are entitled to know what are the likely risks involved in their treatment, before proceeding. In most countries, all adults are assumed to be competent to offer consent, unless they are *unable* to take in and/or retain information about their care and treatment; understand the information; and weigh up the information as part of a decision-making process.

In general when people are invited to give *informed consent* for ECT they should:

- know *who* is recommending the treatment; why this is the treatment of choice; what alternatives are available; and what are the risks and benefits involved in the treatment;
- receive a full explanation of the ECT procedure itself;
- be informed about the *likelihood* and *severity* of all risks related to the anaesthetic and muscle relaxants used in ECT, and their short- and long-term effect;
- be told about the possibility of emergency medical intervention should any complications occur during the time the person is under the anaesthetic;
- understand that his or her consent is voluntary and can be withdrawn at any time without any penalty;
- be encouraged to ask questions, at any time (before, during and after) about the ECT procedure and know the formal identity (and authority) of the person answering those questions; and
- be told what restrictions might need to be placed on the person's behaviour before, during and immediately after the administration of the ECT.[54]

In principle, such conditions should apply to *any* (all) offers of care and/or treatment. At the same time, it is the professional's responsibility to help the person to weigh up all the potential contradictions likely to exist within such 'information', ensuring at all times that the person is the final arbiter; and is not subtly coerced, or manipulated (see Chapters 12, 13 and 15).

In the United Kingdom, the National Institute for Clinical Excellence (NICE) advised staff to highlight the potential for a resulting cognitive impairment during the consent process. The patient should be made aware that ECT may have serious and permanent effects on both memory and non-memory cognition.[55]

The process for obtaining informed consent is usually the responsibility of a senior member of the medical team – for example a Consultant Psychiatrist. Bray[56] noted that:

The Capacity Act 2005 is clear that except in an emergency (where a person will be sectioned under the Mental Health Act) ECT may not be given to anyone who has capacity to refuse consent, and may only be given to an incapacitated person where it does not conflict with any advance directive, decision of a deputy or of the Court of Protection.[57]

However, where other members of the team, such as nurses, doubt the wisdom of any proposed course of treatment – such as ECT – it is their professional duty to register their objections. For many nurses, this may not be easy, as it risks disrupting team cohesion. However, as Kashka and Keyser noted: 'the reluctance of the staff nurse to intervene also illustrates the need for ethical groundedness of nurses at all levels'.[58]

Conclusion

ECT remains the most controversial form of psychiatric treatment. It has virtually been abolished in Italy, where it first caught the psychiatric imagination; and is available in Germany and Belgium only in specialist centres.[59] Finland, once recording a high use of ECT with inpatients (14 per cent), has seen this drop off to 2 per cent. In the Irish Republic, just over one-third of approved centres actually use ECT, and the Irish psychiatrist Pat Bracken has led a campaign[60] to remove the existing clause within Irish mental health legislation, which allows for *involuntary* ECT.[61] In the USA, once the electroshock capital of the world, ECT is not used at all in more than one-third of the 317 US metropolitan areas.[62] In the remainder, the use of ECT varied enormously, suggesting local 'enthusiasm' rather than anything resembling a policy based on the 'best available evidence'.

This chapter has focused, of necessity, on the potential for brain damage involved in ECT. After all, its brain-damaging was one of its attractive features for early American practitioners.[63] For all who receive it, ECT produces memory loss around the time of the treatment, which may persist over a long period for many 'patients'. Also, as Johnstone found, the nature of the 'treatment' can be highly disturbing, generating feelings of humiliation, failure, worthlessness and a powerful sense of being abused and assaulted.[64] Any 'benefit' gained from ECT is likely to be short-lived, lasting only a few days (hence the need to repeat the procedure, *ad nauseam*). Neither does it prevent suicide, as has often been claimed.[65,66] Indeed, among the many 'celebrities' given ECT was the writer, Ernest Hemingway. A few days before he killed himself, soon after receiving ECT, Hemingway said: 'What is the sense of ruining my head and erasing my memory, which is my capital, and putting me out of business? It was a brilliant cure, but we lost the patient'.[67]

The New Zealand psychologist, John Read, noted that where its use is not actually banned, the use of ECT is very much in decline. In England its use has fallen by almost 60 per cent in 20 years. If the annual reduction is sustained, ECT will disappear in England by 2013.[68]

Despite the contemporary vogue for 'evidence-based medicine' there have been very few studies, which have compared ECT with 'simulated ECT' (everything except the shock): representing an 'active' versus a 'placebo' intervention. The justification for *not* conducting such a comparison has long been that it would be unethical not to offer all patients a treatment, of *proven efficacy*. 'The *assumption* that ECT is effective is used to justify not evaluating whether it *is* effective'.[69]

Perhaps the real reason why practitioners are so protective of ECT is self-protection in disguise. More importantly, in a society where people routinely avoid electric shocks (and epileptic seizures, if they can) it is difficult to view passing an electric current through the brain – the repository of all human consciousness – as anything less than barbaric. Read observed:

> To acknowledge the true risk of death or the real extent of brain damage is virtually impossible for those who prescribe ECT. It would expose them to moral condemnation and serious legal and financial consequences. They need to believe the treatment is safe and effective.[70]

I suggested at the outset that the ethical problems associated with ECT are straightforward: if people *wish* to have such a 'treatment', however dubious its effectiveness and however dangerous its effects, they should be free to ask for it. The real ethical problems arise when we consider the role of professionals in responding to such requests; especially where they *suggest* ECT as a 'treatment option'.

Where ECT is under consideration as part of the care treatment plan for an individual 'patient', *all* mental health professionals might consider, the following questions:

- Given what you know of the *person* (and the person's problems) how confident are you that a course of ECT is the *most appropriate* 'response' *at this time*? On what evidence do you base your professional judgement?
- How would you decide that a course of ECT represents a *better* (i.e. safer, more effective, more meaningful) response than any alternative? What evidence would you bring to bear in making such a judgement?
- How confident are you that the person has been informed fully of *all* the possible physical and psychological problems (including death) which might be associated with the administration of ECT, as well as a *realistic prediction* of its benefits, before giving 'informed consent'?
- If you are in any doubt that all such information has been part of the process of informed consent, what would you be willing to do to address this?
- If you believe that ECT is *not* an appropriate treatment for a person, what action will you take?

Some readers may take the view that this chapter is in some sense opposed to the use of 'ECT'. In conclusion, I would like to repeat my initial comments. I am *not* in favour of banning ECT. Indeed, I believe that if people genuinely wish to have such a course of treatment, for whatever reason, they should be free, at least, to request it. However, there should be no obligation placed on others, to administer such 'treatment'. If freedom is to mean anything it must involve freedom for everyone.

However, if mental health professionals have *any* doubts about the validity of ECT as a psychiatric 'treatment', or any concerns about the 'trade-off' between any expected 'benefits' and the possible 'costs' – risk of death, memory loss, other cognitive dysfunction or emotional distress related to the ECT process – in my view they *must*, ethically, decide what course of action they should take.

Even those who are not directly involved in ECT are ethically compromised. Much of the organized opposition to slavery, racial discrimination, sex discrimination, 'homophobia' and various other 'civil rights' involved persons who had *no* direct association with situations that were viewed, at the time, as social 'wrongs'. This did not appear to offer them a 'get out' clause.

In 40 years in the mental health field, I have never been involved in any aspect of the administration of ECT. One of my critics argued that, as a result, my views were: 'typical of those written by professionals, one or more steps removed from direct patient care or personal experience'.[71] I would hope that I would not need to be a victim of persecution or discrimination or any other act of barbarism to know that it was, *indeed*, an act of barbarism. Many of the ethical positions we need to take are based not on direct experience, but on empathy, sympathy and fellow-feeling. At least, I hope that is the case.

Notes

1   ECT continues to be called electroshock therapy (EST) in the USA.
2   For a comprehensive review of ECT, its background and effect on recipients, see: Bray J The nurse's role in the administration of electroconvulsive therapy. In P Barker (Ed.) *Psychiatric and Mental Health Nursing: The Craft of Caring*. London: Arnold, 2009.
3   Department of Health. *Electroconvulsive Therapy: Survey Covering the Period from January 1999 to March 1999*, London: Department of Health, 1999.
4   Valenstein ES *Great and Desperate Cures: The Rise and Decline of Psychosurgery and Other Radical Treatments for Mental Illness*. New York, NY: Harper Collins, 1987.
5   For a detailed account of the history of 'iatrogenic epilepsy', see: Szasz TS *Coercion as Cure: A Critical History of Psychiatry*. London: Transaction Publishers, 2007.
6   Szasz ibid. p. 126.
7   Physician-induced seizures.
8   Jones K Insulin coma therapy in schizophrenia. *Journal of the Royal Society of Medicine* 2000: 93, 147–9.
9   Schilder P Notes on the psychology of metrazol treatment of schizophrenia. *Journal of Nervous and Mental Disease* 1939: 89, 133–44.
10 Cerletti U Old and new information about electroshock. *American Journal of Psychiatry* 1950: 107, 87–94.
11 Cerletti ibid.
12 Szasz op. cit. p. 132.
13 A condition where oxygen is deficient in brain tissue.
14 Fink M *Electroshock: Restoring the Mind*. Oxford: Oxford University Press, 1999.
15 Freeman H Taking the horror out of shocks. *Nature* 1999: 401, 327.
16 http://www.ect.org/category/ect-side-effects/page/3/ (Accessed: 21/03/10).
17 Sterling P ECT damage is easy to find if you look for it. *Nature* 2000: 403, 242.
18 Sterling ibid.
19 Sament S Letter to the Editor. *Clinical Psychiatry News* 1983, March 11th.
20 Rami-Gonzalez L, Bernardo M, Boget T, Salamero M, Gil-Verona JA, and Junque C Subtypes of memory dysfunction associated with ECT: Characteristics and neurobiological bases. *Journal of ECT* 2001: 17, 129–35.
21 UK ECT Review Group Efficacy and safety of ECT in depressive disorders. *Lancet* 2003: 361, 799–808.
22 Read J Electroconvulsive therapy (Ch. 8). In J Read, L Mosher and R Bentall (Eds.) *Models of Madness*. London: Routledge, 2004, p. 92.
23 Freeman W Brain-damaging therapeutics. *Diseases of the Nervous System* 1941: 2, 83.
24 Harsanyi, D *Nanny State: How Food Fascists, Teetotaling Do-Gooders, Priggish Moralists, and Other Boneheaded Bureaucrats are Turning America into a Nation of Children*. New York, NY: Random House, Inc., 2007.
25 This situation is now changing as ECT becomes a more highly specialized form of 'treatment', administered by specially prepared staff.
26 Mind Freedom International fought a long campaign on behalf of a Minnesota man – Ray Sadford – who wanted to refuse the state-order 'electroshock'. Details of his successful campaign, and also the significant amount of opposition Ray and Mind Freedom encountered, can be found at: http://www.mindfreedom.org/ray-sandford-minnesota/web-of-links/?searchterm=Ray%20Sandford (Accessed: 29/03/10).

27 Morgan RF *Electroshock: The Case Against.* Toronto, Ontario: IPI, 2005.

28 Breggin P *Electroshock: Its Brain Disabling Effects.* New York, NY: Springer, 1979.

29 Frank LR *The History of Shock Treatment.* San Francisco, CA: Frank, 1978.

30 MIND *Shock Treatment: A Survey of People's Experiences of ECT.* London: MIND, 2001.

31 We should not forget that other psychiatrists are completely opposed to the use of ECT.

32 http://www.healthyplace.com/bipolar-disorder/treatment/ect-electroconvulsive-therapy-for-bipo-lar-disorder/menu-id-67/

33 Challiner V and Griffiths L Electroconvulsive therapy: A review of the literature. *Journal of Psychiatric and Mental Health Nursing* 2000: 7, 191–8.

34 Milstein V, Small JG, Small IF, and Green GE Does electroconvulsive therapy prevent suicide? *Journal of ECT* 1986: 2, 3–6.

35 Sharma V Retrospective controlled study of inpatient ECT: Does it prevent suicide? *Journal of Affective Disorder* 1999: 56, 183–7.

36 Black D, Winokur G, Mohandoss E, Woolson RS, and Nasrallah A Does treatment influence mortality in depressives? A follow up of 1076 patients with major affective disorder, *Annals of Clinical Psychiatry* 1989: 1, 165–73.

37 http://www.schizophrenia.com/family/ect1.html (Accessed: 29/03/10).

38 http://www.rcpsych.ac.uk/mentalhealthinfo/treatments/ect.aspx (Accessed: 29/03/10).

39 Greenhalgh J, Knight C, Hind D, and Walters S Clinical and cost-effectiveness of electroconvulsive therapy for depressive illness, schizophrenia, catatonia and mania: Systematic reviews and economic modelling studies, Health Technology Assessment 2005: N0 9 http://www.hta.ac.uk/execsumm/summ909.shtml (Accessed: 29/03/10).

40 Burstow B Electroshock as a form of violence against women, *Violence Against Women* 2006, 12: 372–92.

41 Orr A and O'Connor D Dimensions of power: Older women's experiences with electroconvulsive therapy (ECT), *Journal of Women and Aging* 2005: 17, 19–36.

42 Orr and O'Connor op. cit.

43 Stek ML, Wurff van der FFB, Hoogendijk WJG, and Beekman ATF Electroconvulsive therapy for the depressed elderly. *Cochrane Database of Systematic Reviews* 2003: Issue 2.

44 Baldwin S and Oxlad M *Electroshock and Minors: A Fifty Year Review*, Westport CT: Greenwood Press, 2000.

45 http://www.timeshighereducation.co.uk/story.asp?storyCode=148627&sectioncode=29 (Accessed: 28/03/10).

46 Barker PJ and Baldwin S Shock story: ECT and children. *Nursing Times* 1989: 86, 52–5.

47 http://www.heraldsun.com.au/news/victoria/child-shock-therapy/story-e6frf7kx-1111118657718 (Accessed: 28/03/10).

48 Johnstone L Adverse psychological effects of ECT. *Journal of Mental Health* 1999: 8, 69–85.

49 Johnstone L ibid.

50 Johnstone ibid, p. 83.

51 Johnstone ibid. p. 84.

52 Abrams R The mortality rate with ECT. *Convulsive Therapy* 1997: 13, 125–7.

53 See: Berg JW, Applebaum PS, Lidz CW, and Parker LS *Informed Consent: Legal Theory and Clinical Practice* (2nd ed.), Oxford: Oxford University Press, 2001.

54 For a detailed discussion, see: Kashka MS and Keyser PK Ethical issues in informed consent in ECT, *Perspectives in Psychiatric Care* 1995: 31, 15–21.

55 NICE *Guidance on the Use of Electroconvulsive Therapy*, Technology Appraisal 59, London: NICE, 2003. See: http://www.nice.org.uk/TA059 (Accessed: 29/03/10).

56 Bray J op. cit.

57 See the Mental Capacity Act: http://www.opsi.gov.uk/acts/acts2005/ukpga_20050009_en_1 (Accessed: 29/03/10).

58 Kashka and Keyser op. cit. p. 21.

59 Eranti SV and McLoughlin DM Electroconvulsive therapy – state of the art. *British Journal of Psychiatry* 2002: 182, 8–9.

60 Bracken P Compulsory ECT is wrong. http://www.psychminded.co.uk/news/news2010/march10/compulsory-ect-is-wrong002.html (Accessed: 29/03/10).

61 http://www.delete59b.com (Accessed: 29/03/10).

62 Hermann RC, *et al.* Variation in ECT use in the United States, *American Journal of Psychiatry* 1995: 152, 869–75.

63 Freeman W op. cit.

64 Johnstone op. cit.

65 Sharma op. cit.

66 Milstein, *et al.* op. cit.

67 Hotchner A *Papa Hemingway*, New York, NY: Bantam Books, 1967, p. 308.

68 Read op. cit. p. 96.

69 Read op. cit. p. 88.

70 Read J op. cit.

71 http://www.psychminded.co.uk/news/news2003/may03/Phil%20Barker,%20a%20psychotherapist%20and%20visiting%20professor%20in%20health%20sciences%20at%20Trinity%20College,%20Dublin,%20writes%20in%20the%20Guardian.htm

15 Medication

Austyn Snowden

The development and the use of psychiatric drugs

Psychiatry as presently understood is barely 150 years old and current concepts of mental health and illness are considerably younger. Prior to the 1950s there were no antidepressants as currently understood, and prevalence of clinical depression was around 100 per million, according to Porter.[1] Prevalence currently runs at around 10 per cent: a 1000-fold increase. The reasons for this are complex, but include, for example, the increasingly rights-based individualism inherent in modern Western societies[2] and inconsistencies in historical definitions of depression.[3] In the pre-prescription era no records exist as to what drugs people took. Even serious episodes warranting hospitalisation offered no clues, as the discharge summary didn't indicate drug treatment as patients were expected to get this for themselves.

Ancient treatment, aligned with ancient concepts of health, included notions of rebalancing an imbalanced organism. Egyptians correlated health of people with the health of the Nile delta and so purged and cut accordingly; and channelling and scraping relieved congestion and encouraged flow. The notion of bile originated here according to Ramsamy,[4] representing both the mud of the river bed and the substance which needed to be removed from the body in times of human madness. The idea of bile was also foundational in Galenic medicine which likewise focused on issues of balance and applied purges and stimulants accordingly. The notion of biochemical imbalance persists. Current understanding is expressed in the language of neurotransmitters, epigenetics and holism, but the themes are remarkably familiar.

Early records from Broadgate Hospital, a Victorian-built asylum where I trained in Yorkshire, show examples of physicians prescribing in the early asylums around 1848.[5] Purgatives were used extensively, especially *croton oil* (a mild laxative in small doses and an external irritant now used in cosmetic skin peels), *calomel* (highly toxic mercury-based laxative), *colocynth* (liver stimulant and diuretic) and *senna*. Sedatives were used for mania, with or without *tonics* or *antimony* (now used by vets as a skin conditioner in ruminants, it is also a component of safety matches) and *saline*. For melancholia healthy digestion was encouraged, again using calomel as a purge. Epilepsy was treated according to severity and status. The healthy got drastic purges with *oleum terebinthinae* (turpentine oil). Less physically well patients got tonics. Paralysis was treated with diuretics. In 'great apathy of the system' *creosote* (carcinogenic laxative and cough suppressant, banned even as a wood preserver) and other stimulants with tonics and counter irritants were prescribed.

Outside of hospital, prescriptions of hyoscine, paraffin or creosote were generally self-administered. After 1906 control of substances considered likely to be abused became subject to increasing legislation. The notion of abuse itself has been the subject of much debate and criticism (see Dally[6]). Nevertheless, the outcome was that *opium* and preparations containing more than 1 per cent were restricted in the 1906 amendment to the Pharmacy Act 1869. The 1920 Dangerous Drugs Act further placed control on *cannabis* and preparations containing *dyhydrocodeine*. *Cocaine* was also banned following stories of 'crazed soldiers' in the First World War. Control of these substances for medicinal use was transferred to the medical profession, and by 1941 most medicines needed a prescription under the Pharmacy and Medicines Act 1941. Extension of this power to all new medicines in the 1950s effectively and fortuitously put psychiatry in charge of an area of health care previously largely ignored by it. The medicines discussed below fell into their hands. In other words, a system designed to protect society from 'addicts' was rolled out to legislate and control all medication management, putting the medical profession firmly in charge. Psychiatry entered the modern era through a combination of legislation and luck.

Understanding of how these remedies worked was limited relative to today, but congruent with the concepts of health of the time. Modern medicine subsumes the notion of chemical receptors. Paul Ehrlich was the first scientist to coin this term to refer to a specific target for a chemical within the body, and proposed the receptor theory of drug action in the early 1900s. This idea of the 'magic bullet' has persisted and largely underpins current cultural understanding of how drugs work.

The big breakthrough in psychotropic medicine undoubtedly originated with chlorpromazine. Henri Laborit is widely credited with first noting its potentially therapeutic effects. Laborit was a surgeon attempting to improve the care of his patients by experimenting with an anti-histamine sent to him by Charpentier in 1952. Laborit wanted a pre-anaesthetic to counter the shock some of his patients endured, and Charpentier knew his anti-histamine had central nervous system depressant effects as a result of animal tests. When Laborit administered Charpentier's new drug he noted an *unusual* calm about his patients. This is where Laborit's skills of observation were key. His patients became oblivious to their surroundings in a state Laborit referred to as 'euphoric quietude'.[7] He eventually persuaded his psychiatrist colleagues to try the drug in their more disturbed patients and they discovered remarkable effects. Previously catatonic or acutely deluded patients appeared to regain an immediate sense of relief from their highly distressing symptoms. More significantly the effects seemed to persist and improve with continued use as opposed to the short-term sedating properties noted in previous anti-histamines. Chlorpromazine was subsequently prescribed for over 100 million people.

This success was not lost on other drug manufacturers, who began urgently developing and testing other anti-histamines and their derivatives. A fortuitous consequence of this activity was the discovery of the first tricyclic antidepressant (TCA) imipramine. Kuhn[8] was expecting to discover antipsychotic effects as imipramine is a cogener of chlorpromazine and very similar in structure. However, these patients didn't become less psychotic, some even becoming more agitated. Those who were also depressed improved in mood, leading Kuhn to hypothesise that imipramine could be an antidepressant. This was supported in subsequent trials. Even more fortunate was the discovery of the first mono amine oxidase inhibitor (MAOI) iproniazid. It was being tested as an antibiotic in tuberculosis. Again this was ineffective in its tested purpose but several patients reported feeling much brighter and more energised, and in some cases euphoric. This clinical effect was noted by Kline[9] and investigated further, resulting in iproniazid being marketed as an antidepressant. Other MAOIs followed.

These and other similar developments in the 1950s and 1960s led to great expectations within the psychiatric community that the underlying pathology of psychiatric conditions would soon be mapped. Unfortunately this optimism was premature, and no more effective treatments have been developed since. Selective serotonin reuptake inhibitors (SSRIs) and the selective norepinephrine reuptake inhibitors (SNRIs) have been developed rationally as a result of these advances but are no more effective than the TCAs. That they are less lethal makes them preferable as a first-line treatment.[10] The same can be said of the atypical antipsychotics compared to the original phenothiazines. With regard to anxiolitics nothing has improved on diazepam despite the effort.

One obvious explanation is the sheer complexity of the science. Another more cynical explanation is economic. Drug companies are extremely sophisticated at marketing. Why would they spend billions searching for alternatives when they already hold recipes for another generation of look-alikes which they can market at great profit?[11] One of the latest examples of this is escitalopram, which is marketed as the effective side of the citalopram molecule. However, escitalopram is in no sense a *new* treatment.

In summary, antipsychotic medication was discovered whilst looking for a pre-anaesthetic agent. Antidepressants arose whilst looking for more antipsychotics, and the first MAOI was discovered whilst looking for a cure for tuberculosis. Drug companies have made substantial profits from these medicines and their influence is sophisticated and self-serving. Psychiatry came to control the administration of these psychotropic drugs due to legislation primarily aimed at restricting abuse of controlled drugs. They just happened to be in the right place at the right time. This is not necessarily good news however. Even back at the beginning of this story one of Laborit's colleagues described chlorpromazine as a 'veritable medicinal lobotomy'.[12] Whilst it is unclear whether this was expressed as a positive or negative development (lobotomy was a treatment staple of the time) it has been evident since their introduction that these drugs are potentially devastating in their effects, and certainly far from the carefully targeted chemicals some are now portrayed to be. In fact, initially this blunderbuss property was celebrated. Chlorpromazine was marketed as *Largactil*, which was an abbreviation of 'large number of actions'. As far as ethics are concerned then, what is the best that can be achieved with these medications, and how can we prevent the worst?

Ideology: to engage with medication or not?

Psychiatric drugs are a predominantly biological intervention. That is, there is a biological change in the recipient which results in a change of state. This change can be measured and efficacy is claimed as a consequence. This is how pharmaceutical companies sell drugs. However, it does not necessarily follow that there is a biological foundation of mental 'illness'. It is important therefore to briefly explore the link between biology and classification of mental health problems in order to contextualise any further discussion.

One hundred years after Kraepelin there is still no solid link between biological cause and effect in psychiatry. For example, for decades schizophrenia has been considered a genetic disorder. Discovering its cause is thought to be only a matter of time.[13] Yet the sixth symposium for the search for the causes of schizophrenia, held in 2009, acknowledged that 'Some of the promising peaks of the genetic landscape, glimpsed from afar over the last decade have turned out, in part, to be cloudy mirages' (p 508).[13]

This is a common theme, in that the same is true in the search for neural correlates of more common mental health problems. There is no biological test for depression and anxiety cannot be scanned for. This has left room for rational opposition to the concept of biological aetiology. For example Healy[11] argues that mental illness as it is currently understood is a construct of Western medicine designed to pathologise any behaviour considered abnormal. The concept of mental illness has been viewed as a metaphor for moral conflict,[11] a strategy for coping in a mad world[1] or a justification of medical power.[15] Administering psychiatric medication is therefore ethically questionable. To support this position critics point out that the American Diagnostic and Statistical Manual (DSM) is developed by consensus as opposed to biology[16] (see Chapter 12). That is, mental illnesses are not objectively measurable entities like myocardial infarction or cancer but creations of psychiatry. For example, specific diagnoses can have entirely different causes, each requiring a different treatment and DSM offers no indication of the treatment necessary.

However, it is debatable as to whether these critics would actually deny the existence of some form of common and classifiable dysfunction, or the probability that there is a correlation between biology and mental health. For example, psychotic experiences similar to those reported by people classified as psychotic can be induced by N-methyl-D-aspartic acid (NMDA) receptor antagonists such as phencyclidine (PCP).[17] Depression can be mimicked when cortisol is depleted, such as in Cushing's disease.[18] Withdrawal from alcohol or benzodiazepines can lead to symptoms of anxiety.[19] These reactions are predictable and demonstrably biological. Surely then there must be a relation between these physical and mental 'events'? Leaving aside the argument that physical and mental events are equivalent[15] there must therefore be a way of interfering biologically to reduce the distress caused. This is the rationale for drug development, and why people take them. However, targeting interventions requires a systematic approach and this requires a system of classification.

One of the problems for a newcomer to the field is the apparent contradiction between treating people as unique individuals capable of their own personal journey of recovery and classifying symptoms for the purpose of objective biological intervention. It is absolutely clear that mental illness is a currently unpopular concept. This is a function of the *Zeitgeist* which dictates that people should not be stigmatised by being pejoratively labelled. However, there are pitfalls in extending this position too far. A visible corollary of adopting this argument without question is the appearance of baffled undergraduate mental health students using the oxymoronic term 'mental health illness' to describe depression for example. The term has even appeared in the *British Medical Journal*[20] and a module entitled *A Sociological Perspective of Mental Health Illness* can be taken at Bradford University, England. I was recently asked to review a paper for a popular nursing journal that unapologetically used the term throughout. One explanation of the emergence of this meaningless concept is to consider it a function of the inadequacy of language to acknowledge the ongoing existence of certain categories of distress within a society which rejects such ideas as politically distasteful.

Undoubtedly the proper focus of nursing care lies with the individual, their human concerns and their perception of the problem rather than directly with the classifiable disorder they are experiencing (p 117).[21] However, diagnoses are also useful when determining the efficacy of medicines, as this falls within the realm of evidence. Drugs have to be judged against objective criteria and classification is necessarily part of that. It is possible to accept the validity of classification for these purposes without extending this into accepting the biological underpinning of 'mental illness'.

It is, however, pertinent to recognise that nurses and doctors have *no* choice in whether they wish to be involved or not in medication management. In terms of ideology then they need to recognise this professional issue and come to terms with it.

Empirical perspective: do drugs work and at what cost?

The mechanism of drug action is complex and it is not simply about biology. The placebo effect appears to be growing.[22] The same inert substance can create a positive or negative (nocebo) effect.[23] A placebo injection is more effective than placebo medicine, and pseudo surgery even more so.[24] Homeopathic 'medicines' are a good comparator in this discussion as they contain no discernible active ingredients and exert no discernible biological effects.[25] Without wishing to get embroiled in this contentious area I base this claim on the following. The magnitude of dilution of homeopathic medicine is such that it is highly unlikely for any tablet to contain even one molecule of the original preparation.[26] Any mechanism of action is therefore not comprehensible in terms of current scientific understanding.[27] Their biological properties can therefore be disregarded. This can be demonstrated empirically by comparing them to placebos in randomised double blind clinical trials, where they fare no better.[26,27] However, they remain popular despite this, to the extent that £12 million was spent on homeopathic treatments by the National Health Service between 2005 and 2008.[28] Whilst there is no evidence for the efficacy of the tablets,[29] some people still appear to benefit from homeopathy as a whole.[26] The healing power of belief should therefore not be underestimated. In fact, it should be celebrated, cultivated and employed as far as possible. This is a significant point to remember when negotiating treatment with somebody.

However, unlike homeopathic 'medicines' many drugs can be shown to be *objectively* superior to placebos (or a similar drug). These double blind randomised controlled trials (RCTs) inform the research community which drugs perform best against largely objective measurements of efficacy. These trials are often repeated and subject to further scrutiny so that the evidence base for any particular treatment is large. For example the Cochrane collaboration often performs systematic reviews of these RCTs to arrive at more definitive conclusions still, by aggregating data from multiple trials. In this way it can be claimed, for example, that escitalopram is an effective antidepressant by analysing data from 4,000 patients.[30] Chlorpromazine improved symptoms and functioning as demonstrated by 13 trials with 1,121 people diagnosed with schizophrenia.[31] Imipramine, venlafaxine and paroxetine were all found to be superior to placebo in treating generalised anxiety disorder across a range of studies.[32] There is a cost however. Unlike inert homeopathic medicines these treatments incur side effects, from the trivial to the life threatening.

The concept of side effect is problematic, in that one man's side effect is another's therapeutic effect. Consider the 'discovery' of Viagra, a vasodilator originally targeted at resolving angina pectoris. In this case Pfizer simply remarketed their chemical. However, side effects of psychotropic drugs can be considerably less marketable. Parkinsonian side effects, akathisia, torsade de pointes, weight gain, diabetes, tardive dyskinesia are well-known side effects of typical and atypical antipsychotics. Benzodiazepines can lead to dependence, with withdrawal symptoms often worse than the original symptoms the drugs were prescribed for. Older TCAs are cardiotoxic in overdose and SSRIs can potentiate serotonin syndrome, especially when combined with other serotonin raising drugs. Lithium toxicity can lead to coma and death. There are a host of 'milder' side effects in that they are less lethal, but all are distressing; for example sexual dysfunction, dry mouth, dizziness, poor concentration or constipation. From an ethical perspective then the dilemma is straightforward: do the gains (potential relief from distress) outweigh the losses (potential iatrogenic harm)? How do we decide?

Choice

A total of 92 per cent of people with mental health needs took prescribed medication in 2006 and 91 per cent of mental health in-patients take two or more psychotropic drugs.[33] Taking a medicine or not should be an individual's choice, in which case clarity of decision making is dependent upon knowledge. Values also play a significant role. For example people should be free to take homeopathic medicines if they wish to, but they should also know that any mechanism of action is not comprehensible in terms of current scientific concepts.[27] The nurse's role here is therefore to facilitate *informed, evidence-based* choice. Quality of this discussion will therefore depend on the values and knowledge of both parties, the professional judgement of the nurse and the quality of the therapeutic relationship between them. It may be right, for example, in some cases for a nurse to support a decision to try homeopathy. For any non-life-threatening condition it is highly unlikely to do any harm. Unfortunately however, some decisions are more complex, in that they involve forced treatment or, more commonly, discussions founded on unequal power and understanding. The professional judgement of the nurse becomes particularly significant in these decisions. How can choice be genuinely facilitated here?

Concordance is currently seen as the best way of managing medication.[31] The term implies complete agreement. This renders the concepts of non-compliance and non-adherence non-sensical as there should be no problems complying or adhering to a regimen you personally generated and agreed. If someone does not adhere to a regimen that arose from a concordant discussion then it is the discussion that was at fault, not the 'non-adherer'. The problem is that concordance as it relates to prescribing is professionally directed and follows consultation and diagnostic guidelines. Certainly the recipients' views are sought and respected but only to the end of prescribing adherence.[35] A prescription is an instruction that alludes to an unequal (non-concordant) relationship. A person has to be told about the script and given directions. It could certainly be argued that implicitly, if not explicitly, the prescribee and the prescriber therefore come to an agreement, a concord. It is clear, however, that this justification is tautological. That is, if concordance can be made into an all encompassing good it loses coherence as a concept and therefore cannot be tested empirically. This has been evidenced in studies attempting to do so where the term is quickly substituted for something more meaningful, such as 'shared decision making',[36] 'adherence'[33] or even 'compliance'.[37]

Latter *et al.*[38] studied mental health nurses managing medication. They found the nurses were quite happy to go along with their patients' beliefs about medication, even to the extent that they reinforced the 'symptoms' the drugs were supposed to minimise, as long as the end result was that people took their medication. When patients' beliefs suggested they would not be taking their medication nurses tried to amend these beliefs. This is not concordance, it is coercion. A more recent study by Latter *et al.*[39] further confirmed that nurses were not as good at practising concordance as they thought they were. There was a clear disparity between nurses' beliefs that they were practising the principles of concordance and their actions. In other words the recipient of the prescription does not really control these discussions at all.

This is against the spirit of recovery and should therefore be rejected if equality cannot be realistically facilitated or approached. An unequal specialist relationship subsumes paternalism and compliance, which is ultimately about following instructions. One apparently reasonable conclusion to this is that mental health nurses may simply reject the (more difficult) task of developing a deep critical understanding of psychiatric medication for the genuinely concordant humanistic approach favoured by the language of the recovery approach. There is a coherent logic to this and it would be a practical solution if it was professionally acceptable, but it is not. The fact is that nurses must understand medicines in order to exercise professional judgement:

> The administration of medicines is an important aspect of the professional practice of persons whose names are on the Council's register. It is not solely a mechanistic task to

be performed in strict compliance with the written prescription of an independent/ supplementary prescriber. It requires thought and the exercise of professional judgement.[10]

It is therefore worth concluding by examining the impact of two recent developments in mental health. The first is advance directives (see Chapter 26). The second is prescribing rights. This shows the positive link between classification and recovery. Through the active development of professional judgement in medicines management a corollary has been shown to be improved choice for service users.

Advanced statements

I began mental health nursing in 1985 in an old Victorian institution.[5] Industrial-sized bottles of chlorpromazine were a feature of every ward, and liberal PRN (pro re nata) doses of this and other psychotropic medicines *were* normal routine. We now have different mental health legislation, and the institution I trained in is a housing estate. Today, there is more focus on prevention and partnership. This agenda at least goes some of the way to recognise that even in compulsory treatment the person's wishes should be respected as far as possible. The principle of reciprocity underpins this. Also, if the situation could be predicted, advanced statements would be a useful method of expressing genuine choice for the individual who was historically powerless in this situation. The positive interpretation Foy *et al.*[11] gave to their study on the uptake of advanced statements is inconsistent with the data. That is, few people actually valued them and many still felt they had no power as these statements can be overridden. Nevertheless, even though the jury is out on advanced statements these small steps are in the right direction (see Chapter 26).

Mental health nurse prescribing

Since 2003 mental health nurses have been able to train as prescribers. Uptake has been inconsistent across the United Kingdom, with many boards and trusts adopting a 'wait and see' approach. In Staffordshire however, the local trust has actively and strategically supported mental health nurse prescribing. There is evidence that care standards have improved as a result (Nolan, 2007, personal communication). There have been 50 per cent fewer errors since the introduction of nurse prescribing. Getting the right medicine to the right person in the right way has improved. This is thought to be because:

- More attention is given to prescribing medicines generally within the trust.
- More nurses are concerned about administration.
- Increased accountability is devolved to nurses.
- Service users are encouraged to ask more questions.

These are familiar themes in the mental health nurse prescribing literature,[12,13] so there appear to be secondary gains to be had from a workforce more engaged with medication management in general. These gains don't simply cement a biological model of ill health. They empower service users.[14] Engaging with any aetiological model of ill health is anathema to many mental health nurses. However, mental health nurse prescribers have shown that in developing competence in advanced medicine management the person remains at the centre of care.[15] Classification, prescribing and monitoring are tools of recovery, just like empathy, autonomy and choice.

Conclusion

This chapter has looked at the history, biology and social developments in medicine management in mental health. It has shown that the ways mental health problems are conceptualised are closely related to a broader societal view. There has been a consistent move towards rights based approaches to care, as evidenced in recent mental health and human rights legislation.

The ethical issues pertaining to medicine management are not only grounded in empirical evidence of treatment efficacy but also grounded in *choice*, a theme developed throughout the later part of this chapter.

Notes

1 Porter R (2002) *Madness: A Brief History*. Oxford: Oxford University Press.
2 Gray J (2002) *Straw Dogs*. London: Granta Books.
3 Healy D (2002) *The Creation of Psychopharmacology*. Cambridge, MA: Harvard University Press.
4 Ramsamy S (2001) *Caring for Madness. The Role of Personal Experience in the Training of Mental Health Nurses*. London: Whurr.
5 Curry R (1991) *Across the Westwood. The Life and Times of Broadgate Hospital Beverley. Mental Health Unit*. East Yorkshire Health Authority.
6 Dally A (1995) *Anomalies and Mysteries in the 'War on Drugs'*. In Porter R and Teich M (eds) (1995) *Drugs and Narcotics in History*. Cambridge: Cambridge University Press.
7 Swazey J (1974) *Chlorpromazine in Psychiatry: A Study in Therapeutic Intervention*. Cambridge, MA: MIT Press.
8 Kuhn R (1957) Uber die behandlung depressiver zustande mit einemiminodibenzylderivat (Treatment of depressive states with an iminodibenzyl derivative). *Schweiz Med Wochenschn* 87: 1135–40.
9 Kline NS (1958) Clinical experience with iproniazid (Marsilid). *Journal of Clinical and Experimental Psychopathology* 19(Suppl 1): 72–8.
10 NICE (2007) *Depression: Management of Depression in Primary and Secondary Care*. NICE Guideline 23 (amended). Available: http://www.army.mod.uk/documents/general/cg23nice_depression.pdf (last accessed 22nd September 2009).
11 Healy D (2004) *Let Them Eat Prozac*. New York, NY: New York University Press.
12 Cunningham Owens DG (1999) *A Guide to the Extrapyramidal Side-Effects of Antipsychotic Drugs*. Cambridge: Cambridge University Press.
13 Kirkbride JB and Scoriels L (2009) Review of the 6th symposium for the search for the causes of schizophrenia, Sao Paulo, Brazil, 3–6 February 2009. *European Archives of Psychiatry and Clinical Neuroscience* 259: 505–9.
14 Foucault M (1965) *Madness and Civilisation: A History of Insanity in the Age of Reason*. New York, NY: Random House.
15 Szasz T (1961) *The Myth of Mental Illness*. New York: Hoeber-Harper; revised edition 1974, Harper and Row.
16 Kutchins H and Kirk H (1997) *Making Us Crazy. DSM: The Psychiatric Bible and the Creation of Mental Disorders*. New York, NY: Simon and Schuster.
17 Javitt DC and Zukin SR (1991) Recent advances in the phencyclidine model of schizophrenia. *The American Journal of Clinical Hypnosis* 148: 1301–8.
18 Drouin J, Bilodeau S, and Vallette S (2007). Of old and new diseases: Genetics of pituitary ACTH excess (Cushing) and deficiency. *Clinical genetics* 72(3): 175–82.
19 Cohen SI (1995) Alcohol and benzodiazepines generate anxiety, panic and phobias. *Journal of the Royal Society of Medicine* 88(2): 73–7.
20 Lovell K, Cox D, Haddock G, Jones C, Raines D, Garvey R, Roberts C, and Hadley S. (2006) Telephone administered cognitive behaviour therapy for treatment of obsessive compulsive disorder: Randomised controlled non-inferiority trial. *British Medical Journal* 333, 833.

21 Barker P (2003) *Psychiatric and Mental Health Nursing – The Craft of Caring*. London: Arnold.
22 Walsh BT, Seidman SN, Sysko R, and Gould M (2002) Placebo response in studies of major depression – variable, substantial, and growing. *The Journal of the American Medical Association* 287: 1840–7.
23 Benedetti F, Lanotte M, Lopiano L, and Colloca L (2007) When words are painful: Unravelling the mechanisms of the nocebo effect. *Neuroscience* 147: 260–71.
24 Iversen L (2001) *Drugs, a Very Short Introduction*. Oxford: Oxford University Press.
25 Baum M and Ernst E (2009). Should we maintain an open mind about homeopathy? *The American Journal of Medicine* 122(11): 973–4.
26 Linde K, Clausius N, Ramirez G, *et al.* (1997) Are the clinical effects of homeopathy placebo effects? A meta-analysis of placebo-controlled trials. *Lancet* 350: 834–43.
27 McCarney RW, Warner J, Fisher P, and van Haselen R (2009) Homeopathy for dementia. *Cochrane Database of Systematic Reviews* 2003, Issue 1. Art. No.: CD003803. DOI: 10.1002/14651858. CD003803.
28 British Broadcasting Corporation (2010) Sceptics Stage Homeopathy 'Overdose'. Available: http://news.bbc.co.uk/1/hi/uk/8489019.stm (last accessed 2nd February 2010).
29 Goldacre B (2009) *Bad Science*. London: Harper Perennial.
30 Cipriani A, Santilli C, Furukawa TA, Signoretti A, Nakagawa A, McGuire H, Churchill R, and Barbui C. Escitalopram versus other antidepressive agents for depression. *Cochrane Database of Systematic Reviews* 2009, Issue 2. Art. No.: CD006532. DOI: 10.1002/14651858.CD006532.pub2.
31 Adams CE, Awad G, Rathbone J, and Thornley B. Chlorpromazine versus placebo for schizophrenia. *Cochrane Database of Systematic Reviews* 2007, Issue 2. Art. No.: CD000284. DOI: 10.1002/14651858.CD000284.pub2.
32 Kapczinski FFK, Silva de Lima M, dos Santos Souza JJSS, Batista Miralha da Cunha AABC, and Schmitt RRS. Antidepressants for generalized anxiety disorder. *Cochrane Database of Systematic Reviews* 2003, Issue 2. Art. No.: CD003592. DOI: 10.1002/14651858.CD003592.
33 Healthcare Commission (2007) *Talking about Medicines: The Management of Medicines in Trusts Providing Mental Health Services*. London: Commission for Healthcare Audit and Inspection.
34 Latter S, Maben J, Myall M, and Young A (2007) Evaluating nurse prescribers' education and continuing professional development for independent prescribing practice: Findings from a national survey in England. *Nurse Education Today* 27, 685–96.
35 Cribb A and Barber N (2005) Unpicking the philosophical and ethical issues in medicines prescribing and taking (Chapter 6) In *Concordance Adherence and Compliance in Medicine Taking*. London: National Co-ordinating Centre for NHS Service Delivery.
36 Clyne W, Granby T, and Picton C (2007) *A Competency Framework for Shared Decisionmaking With Patients Achieving Concordance for Taking Medicines*. National Prescribing Centre, Keele. Available: www.npc.co.uk/pdf/prescribers/resources/competency_framework_2007.pdf (accessed 27 July 2010).
37 Van Eijken M, Tsang S, Wensing M, de Smet PAGM, and Grol RPTM. (2003) Interventions to improve medication compliance in older patients living in the community. *Drugs and Aging* 20(3): 229–40.
38 Latter S, Yerrell P, Rycroft-Malone J, and Shaw D (2000) Nursing, medication education and the new policy agenda: The evidence base. *International Journal of Nursing Studies* 37(6): 469–79.
39 Latter S, Maben J, Myall M, and Young A (2007) Perceptions and practice of concordance in nurses' prescribing consultations: Findings from a national questionnaire survey and case studies of practice in England. *International Journal of Nursing Studies* 44(1): 9–18.
40 Nursing and Midwifery Council (2008): *Standards for Medicine Management* (Version 1, August 2008). Nursing and Midwifery Council.
41 Foy J, MacRae A, Thom A, and Macharouthu A (2007). Advance statements: Survey of patients' views and understanding. *The Psychiatrist* 31: 339–41.
42 Hemingway S and Harris N (2006) The development of mental health nurses as prescribers: Quantifying the emergence. *Mental Health Nursing* 26, 14–16.

43 McCann TV and Clark E (2008) Attitudes of patients towards mental health nurse prescribing of antipsychotic agents. *International Journal of Nursing Practice* 14, 115–21.

44 Jones M and Jones A (2008) Promotion of choice in the care of people with bipolar disorder: A mental health nursing perspective. *Journal of Psychiatric & Mental Health Nursing* 15, 87–92.

45 Snowden A (2010) Integrating medicines management into mental health nursing in UK. *Archives of Psychiatric Nursing* 24(3): 178–88.

Section 3 – Ethical dilemmas

Phil Barker

Psychiatric history hovers, like a threatening shadow, over much of contemporary mental health practice. The past fifty years has witnessed much tinkering with the language of 'mental health' and 'mental illness', both in terms of definitions of the phenomena associated with 'madness' and the kind of responses needed, in the name of care and treatment.

In one sense, not much has changed. Despite all the 'neuroscientific' talk and the countless neurochemical hypotheses, there remains no evidence that what has long been called 'mental illness', is any more than ways that people behave, which are disapproved of – either by the people themselves, or by others. Indeed, as has been said, repeatedly, before, such 'mental' illnesses, would be 'physical' illnesses, and would be the preserve of neurology or endocrinology. Today, the most well-known forms of 'treatment' remain, essentially, ways of managing something which no one really understands. That much has not changed in over a hundred years. Not surprisingly, all this uncertainty carries considerable implications for all the different ways that professionals might need, or be expected to relate to the people in their care.

1   *What's in a name?* What once was called 'madness' became, with the passage of time 'lunacy', which then became 'mental illness'. With the increasing professionalization of psychiatric medicine, there developed a need to give formal names to all such 'illnesses'. Today, there are literally hundreds of names for 'psychiatric disorders', necessary to gain access to care and treatment.

> In what way are these any more than banal, circular definitions of patterns of personal, interpersonal or social behaviour?
> What *exactly* do these diagnostic labels refer *to*, beyond the manner in which someone behaves, towards themselves or others?
> What are the legal, social and political implications of assigning a psychiatric diagnosis to a person?

2   *What are the chances of an honest and open relationship?* All the services provided by mental health professionals are expressed through their relationships with the person in their care. Some disciplines rely more on such relationships than others, but little can be done in the name of mental health care without some form of interpersonal communication – especially listening and talking.

> To what extent does the obvious power imbalance limit the chances of professionals relating *honestly*, *openly* and *confidentially* to the person in their care?

Given that most professionals are accountable to colleagues, employers, society or a professional body, why should any person in care ever *trust* the relationship?

3   *What are you aiming for – care or control?* Everyone has the capacity to be 'difficult', in their dealings with themselves but especially in relation to other people. People with so-called 'mental health problems' are, perhaps by definition, difficult. They find it difficult to live with themselves, live out their lives or live with the various people they encounter. It is hardly surprising that they should exhibit some of their distress, despair, disappointment or disenchantment in the presence of others. If this was to happen on a Saturday night at the social club, or in the street on a Sunday afternoon, people would turn a blind eye, or work out a way to respond, with the least upset and embarrassment.

What would you do if someone became upset or disturbed in everyday life?
Does the history of restraint and coercion, and all the associated policies and directives, act as a restraint on our capacity to think of creative alternatives?
At what point in 'containing' a difficult situation, do you move in the direction of trying to understand what it might be about?

4   *Given what I know, should I encourage people to take psychiatric drugs or receive ECT?* Most people, and especially their families and society at large, expect people with a 'psychiatric disorder', to be prescribed psychiatric drugs or receive some more radical therapy. Clearly, however, there is much dispute over how appropriate or effective such drugs might be, and whether or not drugs and treatments like ECT, carry a risk of serious harm.

How would you help people make a truly *informed choice*, regarding any psychiatric treatment, free from all possible sources of influence or 'misinformation'?
What would you do, if someone rejects an offer of drug treatment, or wishes to discontinue treatment, and this decision runs contrary to the views of professional colleagues or the person's family?

Section 4

The human context

Section preface

Phil Barker

Fifty years ago, almost all psychiatric services were delivered in psychiatric hospitals. Today, most of these have been demolished, replaced by smaller 'mental health units' and scattered around the 'natural community'. Many other forms of care, support and therapy of different kinds are delivered by a range of agencies, many based within the private, charitable or non-governmental sectors. The nature of the services on offer has changed, in part as a response to changing philosophies. However, the way we think about 'mental health' is a function of changing social attitudes.

In Section 4 a profile of some very different care settings is offered, alongside a consideration of some of the key social and cultural issues, which either have changed the face of traditional psychiatric care, or signal the wider concerns of society at large.

Despite the 'community care' revolution of the past 50 years, most people who experience a seriously disabling or disruptive 'breakdown' will be offered short-term, intensive care and treatment in an *acute care setting* – so called, because of the acute nature of their problems. Some, who might not wish to avail themselves of such an offer of help, might well find themselves 'committed' by law. The names and the settings, if not also the mix of people, may have changed but the function of the service remains much the same: trying to enable people to return to life in the natural community as quickly as possible.

A significant number of people, who either possess a psychiatric diagnosis or who appear to be psychiatrically disordered, will become involved with the law; mainly through commission of a crime. *Forensic* psychiatric services were developed specifically to address the needs of this ill-defined population and are provided across a wide range of situations, from court diversion schemes to high-security hospitals.

People have used alcohol and drugs for thousands of years, often as part of ritual or ceremony. It seems obvious that people take such substances because of their effects. The idea that they are unable to resist such substances became enshrined in the concept of *addiction* only recently. In these highly addictive times, it has become a hotly contested idea.

The needs of two specific populations – *younger people* and *older people* – have become the focus of much attention in recent years; partly because of lack of attention in the past, and partly because of increased awareness of the kind of 'mental health' problems, experienced by, and peculiar to, each group.

Although every society and culture can provide examples of 'madness', what such states mean varies enormously. Indeed, anthropologists have repeatedly noted that Western ideas of 'psychiatric disorder' often do not find a match in other cultures. As most modern societies are now described as 'multicultural' or 'multiethnic', it is important to consider the role played by ideas of *race* and *culture* in the construction of 'psychiatric diagnoses' and the perceived need for 'psychiatric treatment'.

Finally, people have killed themselves, for all sorts of reasons, down the ages. The concept of *suicide* – or self-killing – is, however, only a few hundred years old. Today, suicide means different things in law, religion, ethics and psychiatry – where arguments have been made, so far unsuccessfully, for viewing it as a manifestation of 'mental illness'. Although psychiatry has, as yet, not transformed self-killing into a 'psychiatric disorder', it has generated a range of theoretical and practical concepts related to the prevention of suicide – which often is seen as a uniquely psychiatric responsibility.

16 Acute care

Jan Horsfall, Michelle Cleary, Glenn E. Hunt and Garry Walter

> No other quality is almost unanimously recognized as being of great importance and yet equally thought to be inapplicable in the real world. This is the conundrum of ethics.
>
> (John Ralston Saul,[1] p. 65)

Introduction

Policy, patient mix, size of the facility, speed of turnover, and numbers of staff and patients constitute the context, goals, and hour-by-hour realities for the people who inhabit acute mental health settings. Context is not a trivial background fixture, but includes acutely mentally unwell patients, busy staff, and a multi-faceted environment that force fluidity and adaptability on all who spend hours there each day. Admissions, discharges, ongoing assessment, and unpredictable interactions and events permeate the milieu as thoroughly as sauce penetrates stew.

People are admitted to acute mental health inpatient units for a variety of reasons. (The abbreviation, 'acute settings' will be used throughout, to refer to all forms of short-term hospital care and treatment.) In a review, Bowers[2] identified the following: *dangerousness* to self or others; *assessment* and *observation* for *diagnostic purposes*; and *treatment by medication*, particularly to ameliorate *positive psychotic symptoms*. Given the potential for danger[3-5] and the fact that nurses are continuous front-line workers, nursing presence is important to all, whether this is acknowledged or not. One may well ask why nurses choose to work in such settings. Nurses may be allocated to the unit; opt for this high adrenalin environment; or find themselves there for a variety of reasons ranging from the pragmatic to the idealistic.

In the view of many contemporary academics, researchers, and some consumer groups, mental health professionals in acute settings are not providing consumer-focused care; not fulfilling professional requirements and not using designated psychological therapies; and social control is their primary *modus operandi* if not *raison d'etre*.[1] (A non-representative shortlist includes the following authors.[6-9]) Rather than accepting claims that overtly, or tacitly, blame those working in these settings, we base this chapter around an outline of the findings of a recent ethnographic study of such nurses in such an acute setting.

Acute settings: practice realities

Deacon and Fairhurst's[10] study of mental health nursing in an acute setting took place mostly in a busy UK inner city acute ward over a period of 20 months and included data gathering over 24 hours per day and 7 days a week. To do justice to the activities under scrutiny, the original data gathering used participant observation, with a special interest in, and focus on, ordinary conversation. These data were reviewed and re-analysed later to uncover previously unrecognised aspects of ward work.

These researchers found that nurses manage multiple agendas including patient groups; the unit as a whole; individual patients; other nurses; and the health care 'team'; ultimately at the behest of the employing institution's policies and goals.[10-12] In other words, nurses in acute settings work to enable other ward participants' interventions, needs, and behaviours to be addressed with the least possible disruptions or contradictions. One of the primary aims of the organisation – in line with national policy agendas – is for rapid patient improvement, a consequence of which is speedy 'throughput'.[13,14] This contributes significantly to the perception that work in acute settings is reactive – inferring that it should not be, as professionals should determine direction and interventions.

According to Deacon and Fairhurst,[10] at crucial times the nurse/s place one patient at the centre of intense personalised support, interactions, and explanations (see also Chapter 5). Along with these focused interventions, nurses also weave anxiety-reducing or humorous remarks into communications with patients in challenging situations, and conversely, weave assessment questions, reminders, or instructional pointers into ordinary activities such as greetings or walking together. Mental health nurses were responsible for a plethora of information facilitation and funnelling.[11,15,16] These include

- recognising, storing, and disseminating pertinent information formally and informally to patients and staff;
- giving others necessary and correct forms;
- locating records for other health professionals for reviews and meetings;
- seeking and clarifying decisions made by others that impinge on patient treatment and freedoms;
- providing a range of reports or feedback to other professionals that are designed for recipient and patient needs (i.e. not from or for a nursing perspective *per se*).[10,17]

If the nurses did not perform as many of these as possible, the unit would not work for patients or any of the other professionals.[15]

Much work in acute settings involves *interpersonal, institutional*, and *policy* factors and these have consequences for ethical practice.[18] This involves triage, liaison, coordination, facilitation, documentation, and discriminating between irrelevant, useful, and essential information. These activities can be invisible[12,15] and incomprehensible unless observers look carefully and aim to understand what they see and hear – this is why ethnographic studies can uncover what authors without awareness and sensitivity cannot pick up.[16]

The limitations of traditional bioethics in acute settings

What characteristics of acute settings provide challenges to traditional bioethics? First, the setting is a group setting, but not a closed group, and not merely a series or aggregate of one-to-one interactions. Those with the power to determine key interventions, such as close observation levels within the arena, are often not physically present.[8,10] Thus, the group does not end at the door to the unit: other external people have interests inside; these include the community, family, carers, neighbours, legislators, and professional organisations, for example.[19] Even one-to-one interactions within the unit are circumscribed by others present,[1] others waiting, knowledge of the past experiences, and expectations for the future. These units consist of fluid interacting elements, rather like an *ecological system* wherein small changes can have unforeseen consequences within an unknown timeframe.[16] Limited resources, policy, professional training, quality audits, etc. impinge, constrain, and make direct and indirect demands on personnel within the unit.

Authors of ethical discussions, explications, and positions commonly outline a range of ethical perspectives, which may include deontology, utilitarianism, principlism, virtue ethics, and ethics of care, often with a particular interest in rules[20,21] (see also Chapters 1 and 2). The principles approach: non-maleficence, beneficence, respect for autonomy and justice feature prominently, no doubt in part because of their apparent clarity and rationality, along with proclaimed flexibility and practicality.[20,22] Principles are not beacons that guide actors to incontrovertibly just decisions; along with other ways of ethical reasoning, the practitioner must at times draw on his/her intuitions, further stretching claims to objectivity.[23] Furthermore, traditional bioethics approaches often assume first, that the potential ethical components of a situation are amenable to delineation and second, that there is a discernible dilemma and some reasonably clear choices.

Over the past few decades, ethical explorations within psychiatry have frequently targeted controversial aspects of practice, including involuntary treatment, community rights versus individual rights, seclusion, violence against others, suicidality, boundary violations, patient competence, conflicts of interest, concerns, and rights regarding medical research[24-28] (see Chapter 2). Saul[1] considers that such a focus on the outstanding events reveals ethical decision-making to be the terrain of heroes and saints (or perhaps devils). The above issues are significant in psychiatry and society, but they are like the dramatic and scandalous parts of a newspaper that can distract from information about changes and events not deemed worthy of headlines, which then remain unexplored and not discussed.

Within acute settings, ethical practice involves quotidian processes such as what is said; how it is said; checking understanding; taking a request seriously; timing a question aptly; questions not asked; information not given; valuing or ignoring patient feelings; discerning subtle behaviour changes; recognising personal worries outside the ambit of psychiatry that impinge on wellbeing; and emotional aspects of safety. This is not unique; outside the unit, ethics also consist of the commonplace minutiae of practical daily life[1] (see also Chapter 1). This is congruent with broad established definitions of ethics as aiming to 'illuminate what we ought to do by asking us to consider and reconsider our ordinary actions, judgements and justifications' (p. xii).[29]

Cultural, social, and professional assumptions are embedded in conceptions of self, normality, and reason, and these underpin psychiatric definitions and discriminations.[21,24,26] Values implicitly contribute to decisions around admission, symptoms, assessment, diagnosis, treatment method, and private or public hospital.[8,16,18,19,26,27,30] There are even more fundamental considerations such as those outlined by Brendel[31]: aetiological models of mental illness 'cannot be determined solely on empirical or theoretical grounds; the model also ought to promote ethical patient care' (p. 48). Ethical care should be embedded in the conceptual infrastructure of psychiatry given that ensuing practical activities (e.g. assessment, treatment, outcome measures) derive from these intellectual foundations.[18] To this end, Brendel[31] endorses the well-established 'stress–diathesis model', given its multi-factorial view of mental illness aetiology.

Hughes and Fulford,[30] in attempting to acknowledge and negotiate values in mental health settings, point out that dealing with the nitty-gritty of an individual patient's situation (casuistry) allows the recognition of values, but the outcome may be that mainstream values, professional values, or those of the majority are most likely to prevail. Conversely, diligent attention to all viewpoints (perspectivism) is probably destined to result in a quagmire of disabling relativism without any focused plan, pathway, or goals. In summary, a range of concerns from macro-social to micro-social and intrapersonal levels of society can impinge on the ethical care of any patient by any health professional. Factors from the macro-social level include, for example, mental health policy, resource availability, under-served populations, the law, health insurance, equity, and human rights legislation. Micro-social level factors include communication, language and negotiation skills, social assumptions, personal preference and choice, confidentiality, cultural identity, self-awareness, and sensitivity to others' responses.[18,32,33] On many occasions, dilemmas and contradictions from any of the above levels can feed in simultaneously to one patient's circumstances *vis-à-vis* psychiatric treatment and care.

Mainstream bioethics in psychiatry tends to claim the terrain occupied by the individual patient and the individual health professional. However, the realities of mental health service provision demand analyses at the organisational, management–administration, group, interpersonal, and intrapersonal levels. This is why the situation is practically difficult, and only focusing on one level or one group will not produce ethical practice in acute settings.

Care ethics and virtue ethics

Ethics of care challenges the atomistic and rationalist assumptions inherent in many traditional ethical schemas by placing relationships and human emotions centre-stage[20,34] (see also Chapter 12). An ethics of care aims to build compassion into the fabric of society and into psychiatry.[31] Care ethics are attractive to practitioners who consider the foundation of their mental health work devolves on therapeutic relationships and the permeation of these by multi-cultural, cross-cultural, and gender differentiated aspects of communication and interaction (see also Chapters 7 and 21).

To enact virtue ethics, practical wisdom – involving clinical experience, awareness of ethical principles, and sophisticated reasoning – must be available to a given health professional for use in a specific situation to achieve a constructive patient outcome.[24,34] Hence, both virtue ethics and care ethics are underpinned by the mental health professional's character and disposition,[20,26,34] raising serious questions about the teachability of virtue ethics.[20]

Grant and Briscoe's[18] discussion of less than satisfactory everyday interactions in acute settings reveals that well-meaning, well-trained, and experienced mental health professionals do not, at times, understand the relevance of patients' needs and concerns to their present wellbeing, recovery, and increasing autonomy. This is in a setting where 'neither the motivation of the staff to help, nor the patients to be helped, is at issue' (p. 174).[18] The scenarios they describe are ordinary and commonplace and involve requests not taken seriously enough, the inappropriate use of a name, and expectations that it is straightforward for all patients to make a request in a group forum. There are no discernible dilemmas, no crises, and no overtly problematic incidents/situations/events. Furthermore, there are practitioners who do not even recognise conflict of interest, alternatives, or the likely consequences of a decision or non-decision for a specific patient.[35]

Care ethics and virtue ethics focus on the *persons* of the actors in a given situation and therefore complement more concrete rules-based ethics.[21,34,36] Or, as Somerville[35] suggests, principle-based ethics locates 'ethics power' external to the decision-maker, which then needs to be balanced by human-based morality (principle-based utilitarianism) that places 'ethics power' within society – thus seeking universal human values. From a practical perspective, is this unwieldy and will it inevitably produce treatment and care that is truly respectful of patients?

Enhancing ethical practice in acute settings

After reviewing the aims of ethics ranging from developing codes, objective rules, or over-riding principles, to having recourse to humanism, justice, and universal values, Johnstone[37] concluded that the role of ethics is to 'motivate moral behaviour, to settle disagreements and controversies between people, and to generally bind people together in a peaceable com-munity' (p. 64). If this intention is taken seriously, perhaps the ethics project in an acute setting is to improve interactions between staff and patients; increase professionals' aware-ness that others may have different perspectives and desires; encourage authentic respect for all involved in patient treatments and their consequences; and to ask, listen, and negotiate more. This sounds very much like patient-centred care – an orientation or belief system endorsed by many professionals and educators. The difficulty appears to be that consumer-focused care is not happening to the degree intended by mental health policymakers and hoped for by patients, and this is noted by even sympathetic researchers.[6,7,8,18,38]

Consumer literature abounds with constructive suggestions for improving professional practice in mental health facilities – much (but not all) of which is as relevant to acute set-tings as to other settings.[4,30] Nursing literature documents the distress of nurses being unable to do what they should be doing, being unable to cope with what they see and hear as students,[39] being overwhelmed by the authority of medical practitioners,[28,40] and the contradic-tions between mental health ideology and actual practice in acute settings.[4,12,15]

Again, we can invoke external factors that impede the delivery of real patient-focused care (even though these can be used as excuses for unprofessional commissions or omissions) and micro-social factors, such as professionals' commitment to respectful and effective col-laboration and dialogue. Neither of these is beyond the traditional territory of mental health education or research.

Despite the myriad of challenges in enacting ethical reasoning and care in complex milieux such as acute settings, it is essential that ethics become central to mental health practice across disciplines; in the first and last instances to provide acceptable helpful and hopeful patient treatment. Given the pace and chaos, and diversity of patients and practi-tioners, a realistic approach needs to be taken to take from a whole-unit perspective to ensure that ethical care is do-able.[41] Values-based medicine is proposed by Hughes and Fulford[30] as a potential way to address these demands. They deem that practitioners must find practical ways to negotiate diverse or conflicting values in mental health settings, and this 'ought to be the bread and butter of psychiatric practice' (p. 1006).[30]

Their orientation highlights values, which may be embedded in all approaches, acknowl-edged or not. Salient aspects of the programme include the following:

- In any decision, the patient's perspective must be heard and not assumed.
- Facts and values must be attended to in all clinical decision-making.
- Decision-making is a collaborative process.
- When values conflict, mutual respect, acknowledgment of differing viewpoints, and negotiation are the way through.[38]

In an effort to encompass contemporary UK policy frameworks, their workbook reiterates familiar principles such as having the consumer at the centre of the service goals, having a recovery focus rather than treatment *per se*, and an authentic multidisciplinary approach. They consider that awareness, reasoning, knowledge, communication, and a valuing of relationships constitute the foundations of mental health practice. The workbook sets out activities that groups of practitioners can work through, preferably together. Woodbridge and Fulford[38] set out ten essential shared capabilities for mental health professionals (see also Chapter 25):

- working in partnership;
- respecting diversity;
- practising ethically (including respecting rights, acknowledging of power differentials, and adhering to professional boundaries);
- challenging inequality (addressing stigma, discrimination, and social exclusion);
- promoting holistic recovery;
- identifying consumers' needs and strengths;
- providing patient-centred care;
- making a difference (drawing on evidence-based practice and taking account of consumer lifestyle preferences and aims);
- promoting safety and positive risk-taking (working through control versus care issues and public/societal expectations *vis-à-vis* consumer and professional values);
- participating in ongoing personal development and learning (a lifelong-learning approach to professional development).[38]

Biting some bullets

These orientations and skills sound deceptively simple, but at the individual practitioner level they demand, at least, the challenges of personal values clarification and increasing self-awareness to facilitate reflective practice.[32] Given this state of affairs, there seem to be three options:

- carry on regardless with the usual mixture of ethical and unethical practice;
- invoke well-rehearsed complex ethical models; or
- look outside traditional approaches and take a whole unit, collaborative consumer-focused orientation.

Perhaps the values-laden question that each practitioner (all disciplines and managers with power or influence on the ward) could begin with is, 'do I want to work with mentally ill patients for their benefit, given their varying needs, values and life choices?'

If ethical care and reasoning were straightforward, intelligent and caring professionals would have come up with clear cut and practicable guidelines to which all workers in a given mental health unit can – and do – adhere. If we believe the literature and research, this is not undoubtedly so. Perhaps the traditional notion of individual practitioners working one-on-one with patients bearing rules in mind, or thinking through abstract ideas from another discipline (philosophy), is a paradigm born in the past when ethicists also assumed settings without the present 'hurl-burly'.

Serious changes in culture are required in acute settings at the unit level to enact authentic cross-disciplinary collaboration and address the above personal and professional values and practice skills to place ethics at the centre of patient care. This will not be easy. Improving the professional culture means working with all of the people involved and inevitably will include administrative changes as well as the model of patient care underpinning the way business as usual is understood and carried out. Thus, staff education is intrinsic to these processes. An essential facet of culture change is that patients are to be respected as people knowledgeable about themselves and their needs.[18] If patients were actually listened to, they could become 'teachers to the staff, helping staff learn better ways of providing care to them during times of crisis' (p. 166).[28]

In conclusion, the primary aim of admission is to benefit the patients who are admitted. In achieving this aim, it behoves all staff and stakeholders to become aware of the various ethical issues and challenges, albeit complex, impacting on such units and treatment processes. Although perhaps daunting, ultimately ethics are nothing but reverence for life.[12]

Notes

1 Saul JR, *On Equilibrium*, Camberwell, Vic, Penguin, 2001.
2 Bowers L, Reasons for admission and their implications for the nature of acute inpatient psychiatric nursing, *Journal of Psychiatric and Mental Health Nursing* 2005, 12, 231–6.
3 Bowers L, Simpson A, Eyres S, Nijman H, Hall C, Grange A, Phillips L, Serious untoward incidents and their aftermath in acute inpatient psychiatry: the Tompkins Acute Ward study, *International Journal of Mental Health Nursing* 2006, 15, 226–34.
4 Deacon M, Warne T, McAndrew S, Closeness, chaos and crisis: the attractions of working in acute mental health care, *Journal of Psychiatric and Mental Health Nursing* 2006, 13, 750–7.
5 Kindy D, Petersen S, Parkhurst D, Perilous work: nurses' experiences in psychiatric units with high risks of assault, *Archives of Psychiatric Nursing* 2005, 19, 169–75.
6 Cutcliffe J, Happell B, Psychiatry, mental health nurses, and invisible power: exploring a perturbed relationship within contemporary mental health care, *International Journal of Mental Health Nursing* 2009, 18, 116–25.
7 Hall JE, Restriction and control: the perceptions of mental health nurses in a UK acute inpatient setting, *Issues in Mental Health Nursing* 2004, 25, 539–52.
8 Hamilton B, Manias E, Maude P, Marjoribanks T, Cook K, Perspectives of a nurse, a social worker and a psychiatrist regarding patient assessment in acute inpatient psychiatry settings: a case study approach, *Journal of Psychiatric and Mental Health Nursing* 2004, 11, 683–9.
9 Mullen A, Mental health nurses establishing psychosocial interventions within acute inpatient settings, *International Journal of Mental Health Nursing* 2009, 18, 83–90.
10 Deacon M, Fairhurst E, The real-life practice of acute inpatient mental health nurses: an analysis of 'eight interrelated bundles of activity', *Nursing Inquiry* 2008, 15, 330–40.
11 Buus N, Negotiating clinical knowledge: a field study of psychiatric nurses' everyday communication, *Nursing Inquiry* 2008, 15, 189–98.
12 Fourie WJ, Mcdonald S, Connor J, Bartlett S, The role of the registered nurse in an acute mental health inpatient setting in New Zealand: perceptions versus reality, *International Journal of Mental Health Nursing* 2005, 14, 134–41.
13 Bowers L, Flood C, Nurse staffing, bed numbers and the cost of acute psychiatric inpatient care in England, *Journal of Psychiatric and Mental Health Nursing* 2008, 15, 630–7.
14 Delaney KR, Johnson ME, Inpatient psychiatric nurses need to speak up, *Archives of Psychiatric Nursing* 2007, 21, 288–90.
15 Cleary M, The realities of mental health nursing in acute inpatient environments, *International Journal of Mental Health Nursing* 2004, 13, 53–60.
16 Jones A, Bowles N, Best practice from admission to discharge in acute inpatient care: considerations and standards from a whole system perspective, *Journal of Psychiatric and Mental Health Nursing* 2005, 12, 642–7.
17 Cleary M, Edwards C, 'Something always comes up': nurse–patient interaction in an acute psychiatric setting, *Journal of Psychiatric and Mental Health Nursing* 1999, 6, 469–77.
18 Grant VJ, Briscoe J, Everyday ethics in an acute psychiatric unit, *Journal of Medical Ethics* 2002, 28, 173–6.

19 Rosenman S, Psychiatrists and compulsion: a map of ethics, *Australian and New Zealand Journal of Psychiatry* 1998, 32, 785–93.

20 Bloch S, Green SA, An ethical framework for psychiatry, *British Journal of Psychiatry* 2006, 188, 7–12.

21 Brendel DH, Introduction: the diversification of psychiatric ethics, *Harvard Review of Psychiatry* 2008, 16, 319–21.

22 Robertson M, Ryan C, Walter G, Overview of psychiatric ethics III: principles-based ethics, *Australasian Psychiatry* 2007, 15, 281–6.

23 Davis JK, Intuition and the junctures of judgment in decision procedures for clinical ethics, *Theoretical Medicine and Bioethics* 2007, 28, 1–30.

24 Crowden A, The debate continues: unique ethics for psychiatry, *Australian and New Zealand Journal of Psychiatry* 2004, 38, 111–14.

25 McDaniel C, Erlen J, Ethics and mental health service delivery under managed care, *Issues in Mental Health Nursing* 1996, 17, 11–20.

26 Radden J, Notes towards a professional ethics for psychiatry, *Australian and New Zealand Journal of Psychiatry* 2002, 36, 52–9.

27 Robertson MD, Walter G, Many faces of the dual-role dilemma in psychiatric ethics, *Australian and New Zealand Journal of Psychiatry* 2008, 42, 228–35.

28 Taxis JC, Ethics and praxis: alternative strategies to physical restraint and seclusion in a psychiatric setting, *Issues in Mental Health Nursing* 2002, 23, 157–70.

29 Beauchamp T, Childress J, *Principles of Biomedical Ethics*, 2nd ed., New York, NY: Oxford University Press, 1983.

30 Hughes JC, Fulford KW, Hurly-burly of psychiatric ethics, *Australian and New Zealand Journal of Psychiatry* 2005, 39, 1001–7.

31 Brendel DH, The ethics of diagnostic and therapeutic paradigm choice in psychiatry, *Harvard Review of Psychiatry* 2002, 10, 47–50.

32 Eckroth-Bucher M, Philosophical basis and practice of self-awareness in psychiatric nursing, *Journal of Psychosocial Nursing and Mental Health Services* 2001, 39, 32–9.

33 Horsfall J, Stuhmiller C, Champ S, *Interpersonal Nursing for Mental Health*, New York, NY: Springer Publishing, 2001.

34 Robertson M, Walter G, Overview of psychiatric ethics II: virtue ethics and the ethics of care, *Australasian Psychiatry* 2007, 15, 207–11.

35 Somerville M, *The Ethical Imagination*, Melbourne, Victoria: Melbourne University Press, 2006.

36 Rudnick A, A meta-ethical critique of care ethics, *Theoretical Medicine and Bioethics* 2001, 22, 505–17.

37 Johnstone M, *Bioethics: A Nursing Perspective*, 3rd ed., Sydney, NSW: Harcourt, Australia, 1999.

38 Woodbridge K, Fulford KW, *Whose Values? A Workbook for Values-Based Practice in Mental Health Care*, London, Sainsbury Centre for Mental Health, 2004.

39 Ewashen C, Lane A, Pedagogy, power and practice ethics: clinical teaching in psychiatric/mental health settings, *Nursing Inquiry* 2007, 14, 255–62.

40 Vuokila-Oikkonen P, Janhonen S, Vaisanen L, 'Shared-rhythm cooperation' in cooperative team meetings in acute psychiatric inpatient care, *Journal of Psychiatric and Mental Health Nursing* 2004, 11, 129–40.

41 Bowles N, Jones A, Whole systems working and acute inpatient psychiatry: an exploratory study, *Journal of Psychiatric and Mental Health Nursing* 2005, 12, 283–9.

42 Schweitzer A, *The Teaching of Reverence for Life*, London, Owen, 1966.

17 Forensic care

Tom Mason

Introduction

This chapter considers the ethics of *adults* in forensic psychiatric care settings and a distinction is drawn between other vulnerable groups in such settings, for example, children or the elderly. However, the group termed 'adult' also includes vulnerable sub-populations such as women, learning disabled, enduring psychoses and some would include certain types of personality disorders. In drawing these distinctions a set of ethical concerns both emerge from within the sub-populations and also overlap with each other. For example, whilst women in forensic care may highlight specific ethical concerns in relation to their gender, sexuality and vulnerability to sexual abuse, learning disabled adults in such services may suggest ethical issues such as disempowerment, lacking a voice and vulnerability to physical abuse as their greatest concerns. Therefore, as each adult sub-population would raise their specific ethical concerns, requiring greater space than allowed in this book, a more succinct approach is offered here. Rather than focusing on the ethics of each sub-population it is intended to review the ethics of adults in forensic care in relation to the service and science of forensic practice. Let us deal with the issue of defining forensic practice before we begin.

Although each discipline would define the term 'forensic' in relation to their own professional group, for example, forensic psychiatry, forensic psychology, forensic psychiatric nursing and so on, our basic understanding of the term 'forensic' relates to a court of law, a legal forum or judicial body. This would suggest that forensic practice would involve the application of therapeutic principles to those who have interfaced with the law at one level or another and who are considered to have either a learning disability, mental health problem or a personality disorder. For our everyday purposes we understand that this forensic practice is undertaken in an array of forensic services including high, medium and low secure psychiatric provision as well as court diversion and community facilities.

Relationship between mental disorder and criminal behaviour

The relationship between mental disorder and crime is largely axiomatic and not clearly established either philosophically, objectively or scientifically. There are fundamentally four positions to outline in this debate:

- A: mental disorder in criminals;
- B: mental disorder in non-criminals;
- C: criminal behaviour in psychiatric patients;
- D: criminal behaviour in non-psychiatric people.

However, riven throughout these positions are issues of the definitional criteria employed, the identification of persons in each of the groups, the clinical orientation of the researchers and both professional and political influences.

Mental disorder in criminals

Assessing mental disorder in criminal populations is fraught with difficulties, particularly in relation to diagnostic criteria. In a study by Gunn *et al.*[1] they reported on 1,365 adult males and 404 young males from 16 prisons in England. These authors reported a primary diagnosis of mental disorder in 37 per cent of prisoners, with substance abuse being 23 per cent, personality disorder 10 per cent, neurosis 6 per cent, psychosis 2 per cent and organic disorder 0.8 per cent. In a review of studies by Blackburn,[2] including mental disorder and crime and mental disorder and violence, a wide range of figures are reported; however, taken overall there is a tendency towards figures of between one-quarter and one-third of all prisoners having some form of mental disorder. More recent figures confirm little change to this status.[3-5] The reports may well be even greater given that some criminals with mental disorder may well be in psychiatric settings or diverted to other facilities. Although it is interesting to note these figures and how they may have been constructed they merely inform us that groups of researchers have identified certain diagnostic criteria, by their own definitional framework *in* a group of criminals who have been captured. They cannot tell us how many criminals with mental disorders there are who have not come before the courts. Nor can they inform us that it is the mental disorder that *caused* the criminal behaviour.

Mental disorder in non-criminals

The fact that mental disorder exists in non-criminals (general population) obfuscates any relationship between mental disorder and crime. From the National Statistics Office in the United Kingdom it is reported that approximately 1 person in 4 are likely to experience a mental health problem in the course of a year, with anxiety and depression (between 8 and 10 per cent of the population experience depression) being the most common. They also report that depression affects 1 in 5 of the older population in community settings and 2 in 5 living in care homes. British men are three times more likely to commit suicide than women and self-harm in the United Kingdom is the highest in Europe.[6,7] Although rates of mental disorder vary across Europe, the United States and Canada, they are reported in all developed countries. Prevalence and types of disorder may differ but where one diagnosis wanes another waxes. Even in non-psychiatrised countries that do not have psychiatrists, a psychiatric system or structured services, mental disorders can still be found.[8] Furthermore, numerous cultures identify specific disorders related to them and these do not appear in other cultures – at least not in their specific form.[9] Thus, mental disorder is a universal phenomenon which does not usually lead to, or cause, criminal behaviour.

Criminal behaviour in psychiatric patients

Crime by psychiatric patients who have shown no previous criminality is an area of increasing research interest but this research to date is inconclusive. This is recognised in the two headlines 'no significant relationship between violent crime and mental illness'[10] and 'link between crime and mental illness identified'.[11] In the majority of writings on this topic the one common theme to emerge is that it is usually a small number of people with a mental disorder who do go on to commit crime. However, there is also a view that under-treated mental disorder will invariably lead to an increase in crime rates.[10,12] Thus, the 'relationship' between mental disorder and crime is statistically small and yet it features large in the eyes of the professionals, public and politicians in the past as much as it does today.[13,14] If we are far from establishing the relationship between mental disorder and crime, and it would appear that we are, we are even further from understanding how this might occur, or the causal mechanism involved.

Criminal behaviour in the non-psychiatric populations

Crime rates in the non-psychiatric general population are also hotly debated with little agreement about methods of reporting crime, collecting the data and collating it. From the Home Office Crime Reduction website it is reported that 'overall levels of crime stable at 11.3 million crimes, rise of crime up by 2 percentage point (statistically significant), violence stable (5% increase but this was not statistically significant), all personal crime stable and all household crime stable'.[15] They also report that domestic burglary, vehicle offences, sexual offences and violence were down whilst robbery and drug offences were up. The British Crime Survey have also reported a downward trend but still claim 10.1 million crimes in 2007/8. They reported that 'nearly three-quarters of these were property crimes … violence against the person accounted for almost one-fifth of all recorded crime'.[16] Finally, the Crimestoppers statistics report that '120 per cent rise in victims of knife crime … credit crunch crimewave … online banking fraud doubles … 1 in 5 think domestic violence is justified … 1 in 3 carry knives'.[17] Despite the lack of clarity of these statistics the overriding point is that there appears to be a considerable amount of crime in non-psychiatric populations.

From the foregoing we are now in a position to outline four possible scenarios in relation to the relationship between mental disorder and criminal behaviour (Table 17.1).

These 'positions' are merely possibilities of generalised ways in which the public may view the relationship between mental disorder and criminal behaviour. The position that is the most common view is 'B' in which a person becomes mentally disordered and commits a crime, which is then viewed as being *caused* by the mental disorder. The most interesting position is 'D' which involves a criminal who develops a mental disorder and *does not* commit a crime, which can be viewed as the mental disorder *preventing* the crime. Both these positions can be accepted if the causal relationship between mental disorder and crime is also accepted.

Tensions between incarceration in prison or referral to secure psychiatric services

Mentally disordered offenders can be found both in the mental health system as well as in the criminal justice system and this section is concerned with how they are placed in one rather than the other. A person who commits an offence, is arrested by the police, charged, remanded (or bailed) and brought before the courts, can be referred to the mental health system at various stages either prior to formal police processing or following it.[18] The police may remove a person considered to be suffering from a mental health problem to a place of safety or in some cases psychiatric nurses visit police stations to assess an arrested person's mental state.[18] Many courts have court diversion schemes which function to divert mentally disordered persons away from the criminal justice system by requesting a psychiatric referral.[19]

Table 17.1 Mental disorder and criminal behaviour relationship outcomes

Person type	Mental disorder	Act	Status	Rationale
A. Non-criminal	Becomes mentally disordered	Does not commit a crime		Considered to be a person with mental health problems either in the community or a psychiatric in-patient
B. Non-criminal	Becomes mentally disordered	Does commit a crime		Considered to be a person who commits the crime because of the mental disorder but equally could have turned to crime despite the mental disorder. Therefore the mental disorder could have caused the crime
C. Criminal	Becomes mentally disordered	Does commit a crime		Considered to be a criminal who commits crime anyway but develops a mental disorder. Therefore, the mental disorder may or may not be related to further crime
D. Criminal	Becomes mentally disordered	Does not commit a crime		Considered to be a criminal who intends to commit further crime but develops a mental disorder and does not do so. Therefore, the mental disorder could have prevented the crime

Once in court a person may be referred for a psychiatric report before or during the trial or at the sentencing stage the judge may consider a Hospital Order. Following sentence to the prison system a prisoner may be transferred to a secure psychiatric facility under the Mental Health Act. Thus, there are many stages at which a mentally disordered offender may be diverted or transferred from the criminal justice system to the mental health system.[20]

Rutherford and Duggan[21] state that 'there are more than 3,500 people in the medium- and high-security hospitals who have been directed there by the courts or prison system' and from the Social Exclusion Unit[22] there is a claim that more than two-thirds of the prison population in England and Wales have two or more mental health problems. The latter is an alarming figure and clearly, if accurate, many of these mentally disordered offenders will go untreated. However, what is less clear is, for those who are directed to the mental health system, how this actually occurs. It has long been suggested that these referrals for psychiatric reports are more serendipitous than strategic and are largely due to the lawyers, barristers and judges having some personal interest in mental health or learning disability issues;[20] the numerous hurdles in place for the remainder ensure that the majority do not get referred. The ethical concerns relating to this include a general acceptance that a psychiatric system is a more humane placement for someone with a mental disorder and this clearly suggests that the large mentally disordered population untreated in prisons is unethical. Furthermore, it is well known that prison itself can cause a person to become mentally disordered due to the stresses within that system[20] and the ethical concern relates to the fact that an offender may well become seriously disordered in jail having arrived there without such mental health problems.

Hospitalisation

Given that hospitalisation, or more accurately 'psychiatrisation', is considered a more humane system of referral for someone with a mental disorder who has committed a serious crime, then we need to examine the nature of this hospitalisation. The hospitalisation will usually involve admission to a high or medium secure psychiatric facility with perhaps a low-security service a possibility at one level or another in the future. Thus, the examination of this forensic referral will focus on three aspects, namely, (a) the efficacy of the 'science' of forensic psychiatry, (b) whether this 'science' is available as treatments and (c) the accuracy of prognoses.

The efficacy of the 'science' of forensic psychiatry

The first point to consider is whether psychiatry itself is a science. Theories of Mind (ToM) are in abundance but with little agreement as to how it works, let alone where it is.[23] The science, if any, will refer to the chemical composition within the structures of the brain, and altering this composition with drugs and observing behavioural changes is about as far as the science stretches.[24] Explanations as to how the changes in chemical composition produce different behaviours remain elusive. What we may know is that some drugs, behavioural approaches, psychological interventions and 'talking therapies' do change some peoples reported mental states and behaviour. However, we know little of the science of how they produce this reported effect. In terms of forensic psychiatry (involving offending behaviour) we are in dire straights indeed as the efficacy of changing criminal behaviour is notoriously difficult.[25]

There may well be many psychiatrists, psychologists, psychiatric nurses and so on, who claim that they do not address the offending behaviour in their treatment philosophies but instead focus on attempting to alleviate the mental state symptoms, stabilise aberrant thinking and/or alter personality traits. However, there are many more in the forensic disciplines who would argue that the focus on recidivism rates, risk assessment and management strategies ensure that the public and politicians insist that offending behaviour is taken account of in treatment approaches. Unfortunately, this double-edged sword involving the 'science' of psychiatry and the 'science' of offending behaviour brought together as forensic psychiatry is a blunt instrument indeed. This is not to say that there are not successes as, on the contrary, as we will see later, the majority of forensic patients do not re-offend. However, *why* they do not or *how* it occurs that they do not is unknown. Thus, the 'science' of forensic psychiatry is at best an inchoate one.

The availability of forensic psychiatric 'science'

Whilst we may conclude that referral to the forensic mental health system is more humane than incarceration in prisons (but questions remain regarding this) we must ask ourselves whether the expansion of forensic secure facilities is matched by the application of treatments for this growing population. It is a simple matter to glance at the contents pages of numerous psychiatric textbooks and produce a 'menu' of treatment approaches. However, transferring these approaches to the forensic domain may be neither appropriate nor effective. Yet, the important ethical question relates to whether these treatment approaches are even available in these forensic facilities. We can be reasonably sure that drugs are available and provide the mainstay of treatment but other approaches and their availability appear thin on the ground. It is fair to say that the main focus is on assessment of risk[26] and the management of violence.[27] However, the actual delivery of treatment approaches is small by comparison.[28,29] It is not surprising that Konrad[30] claims this to be a case of 'forensic psychiatry in dubious ascent'.

Prognoses (or re-offending or recidivism)

An anecdote goes that in the early 1960s Dr Patrick McGrath, the then Medical Director of Broadmoor Hospital, claimed on TV that he could safely release two-thirds of his patients in Broadmoor but unfortunately he did not know which two-thirds. What he was foretelling the audience was that research on follow-up studies would largely show that approximately two-thirds of released forensic patients did not re-offend.[31] Of course, there are different reported rates of recidivism by diagnostic category as there are by gender, offence type, length of stay and length of follow-up period. The 'first generation' of clinical predictions of dangerousness emanated from the United States[32] but now they feature across the developed world.[2] Risk assessment approaches now focus on an array of factors. For example, behavioural and personality differences[33]; specific offences such as homicide[34]; fratricide[35]; amnesia[36] and the impact of rehabilitation.[37] Recent follow-up studies from a medium secure unit reported almost half (49 per cent) of discharged patients were reconvicted, with two-fifths (38 per cent) readmitted to secure psychiatric care.[38] In another study Maden[39] reported a re-offence rate of released forensic psychiatric patients as one-third of men and 15 per cent of women. Of note in these two recent reports is the fact that between a half and two-thirds did not re-offend, which is similar to the situation in the 1960s.

In forensic psychiatry, prognoses are made in relation to both the prediction of relapse of their mental state and the risk of re-offending despite the issues of causal relations outlined above. It is not the fact that the rates of relapse cause such concern but the re-offending that creates victims which causes public and political outcry. Again, it is not these rates that is alarming but the fact that we do not have the 'science' to more accurately identify which patients fit into which groups that causes the ethical concerns in the false negatives and false positives.

Ethics of false negatives and false positives

In all branches of medicine giving accurate prognoses, or predictions, is a goal to be strived for and in forensic psychiatry it is invariably re-offence that most people's attention is focused on. However, predictions are just that, estimates of the likelihood of an event happening, or not happening, in the future. These events, in forensic psychiatry, predominantly involve the risk to others and can be both negative and positive. Whilst the science of actuarial prediction of offending is complex there are four fundamental outcomes:

- False negatives – When a person does recidivate when predicted he will not (predictor incorrectly predicts the outcome).
- False positives – When a person does not recidivate when predicted that he will (predictor incorrectly predicts the outcome).

- True negatives – When a person does not recidivate when predicted he will not (predictor correctly predicts the outcome).
- True positives – When a person does recidivate when predicted he would (predictor correctly predicts the outcome).

Although this may be hypothetical in forensic practice as a patient predicted to re-offend would likely be detained indefinitely; however, in the prison system they would be released.

Clearly, in ethical terms, it is the former two outcomes that cause us the greatest concern in forensic care as the latter two are correct predictions. However, it is worth considering the complex ethical dilemmas involved in the last outcome of the true positive in which a person may be indefinitely detained as dangerous and forensic psychiatry being unable to change this condition. In this situation it would certainly have been a more desirable referral to prison under a set sentence for the patient – if not for the future victim. Of course, this would be qualified if the offender was re-captured and returned to prison.

There are four other terms that ought to be mentioned in relation to the prediction of offending. The first is the *predictor*, which is information to identify risk factors that have occurred in the individual, such as paedophilia. The second is the *criterion of interest*, which is future behaviours associated with the predictor, such as the paedophile frequenting schools to watch the children. The final two are the *efficiency* of a predictor to predict beyond chance and the *base rate*, which refers to the frequency of the criterion in the population of interest (paedophiles).

False negatives

Whether patients in forensic care are assessed by actuarial or clinical risk assessment approaches it will be concluded that some will be considered as 'safe'. That is, that they are predicted to not re-offend. In some of these cases the patient will actually re-offend and may cause harm to others. The prediction is incorrect. This outcome has long been of concern in forensic care with follow-up studies a constant stream in the academic journals. For example, we have many studies on the predictive validity of psychopathy,[10] the psychopathy checklist[11] and dangerous severe personality disorder.[12] Furthermore, we have numerous studies on the efficiency of risk assessments for severe mental illness,[13] violence[14] and substance abuse.[15] Comparative studies have been undertaken between males and females,[16,17] between forensic and non-forensic patients[18] and between inpatients and outpatients.[49,50] Yet, despite this intense activity false negatives continue to occur.

The ethical implications for false negatives are threefold. First, they create victims which may involve minor or major injury and even in some cases death. This is further compounded by the emotional pain and suffering of family and friends of the victim. Second, false negatives may cause further incarceration for the offender and whilst for some members of the public they may not consider this an ethical difficulty for others it is justifiably an ethical concern. Finally, there are ethical implications for the professions involved in false negatives and we continue to question our interventions and their efficacy.

False positives

In forensic care predicting re-offending, or dangerousness, is a central focus and concluding that a patient is considered to be an ongoing threat will usually ensure that they continue to be detained involuntarily. However, we know from the follow-up studies, particularly in relation to the Baxstrom studies (a case in United States when 1,000 secure psychiatric patients were ordered to be released by a court), that a proportion are in fact 'safe' to be released. Thus, at any one time throughout the forensic services a number of patients are not a danger to others and could be transferred to lesser security services or released into the community. But, like Dr McGrath above, unfortunately we do not know which ones. The ethical concerns in this scenario are clearly twofold. First, it is a question of civil liberties as the patient is detained when they are in fact 'safe'. This is highly undesirable and had they received a prison term they may well have been released. Second, it must surely be a question of professional ethics and hopefully we salve our consciences in this domain by striving towards an improvement in forensic psychiatric science, with all that this entails, better treatments and better prognoses.

Conclusion

In dealing with the ethics of forensic care there is a need to lay bare the difficult areas of our practice, which may be an uncomfortable enterprise. Certainly, the lack of an established relationship between a mental disorder and criminal behaviour is a major concern given the fact that this belief is a central tenet to the practice of forensic psychiatry. Whilst, for most people, a referral to the mental health services rather than to the prison system is considered a more humane one, ethical tensions arise when detention in the latter far exceeds a sentence in the former. This is further compounded when treatment efficacy is scrutinised in relation to outcome studies. Finally, the ethics of false negatives and false positives continue to cause concern which is evidenced by the research efforts in follow-up studies, risk assessment techniques and predictive approaches. Whilst these difficulties do cause us concern, professional accountability provides the impetus to clinical developments and research in these areas.

Notes

1 Gunn, J., Maden, A. and Swinton, M. Treatment needs of prisoners with psychiatric disorders. *British Medical Journal.* 1991: 303: 338–41.

2 Blackburn, R. *Psychology of Criminal Conduct: Theory, Research & Practice.* Chichester: Wiley, 1993.

3 Butler, T., Allnutt, S., Cain, D., Owens, D. and Muller, C. Mental disorder in the New South Wales prisoner population. *Australian and New Zealand Journal of Psychiatry.* 2005: 39 (5): 407–13.

4 Butler, T., Andrews, G., Allnutt, S., Sakashita, C., Smith, N.E. and Basson, J. Mental disorders in Australian prisoners: a comparison with a community sample. *Australian and New Zealand Journal of Psychiatry.* 2006: 40 (3): 272–6.

5 James, D.J. and Glaze, L.E. Mental health problems in prison and jail inmates. *US Department of Justice Bureau of Justice Statistics, US.* September Report, 2006, pp 1–12.

6 Office for National Statistics. *Psychiatric Morbidity Report.* London: Office for National Statistics, 2001.

7 National Institute for Clinical Excellence. Men are more likely than women to have an alcohol or drug problem, 2003. www.mentalhealth.org.uk/information/mental-health-overview/statistics/ (accessed 2/07/2009).

8 Haslam, N. Folk taxonomies versus official taxonomies. *Philosophy, Psychiatry & Psychology.* 2007: 14 (3): 281–4.

9 Mattelaer, J.J. and Jilek, W. Koro – the psychological disappearance of the penis. *The Journal of Sexual Medicine.* 2007: 4 (5): 1509–15.

10 Grohol, J.M. No significant relationship between violent crime and mental illness, 2009. http:// psychcentral.com/blog/archives/ (accessed 2/07/2009).

11 Bonfiglioli, C. Link between crime and mental illness identified, 2009. www.schizophrenia.com/news/crime1.html (accessed 2/07/2009).

12 Sestoft, D. Crime and mental illness: it is time to take action. *World Psychiatry*. 2006: 5 (2): 95.

13 Guze, S.B., Goodwin, D.W. and Crane, B. Criminality and psychiatric disorders. *Archives of General Psychiatry*. 1969: 20 (5): 583–91.

14 Koenigsberg, D., Balla, D.A. and Lewis, D.O. Juvenile delinquency, adult criminality and adult psychiatric treatment: an epidemiological study. *Child Psychiatry and Human Development*. 2005: 7 (3): 141–6.

15 Home Office Crime Reduction. Helping to reduce crime in your area, 2009. www.crime reduction. homeoffice.gov.uk/sta_index.htm (accessed 2/07/2009).

16 British Crime Survey. Crime: crime figures decline, 2009. http://rds.homeoffice.gov.uk/rds/bcs1.html/ (accessed 23/09/2010) .

17 Crimestoppers. Latest crime statistics, 2009. www.crimestoppers-uk.org/crime-prevention/latest-crime-statistics (accessed 2/07/2009).

18 Mulder, C.L., Koopmans, G.T. and Selten, J-P. Emergency psychiatry, compulsory admissions and clinical presentation among immigrants to The Netherlands. *The British Journal of Psychiatry*. 2006: 188: 386–91.

19 Hartford, K., Carey, R. and Mendonca, J. Pretrial court diversion of people with mental illness. *The Journal of Behavioral Health Services and Research*. 2007: 34 (2): 198–205.

20 Peay, J. Mentally disordered offenders. In: M. Maguire, R. Morgan and R. Reiner (Eds.) *The Oxford Handbook of Criminology*. London: Clarendon Press, 1994. pp. 1119–60.

21 Rutherford, M. and Duggan, S. Forensic mental health services: facts and figures on current provision. *The British Journal of Forensic Practice*. 2008: 10 (4): 4–10.

22 Social Exclusion Unit. *Mental Health and Social Exclusion*. London: Office of the Deputy Prime Minister, 2004.

23 Bentall, R. *Reconstructing Schizophrenia*. London: Routledge, 1992.

24 Saxe, R. and Baron-Cohen, S. *Theory of Mind: A Special Issue of Social Neuroscience*. London: Psychology Press, 2007.

25 Schopp, R.F., Wiener, R.L., Bornstein, B.H. and Willborn, S.L. *Mental Disorder and Criminal Law*. Springer: New York, 2008.

26 Nichols, T.L., Brink, J., Desmarais, S.L., Webster, C.D. and Martin, M-L. The short-term assessment of risk and treatability (START). *Assessment*. 2006: 13 (3): 313–27.

27 Clark, T. and Rowe, R. Violence, stigma and psychiatric diagnosis: the effects of a history of violence on psychiatric diagnosis. *Psychiatric Bulletin*. 2006: 30: 254–6.

28 Kaltiala-Heino, R. and Kahila, K. Forensic psychiatric inpatient treatment: creating a therapeutic milieu. *Child and Adolescent Psychiatric Clinics of North America*. 2006: 15 (2): 459–75.

29 De Jonge, E., Nijman, H.L. and Lammers, S.M. Behavioural changes during forensic psychiatric treatment: a multicenter study. *Tijdschr Psychiatr*. 2009: 51 (4): 205–15.

30 Konrad, N. Forensic psychiatry in dubious ascent. *World Psychiatry*. 2006: 5 (2): 93.

31 Bailey, J. and MacCulloch, M. Patterns of reconviction in patients discharged directly to community from a special hospital: implications for after-care. *Journal of Forensic Psychiatry*. 1992: 3: 445–61.

32 Steadman, H.J. and Keveles, G. The community adjustment and criminal activity of the Baxstrom patients: 1966–1970. *American Journal of Psychiatry*. 1972: 129: 304–10.

33 Hornsveld, R.H.J., Cuperus, H., De Vries, E.T. and Kraaimaat, F.W. An evaluation of behavioural and personality differences between native and non-native male adolescents in the Netherlands ordered into treatment in a forensic psychiatric outpatient clinic and their non-violent peers. *Criminal Behaviour and Mental Health*. 2009: 18 (3): 177–89.

34 Tiihonen, J. and Hakola, P. Psychiatric disorders and homicide recidivism. *The American Journal of Psychiatry*. 1994: 151: 436–8.

35 Bourget, D. and Gagne, P. Fratricide: a forensic psychiatric perspective. *Journal of the American Academy of Psychiatry and Law*. 2006: 34 (4): 529–33.

36 Bourget, D. and Whitehurst, L. Amnesia and crime. *Journal of the American Academy of Psychiatry and Law*. 2007: 35 (4): 469–80.

37 Lindqvist, P. and Skipworth, J. Evidence-based rehabilitation in forensic psychiatry. *The British Journal of Psychiatry.* 2000: 176: 320–3.

38 Davies, S., Clarke, M., Hollin, C. and Duggan, C. Long-term outcomes after discharge from medium secure care: a cause for concern. *The British Journal of Psychiatry.* 2007: 191: 70–4.

39 Maden, A. A third of men and 15% of women discharged from medium secure forensic psychiatry services in the UK re-offend. *Evidence-Based Mental Health.* 2007: 10 (4): 128.

40 Dolan, M. and Doyle, M. Clinical and actuarial measures and the role of the psychopathy checklist. *The British Journal of Psychiatry.* 2000: 177: 303–11.

41 Bolt, D.M., Hare, R.D. and Neumann, C.S. Score metric equivalence of the Psychopathy Checklist-Revised (PCL-R) across criminal offenders in North America and the United Kingdom: a critique of Cooke, Michie, Hart and Clark (2005) and new analyses. *Assessment.* 2007: 14 (1): 44–56.

42 Feeney, A. Dangerous severe personality disorder. *Advances in Psychiatric Treatment.* 2003: 9 (5): 349–58.

43 Lamberti, J.S., Weisman, R. and Faden, D.I. Forensic assertive community treatment: preventing incarceration of adults with severe mental illness. *Psychiatric Services.* 2004: 55 (11): 1285–93.

44 Dernevik, M., Grann, M. and Johansson, S. Violent behaviour in forensic psychiatric patients: risk assessment and different risk-management levels using the HCR-20. *Psychology, Crime and Law.* 2002: 8: 93–111.

45 Richards, H.J., Casey, J.O. and Lucente, S.W. Psychopathy and treatment response in incarcerated female substance abusers. *Criminal Justice and Behavior.* 2003: 30 (2): 251–76.

46 Hoptman, M.J., Yates, K.F., Patalinjug, M.B., Wack, R.C. and Convit, A. Clinical prediction of assaultive behavior among male psychiatric patients at a maximum-security forensic facility. *Psychiatric Services.* 1999: 50: 1461–6.

47 Putkonen, H., Komulainen, E.J., Virkkunen, M., Eronen, M. and Lonnqvist, J. Risk of repeat offending among violent female offenders with psychotic and personality disorders. *The American Journal of Psychiatry.* 2003: 160 (5): 947–51.

48 Linhorst, D.M. and Scott, L.P. Assaultive behavior in State Psychiatric Hospitals: differences between forensic and non-forensic patients. *Journal of Interpersonal Violence.* 2004: 19 (8): 857–74.

49 Doyle, M. and Dolan, M. Predicting community violence from patients discharged from mental health services. *The British Journal of Psychiatry.* 2006: 189 (6): 520–6.

50 Linaker, O.M. and Busch-Iversen, H. Predictors of imminent violence in psychiatric inpatients. *Acta Psychiatrica Scandinavica.* 2007: 92 (4): 250–4.

18 Addictions

Jeffrey A. Schaler

Introduction

All drugs have effects on the body, and we can often measure these effects. The immediate effects of drugs in altering the quality of subjective experience can also be measured. We can, further, examine how mood-altering drugs get into the body. In some cases drugs get into the body by accident or because someone puts them there. None of this is uncontroversial.

Alternatively, someone may put drugs into his or her own body. What motivates the drug consumer is much more disputed. Some people, including myself, believe a person makes a *choice* to take a drug. There is no single reason why people make such choices, which reflect the values, preferences, and goals of each individual drug consumer; just as there is no single reason why people choose to watch TV. Others, whose views are echoed by most politicians, journalists, social workers, and mental health professionals, believe people take certain types of drugs because they have 'lost control' over their actions. They are in the grip of some involuntary affliction – a type of mental illness.

This chapter defines and describes what addiction *is* and what it *isn't*, and how the different ways of explaining addiction based on accurate and inaccurate definitions influence policy decisions in legal, clinical, social, and public policy realms.

Historical perspectives on addiction

The history of ideas about addiction involves two related contexts. The first has to do with the *meaning* of addiction and key controversies about defining, describing, explaining, and implementing policy for drugs and addiction. The meaning of addiction has often been vague or incoherent. Since alcohol is a drug, we will consider it here within the context of drug addiction.

The second has to do with the meaning of chronic drug use before the term 'addiction' was applied to this behaviour and the attribution of problems associated with drinking and drug use. Most of our ideas about addiction are historically derived from ideas first conceived in relation to the consumption of beverage alcohol. Alcohol is used more widely around the world than any other mood-enhancing drugs, and because it has generally been legal, it has been easier to study its use. Currently, illegal drugs such as marijuana, opium, cocaine, and various hallucinogens have been legal much longer than they have been illegal, but in recent decades have generally been illegal, which has hampered research into their use.

Ideas originally developed to describe alcohol addiction have been generalized to apply to all drugs that some people consume for their mood-altering effects, which the authorities consider undesirable. 'Addiction' has become an all-inclusive term: used the same way with different drugs and different behaviours, which are considered socially deviant and socially harmful. Indeed, 'addiction' is now applied to such behaviours as gambling, shopping, or sex and is commonly spoken of as a *disease*, which can be treated. Many people insist that addiction is 'an illness, just like cancer or diabetes'.

Taking the disease metaphor literally leads to confusion. According to the proponents of the disease model of addiction, addiction is a form of self-destructive, involuntary behaviour. Just as a person cannot will away cancer or diabetes, they cannot will away their addiction. Yet the only treatment is to engage in *conversation* with the addict; for example, with a counsellor or therapist. This immediately casts doubt on the claim that addiction is just like any other illness.

Unless they are faith healers, normally judged to be charlatans or frauds, we do not expect doctors to 'treat' cancer or diabetes by exchanging words with the patient. If treatment consists in persuading the addict to adopt a different outlook, by getting him to question his or her values, goals, and preferences, then the claim that addiction is *involuntary* is undermined. How can we expect to cure an involuntary disease by persuasion or by an odyssey of self-discovery?

Of course, some people do terminate or moderate their consumption of drugs following treatment. But in fact most people eventually terminate or moderate their consumption of drugs with or without treatment. There is no evidence that treatment makes any significant difference. Treatment methods have not changed much over the years that addiction has been regarded as a treatable disease. The efficacy of treatment remains about the same as leaving people to their own devices. New approaches to therapy just do not make that much difference when it comes to treatment success. One famous study found that a year of the most comprehensive treatment was no more effective than a 'simple dose of advice' in reducing problems associated with drinking alcohol.[1-3]

Addiction to a drug is not *literally* a physical illness. In some cases it may cause literal physical illnesses, but so may swimming, operating machinery, or performing in a circus. 'Addiction' does not refer to a cellular abnormality, as do all real diseases; the term refers to unacceptable behaviour. Behaviour means mode of conduct or deportment. Involuntary behaviour is a contradiction. Involuntary movements of the body usually refer to reflex actions, convulsions, or seizures. There is no volition present in a reflex.

According to some, the reasons people become addicted are irrelevant to trying to persuade them to abstain or reduce their use of a drug.[4] To others, the reasons why people use drugs are important to understand in order to help a person give up drugs. Any behaviour can be stopped or moderated when this becomes important enough to a person. All people who stop using drugs (other than by being coercively prevented) do so in the same way. They make a decision to do so because they *want* to. People have always been able to control their behaviours. Whether or not they *will* control their behaviours to the liking of others is a different story.

Drug prohibition and its repeal

Drug prohibition is relatively new but it has grown to enormous size and far-reaching scope. If prohibition were repealed, the majority of people in prison for illegal possession, purchase, and consumption would no longer exist as a criminal class, a class that constitutes the *majority* of people in US prisons.

In the existing system of drug prohibition, two groups of people who allegedly oppose one another as adversaries each have a stake. 'Drug warriors', those whose job it is to enforce laws concerning prohibition, make their livelihoods from the system, as do illegal drug dealers. Illegal drug dealers gain from prohibition because removing the obstacles to drugs on the free market would take the wind out of the sails of the black market. The violence associated with the illegal drug trade is primarily among dealers and due to prohibition. Free market competition, higher quality control, and lower prices which repeal would bring are the last thing illegal drug dealers want to see happen.

But wouldn't illegal drug dealers gain from the removal of government harassment? This misunderstands the nature of government intervention in the market. The people who have an advantage in supplying an illegal service are generally different kinds of people from those who would supply it if it were legal. Your corner liquor store today is probably run by people very different in character from Al Capone's soldiers, because they need different skills to survive in a different environment. Making any activity illegal will always associate it with other kinds of illegal activities, including violence. The skills needed to sell drugs under prohibition are different from the skills needed to sell drugs legally in the corner pharmacy. So the individuals now supplying illegal drugs would probably be outcompeted and displaced by less violent, more risk-averse suppliers.

Put differently, the prospect of big financial rewards along with the risk of being shot by rivals or spending years in prison is a package that appeals to a certain type of person. More modest rewards along with far less risk of being shot or jailed are a package that would appeal to a different type of person. Prohibiting an activity is akin to issuing a licence for that activity. The essential effect of a licence is that competition is restricted, so that only some people are able to pursue that line of work and can reap a monopoly profit from doing so. In drug prohibition, peaceful and law-abiding suppliers are kept out, leaving only the criminal elements who pay their 'licence fee' in the form of increased risk of being shot or imprisoned.

Thus, in a strange way, drug warriors and illegal dealers are in bed together. Most members of both groups – not necessarily all – would lose their livelihoods following repeal. They both tend to favour prohibition, because they both benefit from the illegality of drugs. Addiction treatment providers share in the investment that prohibition brings, though not all of their jobs would be eliminated by repeal. There would still be a market for consensual therapy, just as some people now go to therapists because they find it difficult to stop smoking or give up other 'bad' but legal habits. Prohibition facilitates coerced or court-ordered attendance in treatment for addiction. Repeal would leave that exclusively to the prerogative of the individual drug user. He would not have to admit to committing a crime in order to get help, if drugs were legal.

I do not use illegal drugs and I have not done so since I was an undergraduate in college about 40 years ago. Like so many young people in their late teens and early 20s, I experimented with most every drug that was illegal. While I have no interest in using currently illegal drugs should they become legally available on the free market, I do believe that prohibition causes more problems than it solves. I strongly support the repeal of drug prohibition because of the harm prohibition causes to society. I don't claim that there are *no* benefits to drug prohibition: merely that the costs considerably exceed the benefits.

For example, the repeal of drug prohibition would clearly have a profound effect on international terrorism. Drug warriors and terrorists alike recognize that the illegal trade in narcotics, based on the cultivation of poppies in Afghanistan, provides the economic means to fund and fuel terrorist activities. The attempt to eradicate poppy production in Afghanistan only increases the money made on the black market. This is just one example of the principle that making an activity illegal associates it with other illegal activities and thereby strengthens those other activities.

Most people who at some point in their lives voluntarily consume large quantities of mood-altering drugs spontaneously quit or moderate after a while. For example, college students who take drugs most often prefer to have a good job and a comfortable lifestyle. This is not possible while they are using drugs excessively, so most will give up the drugs or moderate their use so that they can live the lifestyle they value.

It is customary to refer to consumption of mood-altering drugs as a problem. But most of the conspicuous unpleasant consequences arise because of prohibition. What remains is a choice of lifestyle which many people, including me, consider unwise, in exactly the same way that we may consider adherence to some religious groups unwise. Religious groups vary in the demands they make upon their members. Most people who are converted to very intense and enthusiastic religious groups leave the group after a short while. The pattern is the same with drug use. Of course, it is sometimes tragic that people can behave self-destructively, but they have many opportunities to do so apart from drugs, and trying to extirpate self-destructive behaviour by force is not the best way to encourage people to become autonomous and critical, so that they are less likely to be self-destructive.

The changing attributions of drunkenness

During colonial days in America, there was no concept of alcoholism or addiction applied to drug consumption. Addiction still meant devotion, attachment, or dedication. The earliest recorded use of the word 'addiction', according to the *Oxford English Dictionary*, is found in the King James Bible (1611), 1 Cor: xvi.15: 'They have addicted themselves to the ministry of the saints.' This quote, like similar ones, illustrates the fact that addiction meant *devotion*, was not particularly applied to alcohol or any other drug, and had no negative connotation. In colonial America, alcohol was called 'the good creature of God'. Its use was encouraged by physicians and ministers alike, for whatever ailed a person.[5] If there was physical pain, or a person felt depressed, physicians and ministers encouraged people to take a drink and drink they did. People consumed substantial quantities of alcohol (vastly greater than Americans do today) without fear of moral judgement or retribution.[6,7]

Neither the drinker nor the drink was blamed for trouble resulting from the consumption of alcohol during the colonial period. What people blamed drink-related trouble on was the *company* a drinker kept. The tavern was blamed, as well as the people he drank with. If he got into fights or someone became hurt as a result of drinking, it was the *place* and the *persons* he drank with that people blamed – not the alcohol.

We may call this a *social interaction attribution*. Trouble was blamed on *who* you drank with and *where* you drank. Problems were *not* blamed on the person himself or the alcohol. There was no notion of involuntary addiction to a drug or belief that one became enslaved to the drug. There was no attribution regarding heredity or something inside a person's body that made him drink.

Gradually, ministers and religious persons began to view the consumption of alcohol as indulging in too much pleasure, participating in an activity of worldly, and therefore sinful desire. Feeling good for physical reasons came to be considered sinful. Trouble that came from drinking was blamed on vice, and abstinence was considered a virtue. Drinking alcohol and being drunk was considered a character flaw, ungodly, like promiscuous sex or masturbation.

Thus, we first had a social interactionist view on trouble brought about from drinking alcohol. But this gave way to a new view of drinking and drunkenness as a kind of fleshly desire. So was born the 'sin model' of drunkenness.

Invention of the disease model

Soon after the Revolutionary War, Benjamin Rush, a physician, known today as the 'father of American psychiatry', a signer of the Declaration of Independence and a highly influential political rhetorician, blazed a new trail in the medicalization of deviant behaviour. Rush claimed that chronic drunkenness was a medical disease.[8] No new medical facts supported this conclusion. Rush did not conduct research to show that chronic drunkenness was a disease. In effect, he *invented* the idea.

Previously, most socially unacceptable behaviours had been attributed to vice and virtue, lack of morality, and man's inherent depravity due to original sin. Applications of the disease concept proliferated. *Lying* was considered a disease. '*Revolutiona*' was a putative disease that caused people to *resist* the revolutionary cause in America. '*Anarchia*' was pronounced the *medical* reason why people did not settle down after the Revolutionary War. Insanity was attributed to masturbation – and dominated views of madness and suicide from Rush's day well into the 1930s.

Homosexuality is a striking instance of a socially unacceptable behaviour labelled a disease. It was only in 1973 that the *American Psychiatric Association* declassified homosexuality as a disease. Homosexuality was declassified as a disease the same way it was first classified: through political rhetoric, invention, and pronouncement, not through the discovery of a physical pathogen or its absence. This is the way it has been for all behaviours labelled diseases. Behaviours were renamed diseases, then placed within the domain of medical treatment, then sometimes removed from this domain when the climate of political opinion favoured toleration of the behaviour in question.[9,10]

The Civil War and its aftermath was a period of much pain and suffering. Alcohol consumption was very high by more recent standards. Even though opium was available, alcohol was the drug of choice. Some people tried to drink their troubles away. In some cases, families became destitute. Children were farmed out to relatives and others, as families simply could not afford to take care of them.

At this time, syphilis was rampant and incurable. Many of the people committed to mental hospitals or insane asylums were suffering from advanced syphilis. The tertiary stage of syphilis involves the destruction of the central nervous system. When it was discovered that syphilis was caused by a bacterium in 1900, this made a strong impression on people's thinking. Here was a clear case where insanity was due to a disease and the disease due to an identifiable physical pathogen. Awareness of this undoubted fact encouraged the belief that other kinds of insane behaviour might be caused by a physiological agent.

The hankering for a genetic, bacterial, viral, or physiological cause of 'mental illness' (disconcerting behaviour), including addiction, was boosted and has remained intense ever since. What is interesting today is that mental illness, including addiction, is still attributed to a physiological disease agent, even though, after all this time, no physiological disease agent has been identified in the overwhelming majority of cases. In those few cases, such as syphilis of the brain, where a purely physical cause has been found, these cases have tended to become part of ordinary physical medicine, no longer attracting the interest of psychiatrists or clinical psychologists preoccupied with supposed 'diseases of the mind'. Advanced syphilis and Alzheimer's, for example, are not considered real 'mental illnesses', precisely because they are physical diseases with identifiable physical causes.

After the Civil War, Protestant religious leaders began to perceive alcohol itself as evil. The Women's Christian Temperance Union and other organizations like the Anti-Saloon League marked a new trend in attitudes regarding alcohol. Alcohol, the substance itself, was blamed or attributed for the problems that resulted from drinking. Alcohol was renamed 'demon rum', 'that engine of the devil', and its manufacture, distribution, and transportation banned through the passage of the Volstead Act.[11]

Prohibition worked in the sense that incidence of cirrhosis of the liver, for example, declined during the approximate 13–14 years *Prohibition* was in force. Some people were induced by its illegality to stop drinking. But *Prohibition* failed in other ways:

1   law enforcement could not control black market crime resulting from the illegality of alcohol;
2   most people still believed they had a right to drink and the government had no business telling them what they could and could not put into their bodies;
3   legislators and other leaders in government became concerned that prohibition was breeding a general sense of lawlessness;
4   the United States was in the middle of a severe economic depression, and political leaders realized that much needed revenue could be gathered by legalizing and taxing sales of alcohol; and finally,
5   many people just did not believe the political rhetoric of prohibitionists. They did not believe that alcohol was a universally addictive substance, something that would make anyone an 'alcoholic'. Most people knew perfectly well that they could drink without serious trouble.

Prohibition was repealed in 1933. However, repeal coincided with yet another important shift in the attribution of trouble brought about through the consumption of alcohol. A new spiritual self-help fellowship of chronic drinkers was founded, Alcoholics Anonymous (AA), and with its establishment came a new perspective on alcohol.

People in AA acknowledged that alcohol was not addictive for most people. However, for a minority of the population (as high as 10 per cent), alcohol was an *irresistible* addiction. For some reason, attributed to some genetic or biological factor that made people with the disease of alcoholism different from the normal population, alcohol consumption unleashed the disease of alcoholism. This disease was characterized by 'loss of control'. For the 10 per cent born with this mysterious biological difference – as yet unidentified – when they consumed alcohol they could not stop. If they took one or two drinks, loss of control was unleashed, and they swallowed drink after drink, usually until they passed out. Regardless of any intention to the contrary, alcoholics could not control their drinking. It was physically impossible for them to have just one or a few drinks and then stop.[12]

Thus, the disease concept was reborn with AA and other derived *Twelve Steps* programmes. Addiction was not universal but confined to a minority. For that minority, heavy drinking was irresistible and involuntary. An alcoholic (a drunk) was fated by his bodily constitution to be always an alcoholic. He could never be cured. The only salvation was for the alcoholic, instead of exerting his will, to renounce his will to 'a higher power' (God), following which the alcoholic must totally abstain from alcohol. In such programmes, the first lesson is to accept that you are helpless and can do nothing to control your disease.

Popularity of the AA theory

The AA theory of alcoholism has become very popular. Movies in which a character who used to be a drunk but has been dry for a while takes 'that one drink' and then automatically takes another 20 and becomes paralytic drunk are familiar enough. Most people probably suppose that there is some scientific support for the AA theory. But among those knowledgeable about research into addiction, the AA claims are controversial, and the full package of AA beliefs about addiction is always rejected.

Ever since AA asserted that 10 per cent of the population was born with the disease of alcoholism, a disease allegedly characterized by loss of control, researchers have been testing the loss of control hypothesis. No research has been able to observe loss of control with any drug. For example, a group of long-time heavy drinkers, classified as the most severe kind of alcoholics, were allowed as much alcohol as they could drink daily and were at the same time given incentives, in the form of better living conditions if they reduced their alcohol consumption. They moderated their drinking when they could gain improved living conditions by doing so. Similar results have been found for marijuana and cocaine. A study of heroin use by Vietnam veterans found that they were in control of their heroin use and could moderate it if they *chose*.

The scientific evidence we have fully corroborates the view that a person's mindset, their values, and the way they experience their environment are the most accurate explanations and predictors of use. The more a person believes he has the power to control or abstain from drugs, the more likely he is going to do what is necessary for him to achieve this goal. Both common sense and research support this truism. Conversely, the more a person believes he cannot abstain or control his behaviour, the less he is going to do to prepare for this. Convince people they are helpless and they will be more likely to act helpless. Convince people they are powerful and they will often demonstrate how powerful they can be. The *Twelve Steps* message is therefore exactly the worst thing to tell people with a drug problem.[13]

Today people who want help often turn to AA (or offspring like Narcotics Anonymous, NA). In AA, a religious conversion experience – conversion to a spiritual 'higher power' – is necessary to achieve and maintain abstinence and sobriety. ('Spiritual thinking' refers to belief in a metaphysical power that can influence personal experience.[14]) While people in AA, eager to please recruits from all religious backgrounds, will say that their 'higher power' can be anything a person wants it to be, there is one exception to this: they will not allow the *person* himself to be his own 'higher power'.

According to AA doctrine, a person has gotten into trouble, unleashing the dormant disease within himself, because he thought he could control his behaviour. This is what the AA historian Ernest Kurtz meant by 'not-God' as a central tenet in AA ideology. In other words, the person thought *he was the higher power*, he thought *he* was God. In order to have a true conversion experience and work the spiritual path of AA, he must realize he is 'not-God', something else is. From this standpoint, alcoholism is rooted in hubris. This is why abstinence is not sufficient in AA. A person must ultimately become 'sober' and get over his 'pride problem'. He must get over thinking he can control his own behaviour and recognize that only God or his 'higher power' can control his behaviour. (A difficulty with this AA doctrine is that it seems to point to the conclusion that once the person has overcome his pride problem and yielded everything to God, the person then ought to be able to drink moderately and responsibly like the normal 90 per cent of the population. But instead AA insists that the person must remain totally abstinent ever after.[15-17])

Psychologically, the focus of treatment is in the exact opposite direction to what extensive research on self-efficacy reveals. According to this research, the more one *believes* he has the power to do what is necessary to achieve responsible drinking or drug use, the more likely he is to do what is necessary to achieve that goal.

As a grassroots self-help organization, AA has many admirable qualities. It provides comradeship and comfort to many who benefit from these things. But AA also perpetuates harmful myths about addiction, and there is no evidence that AA has ever made any difference to the aggregate number of people who drink or don't drink. In this, AA is on a par with all other currently known treatment programmes.

How the disease metaphor misleads us

Today, people say that drinking alcohol is the same as having a disease like diabetes, heart disease, or cancer. The analogy is far from accurate or reciprocal. Normally, people with real disease receive medical treatment by consent only. Even when death is inevitable without treatment, a patient has the right to refuse any and all medicine or treatment. (see Chapter 2) This is generally not true when people have metaphorical diseases. Despite the fact that so many people say that behaviour can be a disease, we can learn a great deal about the two by studying the difference.

As a point of reference, the word 'patient' refers to a socially assigned role. Being a patient does not mean that a person is sick or has a disease. Some people are very ill and refuse to be patients. Christian Scientists, for example, believe that sickness and suffering are illusions produced in the mind by bad thoughts. They often refuse to adopt the role of patient, even when they do have diseases. Some people are patients and are not sick. Consider a malingerer, a person diagnosed with Munchausen's Syndrome and someone who wants to commit suicide.

There are three conditions where treatment of literal physical illnesses proceeds ethically and legally without consent today:

1   when a patient is literally unconscious, we treat him because he does not have the capacity to refuse treatment;
2   when a patient is literally a child we treat him against his wishes because he does not comprehend the consequences of refusing treatment; and
3   when a patient is literally contagious, we treat him to protect others.

When it comes to behaviour that is purportedly a threat to self and others, mental health workers in the United States have adapted these three conditions to justify treatment without consent. This is just as true for people labelled mentally ill as it is for people labelled alcoholic or addicted.

1   The patient is said to be metaphorically unconscious. He lacks insight into his 'disease'.
2   The person suffering with a form of mental illness called addiction is said to be a metaphorical child. He doesn't take care of himself, because he is addicted. He must be protected from himself.
3   The drug addict is said to be metaphorically contagious, that is, because of his disease, in this case addiction, he is allegedly more prone to hurt others.

Despite the fact that we cannot predict who is likely to harm himself or others, the US Supreme Court has upheld the right of state authorities to deprive individuals said to be suffering from mental illness of their liberty in the name of clinical treatment for their disease. This mistaken reasoning is one which subverts the Constitution. The US Bill of Rights states that the government cannot deprive a citizen of due process or equal protection of law without a fair and speedy trial. A person must be accused (indicted) and found guilty (convicted) of a crime in order to be deprived of liberty. Proper procedures assuring fairness must be followed.

When it comes to treating people for mental illness, and all its various derivatives, like drug addiction, none of that now matters to American courts. The drug addict is said to be metaphorically unconscious, metaphorically a child, and metaphorically contagious – drug addicts are supposedly contagious because they can spread their addiction disease and infect others or they can hurt others because of their disease. As a result, they must be either put in jail or coerced into treatment (which means having one's values, purposes, and goals changed through *conversations* with a therapist).

Can we handle the truth about drugs?

Drugs are neither good nor bad; neither safe nor dangerous. The applicability of these terms depends entirely on *how* one uses the drugs in question, for what purpose, and with what consequences. When someone says 'drugs are a problem', we must ask the question: 'A problem according to whom?' Heroin, for example, is one of the most effective drugs for reducing pain. In some countries, heroin is the preferred drug for reducing the pain associated with terminal illness. In the United States, the drug is considered too 'dangerous' for that purpose, even when a person has only months to live. The person who has 3 months to live might get addicted to heroin!

Many people have become so confused by anti-drug propaganda that they tend to believe 'dangerous', 'safe', 'good', and 'bad' are chemical properties of illegal or prescription-only drugs, identifiable by chemical analysis. When it comes to the 'science' of addiction and addictive drugs, we generally find politicized science and science fiction. This masquerade concerning science is designed to strengthen prohibition and anti-drug activities on the part of the state and to secure jobs and income for drug warriors and drug treatment providers. It is money wasted that could be used to fight real crime, not victimless crimes, and real diseases like cancer and heart disease.

Consider the following points about the difference between behaviour and disease. A behaviour is voluntary, a disease is not. Behaviour refers to mode of conduct and cannot be found in a body after death. A disease refers to a cellular abnormality or a lesion, and this can be found in a corpse. Behaviours refer to something that people do. They are expressions of personal values, morals and ethics. Diseases are something that people have. They are physical changes in tissues, and they are not expressions of values, morals and ethics. We change our behaviours by exercising our free will as moral agents. We can neither will the onset of a disease, nor can we will it away. Willpower and choice have nothing to do with disease. Drinking too much alcohol is a behaviour that can result in cirrhosis of the liver. But drinking is a behaviour, not a disease, and cirrhosis is a disease, not a behaviour.

The same is true for smoking. Purchasing, lighting, and inhaling smoke from a burning cigarette is a behaviour. Chronic obstructive pulmonary disease, cancer, and emphysema are all diseases. Smoking is a behaviour, not a disease, and cancer is a disease, not a behaviour. The difference is important to clear thinking about addiction. Addiction has come to mean something prescriptive, not descriptive. It is used to say that a person is doing too much of something, according to the values of others. Addiction has become a value judgment about social conformity, not the objective description of a fact.

Attributions, descriptions, and explanations

Descriptions of behaviours and diseases are different from explanations of behaviours and diseases. Explanations are different from descriptions; however, people often confuse the two, just as they often confuse signs with symptoms. For example, if you ask someone, what is depression or schizophrenia, many are inclined to say 'a chemical imbalance in the brain'. That is an explanation, not a description.

People argue about the most accurate explanations for addiction. However, the empirical facts speak for themselves: Mindset, individual values, and how people experience their environment are more accurate predictors of drug use than the chemical properties of drugs, genetics and biological changes that occur through use characterized by withdrawal and tolerance. No two people are identical. No two people use drugs for the exact same reason, in the exact same way, and with the exact same results.

It is claimed that cigarette smokers continue to smoke because they are addicted to nicotine. If this were true, nicotine replacement therapy would work. If cigarette smokers were just nicotine addicts, they could pop nicotine pills and eliminate the increased risk of lung cancer along with nearly all the other deleterious health effects of smoking. If smokers don't stop smoking by switching to other means of ingesting nicotine, there must be something about the experience of smoking, over and above the ingestion of nicotine, which they find enjoyable and rewarding. It may be the ritual or ceremony of smoking or the physical excitement as smoke hits the lungs.

The disease model, as an explanatory paradigm, first suggested by Rush, refined by prohibition, and developed by AA, is philosophically deterministic: 'something' allegedly *causes* a person to use a drug, to seek out and change the way he feels, and perceives himself and the world. Man is no longer considered a moral agent responsible for his actions and their consequences. It is more accurate to look at drug use as a choice – people choose to use drugs for reasons that are important to them. Naturally, a choice may be foolish or ill-advised. But a bad choice is still a choice.

Some policy implications

When it comes to legal arenas, addiction is exculpatory when viewed as a disease. Criminal acts are said to stem involuntarily from the addiction-disease state. If addiction is involuntary, then acts stemming from addiction status are also involuntary. This is the key to understanding a disease-model defence. Diseases have symptoms that stem from disease status. The two are inseparable. Thus, if the disease is involuntary, as all diseases are, then the symptoms that stem from the disease are involuntary, too. Celebrities and others guilty of obnoxious behaviour are aware that they may be forgiven or treated leniently if they proclaim that their behaviour stems from a disease.

Criminal acts that are said to stem involuntarily from addiction-disease status are equally inseparable and involuntary. Criminal acts stemming from disease status are the inseparable and involuntary symptoms or signs of a disease, like sneezing, having a fever, and perhaps most similarly to a seizure or a convulsion that stems from epilepsy. This is how attorneys try to persuade judges and juries that criminal acts by addicts are not immoral, not unethical, and most important, not voluntary. In order for a person to be found guilty of a criminal act, two elements must be present: *mens rea* (guilty mind; intent) and *actus reus* (the criminal act). Addiction, like all mental illness, allegedly undermines *mens rea*.

Another serious policy issue is raised by the increasing reliance of the legal system on treatment programmes, especially *Twelve Step* programmes like AA, as all such programmes, and most obviously AA, are religious. They are mostly religious in the narrow sense that they refer to a spiritual realm, but they are all religious in the broader sense that they seek to overhaul a person's fundamental values. When the state coerces persons into AA because they have harmed someone else, usually through drunk driving, or because they are said to be a danger to themselves or others because of drinking and drug use, the religious nature of treatment becomes constitutionally dubious.

Church and state are legally separate. If the state orders a person into something the courts deem a religious activity, in my country, a violation of the First Amendment to the US Constitution has occurred. The majority of treatment programmes in the United States. meet the court's criteria for religious activities. Several state courts have now ruled that AA is a religious organization. Since AA is such an integral part of treatment for addiction throughout the United States, it is likely that the state's involvement in treatment for addiction could prove to be unconstitutional.

The relevant portion of the First Amendment reads, 'Congress shall make no law respecting an establishment of religion, or prohibiting the free exercise thereof …' The free exercise clause is invoked generally when a person objects to being forced to believe in the ideology of AA and disease-model forms of treatment. This is because a person must admit that he has a disease in order to be viewed as progressing successfully through treatment. The effect may be that some individuals are punished because they dissent from the belief system promoted by psychiatrists, counsellors, and therapists.

In this way, disease-model-based treatment programmes are a problem masquerading as a solution. Even if a person enters AA or a disease-model-oriented treatment voluntarily, the establishment clause violation is called into question when the state subsidizes or 'touches' an activity deemed religious. The state must remain neutral in relation to religion, and neither condemn nor encourage entanglement with a religious programme.[18]

Any number of types of psychotherapy could be used to help a person learn to drink or use drugs responsibly, or, as is usually the case, to become abstinent. Most treatment programmes in the United States are abstinence oriented. However, the theory that a person can only cease to be addicted by total abstention, and not by moderating his drug consumption, is a false theory, disproven by research. Disease-model-based ideology governing treatment is derived from the belief that people addicted to drugs cannot control their behaviour, and can never learn to control their behaviour, when it comes to drug use. Treating behaviour is different from treating a disease. Treating behaviour is either a matter of eliciting the person's voluntary co-operation in rethinking their goals, values and habits, or it is a matter of coercion. This is not true when it comes to treating a real disease.

In the realm of social and public policy, rules for behaviour are laid out in an enforcement venue. For example, consider a restaurant that has a no smoking policy and another that allows smoking. In the past, owners of private property set the rules regarding smoking and no smoking behaviour. Today, in the name of public health, private establishments are increasingly forced to comply with coercively imposed regulations, where the state dictates rules regarding smoking and drinking, regardless of what establishment owners say. The state adopts a paternalistic attitude towards adult citizens, treating them as if they were a threat to themselves. More often than not, it seems that adults embrace this paternalism on an abstract, political level. But when it comes to actually depriving them of freedom in a concrete situation, they may object. At that point it is usually too late.

What then must we do?

Prevalent ideas about addiction are fraught with confusion, contradiction and inconsistency. Historically, various forces within and without the individual have been involved in explaining and blaming the drinking and drug-taking habit. Despite the blatant inaccuracies of so many of these attributions, and the attempt at various points in history to help people disingenuously by reducing stigma through the medicalization of behaviour, viewing addiction as a voluntary behaviour rather than a disease is a key to understanding the truth about why people choose to use drugs and what the consequences of various accurate and inaccurate policy ideas are.

We do well to keep in mind the difference between what drugs *do* to the body and how drugs get *into* the body. Behaviours are choices, the expression of a person's morality. As such, it is clear that we are dealing with an ethical phenomenon when we approach the topic of addiction. The disease concept applied to a behaviour is a mistake with serious consequences. Behaviour remains behaviour, even when people call it disease.

From a legal viewpoint, I advocate the complete repeal of drug prohibition. I also recommend that individuals are held fully responsible for their voluntary actions. If a particular drug taken by an individual makes that individual more likely to behave violently that individual ought to be held accountable for his violent behaviour. If he claims that he could not avoid being violent having taken the drug, then it follows that he ought not have taken the drug. Taking the drug can then be seen as part of the premeditation of his unlawful actions.

Repeal of drug prohibition would not eliminate all regulations restricting drug consumption. If an airline wants to insist that its pilots do not consume certain drugs, it can forbid them to do so, on pain of dismissal, and the same goes for any department of the military. It is also legitimate for a hotel, a restaurant, a casino, or a mall to require its guests not to consume certain drugs on the premises or for government bodies which regulate streets and highways to control the use of drugs thereon, just as they now control nudity, excessive noise, or driving under the influence of alcohol.

Government should stop using its income to pay for addiction treatment and should not require that healthcare insurance cover addiction treatment. In the United States government support runs the risk of violating the First Amendment. Second, there is no evidence that any kind of addiction treatment is any more effective than doing nothing; the research suggests not. Third, supplying offenders with expensive treatment without charge feeds their narcissistic sense of entitlement and is an unjust imposition on taxpayers. At the same time, individuals should be entirely free to patronize any kind of 'addiction treatment' they want – at their own expense.[19]

Notes

1 Schaler, J. A. (2000) *Addiction Is a Choice*, Chicago, IL: Open Court.
2 Fingarette, H. (1988) *Heavy Drinking: The Myth of Alcoholism as a Disease*, Berkeley, CA: University of California Press.
3 Edwards, G., Orford, J., Egert, S., Guthrie, S., Hawker, A., Hensman, C., Mitcheson, M., Oppenheimer, E., and Taylor, C. (1977) 'Alcoholism: a controlled trial of "Treatment" and "Advice"', *Journal of Studies on Alcohol*, *38*, 1004–31.
4 Milam, J. R., and Ketcham, K. (1983) *Under the Influence: A Guide to the Myths and Realities of Alcoholism*, New York, NY: Bantam.
5 Fingarette, op. cit.
6 Levine, H. G. (1984) 'The alcohol problem in America: from temperance to alcoholism', *British Journal of Addiction*, *79*, 109–19.
7 Levine, H. G. (1978) 'The discovery of addiction: changing conceptions of habitual drunkenness in America', *Journal of Studies on Alcohol*, *39*, 143–74.
8 Szasz, T. (1970) *The Manufacture of Madness: A Comparative Study of the Inquisition and the Mental Health Movement*, New York, NY: Harper and Row.

 9 Conrad, P., and Schneider, J. W. (1992) *Deviance and Medicalization: From Badness to Sickness.* Expanded Edition, Philadelphia, PA: Temple University Press.

10 Schaler, J. A. (2004) 'Giving Marmor credit for the idea that homosexuality is not an illness is undeserved', *British Medical Journal*, 21 February, Letter.

11 Gusfield, J. R. (1963) *Symbolic Crusade: Status Politics and the American Temperance Movement*, Urbana, IL: University of Illinois Press.

12 Jellinek, E. M. (1960) *The Disease Concept of Alcoholism*, New Haven, CT: Hillhouse Press.

13 Schaler, J. A. (1996a) 'Thinking about drinking: the power of self-fulfilling prophecies', *International Journal of Drug Policy*, 7, 187–92.

14 Schaler, J. A. (1996b) 'Spiritual thinking in addiction treatment providers. The spiritual belief scale', *Alcoholism Treatment Quarterly*, *14*, 7–33.

15 Kurtz, E. (1988) *A.A.: The Story. Revised edition of Not-God: A History of Alcoholics Anonymous*, New York, NY: Harper and Row.

16 Schaler (1996b) op. cit.

17 Schaler, J. A. (2005) 'Just one sip for Sipowicz to slip', In G. Yeffeth (ed.) *What would Sipowicz Do?: Race, Rights and Redemption in NYPD Blue*, Dallas, TX: BenBella Books, pp. 63–71.

18 Schaler (2000) and Schaler (2005) op. cit.

19 Alexander, B. K. (2008) *The Globalisation of Addiction: A Study in Poverty of the Spirit*, Oxford: Oxford University Press.

19 Younger people and mental health care

Tim McDougall

Introduction

This chapter discusses the role of the mental health professional in supporting children and young people with mental health problems. After a summary of how mental health problems affect children and young people, a brief description of what services are available to help them, issues of consent, competence and capacity and confidentiality are discussed. Working with children and young people who have mental health problems generates a range of ethical and moral concerns associated with decision making and the journey a dependent child makes to become an independent young adult. Issues such as age of the child or young person, their developmental understanding of the issues involved and the views of their parents or carers must always be taken into consideration. This is not always a straightforward process and mental health professionals often require guidance to make competent care and treatment decisions. Although the chapter is based around a consideration of UK mental health care, it is assumed that the principles have a much wider international relevance.

Background

There are nearly 12 million children under 18 living in England and as many as 1 million will have a mental health problem serious enough to require specialist help.[1] This is in addition to many more young people with significant mental health needs, including children in need, looked after children and disabled children, all of whom are at heightened risk of developing mental health problems and disorders. Rates of mental disorder rise steeply during late adolescence and early adulthood and many mental health problems persist into adulthood, affecting people for their whole lives.

Children's emotional health and psychological wellbeing

The terms 'mental health needs' and 'mental health problems' are often used interchangeably. This can be misleading. Mental health, or 'emotional wellbeing' as it has become increasingly known in children's services, is used to refer to psychological building blocks such as emotional resilience, good self-esteem and the skills to resolve conflict and cope in the face of stress and adversity. All children should have the opportunity to develop good mental health and emotional resilience, and this is fundamental to their overall health and wellbeing.

In comparison, the terms mental health problems and mental disorders refer to difficulties or problems that impact negatively on wellbeing and which require resolution. Mental health problems are often not serious and are transient in nature. Whilst they can interfere with a child's development and functioning, they are distinguished from mental disorders as being less severe, less complex and less persistent in nature. Mental health problems and disorders manifest in children's behaviour, how they feel and what they tell us.

The definition and classification of mental disorder in childhood is an area of debate and uncertainty amongst professionals and the general public. As Mitchell[2] points out, unusual behaviours, emotions or thought processes are included in formal classifications of mental disorder. These occur in a socio-cultural context and during the developmental phases of childhood and adolescence. Indeed, where normal childhood behaviour stops and mental disorder starts is an area of considerable international controversy and debate. For example, the cardinal features of attention deficit hyperactivity disorder (ADHD) are hyperactivity, impulsivity and inattention. However, many argue that being hyperactive, impulsive and inattentive is developmentally normal and just part of being a child.

There is no doubt that clinical thresholds for mental disorder are socially and culturally influenced and determine how a child or young person's functioning is viewed as impairing or otherwise.[3] However, there has been growing concern about an emphasis on a bio-medical model of understanding and explaining children's behaviour.[1] This, critics argue, is a product of Western society where children and young people are all too often labelled as having psychiatric disorders, behaviour problems and special educational needs.[5] Psychiatric diagnoses are also potentially stigmatising. Categorical rather than multi-dimensional systems of diagnosis are commonly used in Europe and North America and emphasise deviation from the 'normal'. However, for children and young people who are concerned about fitting in, psychiatric diagnosis may be unhelpful and potentially harmful to their self-image and relationships with others.

Why is the mental health of children and young people important?

The emotional health and psychological wellbeing of children and young people is a key plank of public health and mental health policy and strategy in the United Kingdom. Internationally, governments are becoming aware that there are numerous reasons to invest now for the future economy and prosperity of their respective countries. Help and support at an earlier stage is likely to be more effective and less costly than that which will be needed over a lifetime if the opportunity for prevention or early intervention is missed.

Research and outcome studies prove clearly that untreated mental health problems place children and young people on developmental trajectories towards a range of negative outcomes. These include educational failure, family dysfunction, poor physical health, crime and anti-social behaviour. Many unresolved mental health problems in childhood persist into adulthood, disrupting personal development, employment, social functioning and economic wellbeing. As well as a range of negative outcomes for the people involved, this places a future burden on the economy through long-term demands on adult mental health services, social services, general health services and the criminal justice system.

What are child and adolescent mental health services (CAMHS)?

Usually referred to by its acronym 'CAMHS', child and adolescent mental health services refers to a network of universal and specialist mental health services that are collectively designed to meet the emotional and psychological needs of children and young people. However, the term CAMHS is used in a variety of different ways and this often causes confusion. Although various attempts have been made to clarify what CAMHS means in practice, debate continues within the professions and services and consensus has not been reached.

The most influential strategy document to set the context in which CAMHS in the United Kingdom have evolved was the National Health Services (NHS) Health Advisory Service (HAS) report, *Together We Stand*.[6] This introduced the now widely used tiered model, explored the role, commissioning and management of CAMHS and recommended a co-ordinated approach to service delivery. Within this framework, CAMHS are described according to a four-tier framework, with each tier characterised by increasingly specialised levels of intervention, care and treatment (see Fig. 19.1).

Frontline professionals in primary, universal or mainstream services at Tier 1 are usually the first point of contact for children and young people. For Tier 1 professionals such as school nurses, health visitors, General Practitioners (GPs) or social workers CAMHS are not their core business and they do not usually have expertise in relation to children's mental health. However, like all professionals charged with the care and welfare of children, primary care workers share joint responsibility for safeguarding and promoting emotional health and psychological wellbeing. They also help prevent mental health problems and disorders and offer support for less-complex difficulties a child may be experiencing. Tier 1 professionals may encounter children and young people who have been traumatised, abused or bereaved, those who harm themselves or others and those with behaviour problems. All are responsible for helping children to develop the building blocks of mental health – good self-esteem, emotional literacy and the skills to resolve conflict in non-destructive and pro-social ways.

CAMHS professionals working at Tier 2 provide training and consultation for Tier 1 colleagues and usually practice through a multi-professional network rather than as part of a multidisciplinary team. Professionals working in services at both Tiers 1 and 2 must be able to access specialist CAMHS for children and young people with more severe, complex or persistent mental health problems. This is for specialist assessment, treatment or management.

Tier 3 CAMHS are local, community-based multidisciplinary teams that include nurses, psychiatrists, psychologists, family therapists, social workers and creative therapists. Tier 3 CAMHS provide a range of assessment and treatment interventions. Sometimes young people have mental health problems that severely impact on day-to-day functioning and quality of life or present the young person or those around them at risk of harm. Tier 4 CAMHS are defined as highly specialised CAMHS and include in-patient child and adolescent units, specialised out-patient services and forensic CAMHS, as well as multi-agency services such as home-based treatment services, community support teams and crisis teams (see Fig. 19.1).

The tiered model is not without fault, and critics argue that it should be dropped in favour of universal, targeted and specialist services, the nomenclature of mainstream children's services. Some mistakenly assume that the higher the tier the more complex the young people receiving services within it are. This is not necessarily the case, and the tiered model should be understood as a way of organising services rather than a way of categorising children and young people who require such services. In addition, the tiered model has been criticised for being too health and illness focused, with insufficient consideration to the broader psychosocial context in which children with mental health problems live their lives.

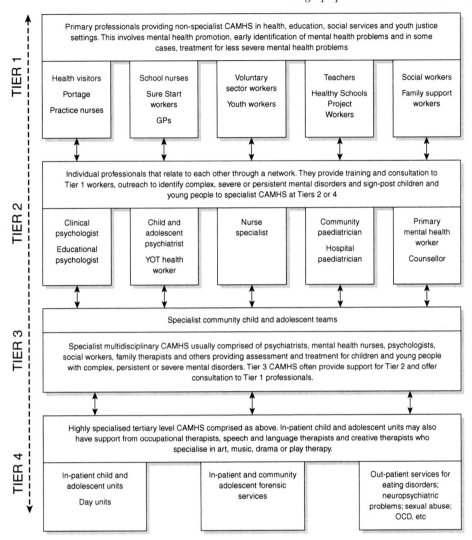

Figure 19.1 CAMHS tiered model of service delivery.[7]

What do CAMHS professionals do?

CAMHS professionals who support children and young people provide holistic interventions. They see the young person as a whole and recognise that their needs, as well as those of their family, are unique. This is not to say that the range of professionals working in CAMHS have the same philosophical, theoretical and therapeutic approach to their work. On the contrary, the background, training and experience of the range of professionals working in specialist CAMHS are broad and varied. Many are skilled at providing psychotherapeutic support, including psychodynamic, cognitive behavioural and family therapy. The holistic approach to care is enabled by well-developed communication skills and ability to engage, creatively and flexibly, with the young person and their family in a number of different ways. The therapeutic approach is tailored to the needs of the individual and family and is usually based on the developmental needs of the child, the available evidence base and the views and choices of all those involved.

Human rights and young people

Human rights in general have been discussed by various authors throughout this book. There are, however, additional considerations for mental health professionals who work with children and young people. Along with the European Convention on Human Rights and the Human Rights Act, the United Nations Convention on the Rights of the Child (UNCRC)[8] provides the overarching human rights framework affecting children and young people.

The UNCRC was the first legally binding international instrument to incorporate the full range of human rights. In 1989 world leaders decided that children needed a special convention because people under 18 years often need special care and protection that adults do not. The leaders also wanted to make sure that the world recognised that children have human rights too.[9] The UNCRC establishes a range of civil and political, socio-economic and cultural rights that apply to all children and young people. Although UK courts have no authority to directly apply the UNCRC principles they can be taken into consideration and have direct relevance to the care and treatment of children and young people. For example, article 37 of the UNCRC states that every child deprived of liberty shall be separated from adults unless it is considered in the child's best interests not to do so. This article was taken into account by the English government when the Mental Health Act 1983 was amended to provide age-appropriate accommodation for children and young people requiring admission to hospital for mental health care (see Chapter 25).

As well as several important articles, there are two guiding principles that professionals who work with children and young people must always take into account in their day-to-day work. First is a need to consider the best interests and views of the child. Second is that decisions in relation to children and young people must be made in a manner consistent with the evolving capacities of the child. This means that as children mature and grow up towards independence, their views and wishes should be given greater weight in the decision-making process. However, there is a general consensus that a child's identity is less firmly formed than an adult's, and that the values, wishes and intentions on which they base their decisions may be less secure.[10]

Balancing human rights with mental health care is not always straightforward. To illustrate, article 19 of the UNCRC entitles children to the right to protection from all forms of violence. States must take measures to protect children from all formals of physical and mental violence, injury or abuse and neglect. This includes a requirement to take measures to protect children from suicide and self-harm. This principle is also enshrined in professional obligations associated with safeguarding, welfare and child protection. This can present mental health professionals with various dilemmas.

For example, many young people choose to self-harm and the mental health professional must consider a range of factors to do with autonomy, choice and privacy and broker these with their professional, organisational and contractual obligations to keep vulnerable young people safe. Perhaps not surprisingly such decisions are often contentious, and mental health professionals sometimes make poorly informed decisions or disagree amongst themselves about whether a decision is reasonable or valid. This contention occurs at a moral, ethical and personal level. Various authors have drawn attention to the impact of individual values, beliefs and attitudes and how these can influence decision making.[11,12]

Children's rights

Along with human rights law, the Children Act 1989 provides the key legal framework governing the care and welfare of all children and young people under 18. The Children Act[13] was passed in order to bring private and public law provisions in a single legislative framework affecting children and families. It attempts to strike a balance between the rights of children, the responsibilities of parents to their child and the duty of statutory agencies to intervene when concerns about the child's welfare requires them to do so.

The welfare principle is of paramount importance when mental health professionals are supporting children and young people with mental health problems. Although the principle has no direct application outside a court setting, the best interests of a child must always be a guiding consideration for organisations' professionals. Importantly, the Children Act refers to children in need and the duty placed on local authorities to safeguard and promote the welfare of children in need. Within the meaning of the Act, a child is in need if he or she is disabled or suffering from a mental disorder of any kind. Whilst the Children Act 1989 has since been amended, most importantly by the Children (Leaving Care) Act 2000,[14] the Adoption and Children Act 2002[15] and the Children Act 2004,[16] the original Act remains in use today and its guiding principles underpin all mental health interventions with children and young people.

Respecting rights

The UNCRC and the Children Act 1989 entitle children to participatory decision-making rights. As children and young people become older and move towards independence their involvement in decision making increases. Whatever the age of the child, it is always important to keep them as fully informed and involved as possible. They should receive clear and detailed information in a format that is appropriate to their age and developmental understanding.

Just as adults are entitled to privacy, dignity and respect, so too are children and young people. Despite these rights and entitlements, young people often report that they are not involved in decisions, frequently have their privacy, dignity and confidentiality compromised and do not feel that professionals respect them.[17] This is unacceptable in modern mental health services and professionals must improve their practice in this area. However, it is important to be clear that the right of children and young people to be involved in decision making does not necessarily mean they make the final decision and their right may be mediated through the law on consent.[18]

Parental rights

The Children Act 1989 defines parental responsibility as 'all the rights, duties, powers, responsibilities and authority which by law a parent has in relation to a child and his property'. Wherever the mental health care and treatment of a child or young person is being considered the person or persons with parental responsibility must be identified and their views sought as appropriate.

The person with parental responsibility is usually, but not always, the child or young person's parent. However, it is important to establish who has parental responsibility and whether this is shared with another parent or the local authority. This is important because they may be able to consent to their child's treatment or authorise admission to hospital if this is deemed to be necessary. It is generally good practice to involve those with parental responsibility even if they do not consent to their child's treatment. The mother of a child will automatically have parental responsibility for her child unless the child has been adopted by someone else. The father has responsibility for his child if he either:

- was married to the child's mother at the time of the child's birth;
- acquires parental responsibility by becoming registered on the birth certificate;
- makes a parental responsibility agreement with the child's mother;
- acquires parental responsibility through a court order.

Step-parents may acquire parental responsibility through a residence order, by adopting the child or being their legal guardian as defined in the Children Act. The local authority can also acquire parental responsibility for a child. This is through a care order and, with restrictions, under an emergency protection order.

Shared parental responsibility

Where more than one person has parental responsibility for a child, each of them may act alone, and without the other, in meeting that responsibility. This means that, for example, mental health professionals can lawfully provide treatment to the child with the authority of one parent, even though both parents have parental responsibility. A person who does not have parental responsibility for a child but has care of the child may do what is reasonable under the circumstances to safeguard or promote the child's welfare. Whether or not the intervention can be considered reasonable depends on the urgency or seriousness of the situation and the extent to which it is practicable to consult a person with parental responsibility.[19] This allows mental health professionals to act in emergencies where treatment is considered necessary; for example, following a serious overdose.

Confidentiality

We have heard that regardless of their age, children and young people have various rights. This includes a common law right to confidentiality which should be generally observed. There are circumstances in which a child or young person's confidentiality can be breached, and this is when there are significant concerns that the child or another child may be at significant risk of harm. Some argue that the potential for breach of confidentiality may clash with the principles of a therapeutic relationship.[20]

Mental health professionals should have a clear understanding of their duties of confidentiality, and any limits to such an obligation should be made clear to the child or young person who has the capacity to understand. This of course presents risks. For example, a child who has been repeatedly let down by adults may struggle to form a trusting therapeutic relationship with mental health professionals and it is therefore crucially important to get the balance right. Where information does need to be shared in the best interests of a child, the amount of information shared should be proportionate to the risk being considered. Generally speaking, information sharing should be a 'needs to know' basis. Where there is a lack of agreement about information sharing, it is likely that article 8 of the European Convention on Human Rights will be applicable.[21] This means that decisions concerning the disclosure of confidential information about a child without their consent require an analysis of whether the proposed sharing of information is a proportionate response to protect the public interest in question.[22]

Issues to do with confidentiality and information sharing frequently arise in day-to-day work with children and young people with mental health problems. For example, mental health professionals may be concerned that sharing information about a young person's self-harming behaviour may breach their right to confidentiality. This is often the case when working with teenagers where the views of the young person and their parents are both important. Whilst it is vital to have a working knowledge of the legal frameworks involved, simply asking the young person and parents about the rules of engagement can often be helpful and need not involve any breach of confidentiality.

Importantly, concerns about confidentiality must not constrain responsible and safe decision making. It is common sense that the parents of a child who has been given emergency treatment in hospital following an overdose are made aware of the risks involved when their child returns home. Parents have a responsibility to keep their children safe and they cannot fulfil their parental roles and responsibilities if they are unaware of the risks that may cause harm to their child.

Decision making

Before embarking on decision making we must be clear about who can decide and what the purpose of the decision is. We have heard that decisions affecting children and young people must be made in their best interests and must aim to be helpful rather than harmful. These principles are enshrined in codes of professional ethics and the duty to do no harm is at one level straightforward. However, well-intended decisions made by mental health professionals can sometimes lead to greater harm than good. For example, admitting a child to hospital following self-harm may not only temporarily keep them safe, but it may also cause disruption to educational, family and social functioning. For these reasons it is always important for mental health professionals to consider the bigger picture and decide on the least restrictive or least disruptive course of action. Sometimes non-intervention can be more helpful than intervention but this should not be an excuse for rationalising services.

The law provides some degree of clarity about who can decide but offers little guidance in the way of ethical inquiry. Due to the various legal frameworks that interact, decision making in relation to children's mental health care and treatment can often be complex and contentious. A number of terms are used when considering the process of making decisions and these include competence, capacity and consent. As Leighton points out, there is no standard or agreed definition of the clinical concept of competence.[23] Children's competence is determined by their maturity and understanding rather than their fixed chronological age. The status of a child is determined by age boundaries and does not represent the level of maturity and understanding that an individual may hold.[24] This means that children may be competent to make one decision but not another.

Additionally, judgements about competency are culturally bound and made in the context of the transitional phase of childhood which is socially constructed and which varies across cultures. Evaluating competency and capacity is a key part of making mental health care and treatment decisions which affect children and young people. In general terms, a person with the ability to consent should be able to:

- understand in broad terms what the treatment is, what it is for and why it is being proposed;
- understand the principle benefits, risks and alternatives to the treatment being proposed;
- understand the likely consequences of not receiving the treatment being proposed;

- retain the above information for long enough to make an informed decision;
- make a choice that is free from external pressure and secondary gain.

Within the framework of UK law, children and young people can do different things at different ages. This is a socio-political rather than psycho-biological issue. For children and young people in England this may seem bewildering. For example, at age 15 they can be sent to prison. At age 16 they can leave school, get married, have sex, join the armed forces or claim benefits. By age 17 they can drive a car or leave home without their parents consent. However, it is not until they are 18 that young people can vote or buy and smoke cigarettes. The law in relation to consent is different according to age and understanding.

Children under 16

Children under 16 can consent to treatment if they are deemed to be competent to do so. Historically, this has been an area of controversy. In 1980 what was then the Department of Health and Social Security (DHSS) issued guidance on the delivery of family planning services. This stated that in certain situations, a doctor (physician) could prescribe contraception for a girl under 16 without the consent of her parents.

The guidance was later challenged in court and the ruling judge concluded that 'the parental right to determine whether or not their minor child below the age of 16 will have medical treatment terminates if and when the child achieves sufficient understanding and intelligence to enable him or her to understand fully what is proposed'. This became known popularly as the test of 'Gillick competence' and the effect was to allow a Gillick competent child under the age of 16 a right to consent to treatment without the necessity to obtain parental consent.[25]

Young people aged 16 or 17

The assessment of capacity and of the ability to make decisions and consent to treatment is different for young people aged 16 and 17. The Mental Capacity Act 2005[26] provides that all people over 16 have the right to autonomy and independent decision making unless it can be shown that they lack capacity. However, it is important to note that competence and capacity varies according to the decision being proposed. A child or young person may be competent to make one decision but not another. Therefore, any assessment of a child or young person's capacity to consent must be 'decision specific'. For example, consent for one thing (such as the assessment of an eating disorder) does not necessarily mean consent for another thing (such as referral for psychological treatment for the eating disorder).

A child or young person's competence evolves as they mature or grow older. In addition, it may fluctuate temporarily as a result of mental disorder such as anxiety associated with traumatic memories of sexual abuse. It is therefore important that the evaluation of consent for treatment is constantly kept under review by mental health professionals.

Summary

To practice ethically and fulfil their professional obligations and codes of practice, mental health professionals must be able to recognise the rights and responsibilities of children, young people and parents. Mental health professionals are accountable for their care and treatment decisions and must therefore be clear about confidentiality and consent and information sharing as it affects children and young people.

The law affecting children and young people with mental health problems is complex and constantly evolving. It is therefore important that professionals understand the legal frameworks within which they work. They should be familiar with human rights legislation, children's rights and mental health law and how these frameworks interact. This is in order to help ensure that mental health practice is lawful, ethical and up to date.

Key points

- Untreated mental health problems place children and young people on developmental trajectories towards educational failure, family dysfunction, poor physical health, crime and anti-social behaviour. Many unresolved mental health problems in childhood persist into adulthood, disrupting personal development, social functioning and economic wellbeing.
- Mental health professionals who support children and young people provide holistic interventions. They see the young person as a whole and recognise that their needs, as well as those of their family, are broad and varied. The therapeutic approach is tailored to the needs of the individual and family and is based on the developmental needs of the child, the available evidence base and the views and wishes of all those involved.
- The European Convention on Human Rights, the Human Rights Act and the UNCRC provide the overarching human rights framework affecting children and young people.
- Just as adults have the right to privacy, dignity and respect, so too do children and young people. Despite this, young people often report that they are not involved in decisions, frequently have their privacy, dignity and confidentiality compromised and do not feel that professionals respect them. This is unacceptable in modern mental health services.
- Care and treatment decisions affecting children and young people can often be complex. It is important that mental health professionals understand the legal frameworks within which they work. They should be familiar with human rights legislation, children's rights and mental health law and how these frameworks interact. This is in order to help ensure that their practice is lawful, ethical and up to date.

Notes

1 Green, H., McGinnity, A., Meltzer, H., Ford, T., and Goodman, R. *Mental Health of Children and Young People in Great Britain*. London: ONS, 2005.
2 Mitchell, M. The diagnosis and management of complex mental illness in young people. In: Harbour, A. (Ed.). *Children with Mental Disorder and the Law: A Guide to Law and Practice*. London: Jessica Kingsley, 2008.
3 Sonuga-Barke, E. Categorical models in child psychopathology: a conceptual and empirical analysis. *Journal of Child Psychology and Psychiatry and Allied Disciplines*, 1998 (39), 115–33.
4 Brady, G. ADHD, diagnosis and identity. In: Newnes, C. and Radcliffe, N. (Eds.). *Making and Breaking Children's Lives*. Ross on Wye, UK: PCCS Books, 2005.
5 Timimi, S. and Radcliffe, N. The rise and rise of ADHD. In: Newnes, C. and Radcliffe, N. (Eds.). *Making and Breaking Children's Lives*. Ross-on-Wye, UK: PCCS Books, 2005.
6 Health Advisory Service. *Together We Stand: The Commissioning, Role and Management of Child and Adolescent Mental Health Services*. London: HMSO, 1995.
7 Figure 19.1 taken from McDougall, T. *Child and Adolescent Mental Health Nursing*. London: Blackwell, 2006.
8 http://www.unicef.org/crc/ (accessed 2010 Feb 7th).

9 Harbour, A. *Children with Mental Disorder and the Law: A Guide to Law and Practice*. London: Jessica Kingsley, 2008.
10 Dickenson, D. and Jones, D. True wishes: the philosophy and developmental psychology of children's informed consent. *Philosophy, Psychiatry and Psychology*, 1996 (2), 287–303.
11 Seedhouse, D. *Values Based Decision Making for the Caring Professionals*. Wiley: Chichester, 2005.
12 Leighton, S. Ethical issues in working therapeutically. In: Vostanis, P. (Ed.). *Mental Health Interventions and Services for Vulnerable Children and Young People*. London: Jessica Kingsley, 2007.
13 http://www.opsi.gov.uk/acts/acts1989/ukpga_19890041_en_1 (accessed 2010 Feb 7th)
14 http://www.opsi.gov.uk/Acts/acts2000/ukpga_20000035_en_1 (accessed 2010 Feb 7th).
15 http://www.opsi.gov.uk/acts/acts2002/ukpga_20020038_en_1 (accessed 2010 Feb 7th).
16 http://www.opsi.gov.uk/Acts/acts2004/ukpga_20040031_en_1 (accessed 2010 Feb 7th).
17 11 Million (Office of the Children's Commissioner for England). *Pushed into the Shadows: Young People's Experience of Adult Mental Health Facilities*. London: 11 Million, 2007.
18 Harbour, 2008. op. cit.
19 National Institute for Mental Health in England. *The Legal Aspects of the Care and Treatment of Children and Young People with Mental Disorder: A Guide for Professionals*. London: NIMHE, 2009.
20 Hunter, M. *Psychotherapy with Young People in Care: Lost and Found*. Hove, UK: Brunner-Routledge, 2001.
21 http://www.hri.org/docs/ECHR50.html#Convention (accessed 2010 Feb 7th).
22 Department for Education and Skills. *Information Sharing: Practitioners Guide*. London: HMSO, 2006.
23 Leighton, 2007. op. cit.
24 Spencer, G. Children's competency to consent: an ethical dilemma. *Journal of Child Health Care*, 2000 4(3), 117–22.
25 Harbour, 2008 op. cit.
26 http://www.opsi.gov.uk/ACTS/acts2005/ukpga_20050009_en_1 (accessed 2010 Feb 7th).

20 Older people in mental health care

Elizabeth Collier and Natalie Yates-Bolton

Introduction

Specialist mental health services for older people are a relatively new development, introduced in the United Kingdom only 20 years ago. Previously, a need for such services was not recognised. Later life mental illness was seen as an inevitable part of ageing and incurable.[1] This was illustrated in the *1952 Diagnostic and Classification Manual* where adjustment reaction of later life (over 65) and 'senile dementia' were the only diagnoses available for older people.[2] From the 1940s various psychiatrists in the United States and the United Kingdom challenged such views, arguing that dementia was not an inevitable part of ageing and that other mental health problems could be experienced.[1] A sufficient body of evidence was not enough to convince the psychiatric community of this until 1980s when the *Diagnostic and Statistical Manual, 3rd edition, Revision* (DSM III-R)[3] noted that the diagnosis of schizophrenia could be given to people in late adult life.

Despite this, from the 1950s several hospitals introduced day centres and other specialist services for older people with mental illness, but no national policy coordinated such developments and indeed it was discouraged.[1] Scotland was the first to open a specialist unit for joint assessments between psychiatrists and geriatricians.[1]

Old age psychiatry became a separate speciality in the United Kingdom in 1988.[5] However, classification of mental illness had only been investigated with people in younger age groups. As Beekman *et al.*[6] noted, understanding of the symptoms of clinical depression had not been developed in the context of older people with the accompanying complexities and implications of ageing processes and physical illness or both. This remains an ethical issue where complex diagnoses are applied to people for whom they have not been developed. In the clinical literature, factors that influence how depressive disorder presents in old age have been highlighted, including the overlap of physical and somatic symptoms and minimal expression of sadness.[7]

Many countries have little specialist help for older people with mental health problems.[8] de Mendonça Lima *et al.*[9] found that only 66 per cent ($n = 11$) of the 17 countries surveyed in Europe had specialist services for older people and only 10 per cent ($n = 2$) taught old age psychiatry. They reported that the World Health Organisation and the World Psychiatric Association collaborated to highlight the 'limited public and professional awareness of stigma and discrimination related issues with regards to the elderly with a mental disorder' (p. 679). They viewed this as discrimination given the frequency of psychiatric disorders in the people who attend primary care services. They state that even for Europe which is in a comparatively better situation in this regards than other WHO regions, programmes and services for elderly persons are under developed. They argued that stigma against older people combines two sets of interrelating issues; presence of mental disorder and the status of older people in a given society where the lower the social status the higher the stigma. In their survey, stigma in relation to psychosis was judged to be greatest, by contrast with clinical depression and Alzheimer's disease.

This is the situation, to varying degrees, around the world where some mental health problems are still not recognised for older people in classification manuals (e.g. eating disorders), despite clinical cases being recognised.[10,11] The main challenge continues to be discriminatory and nihilistic attitudes towards older people who need mental health care. This prevents the development of equitable and fair services. This is reflected in policy across the international community where several consistent themes have emerged in tackling older people's health. This includes challenging age discrimination; independence; promoting mental health; healthy living and integrated services.[12] This reflects a *population* approach to health care that considers the majority of people. Older people in contact with mental health services, however, remain a minority.

Who are 'older people'?

The previous discussion assumes that we all know *who* we are referring to when we talk about older people; 65 years of age tends to be used as a cut-off for delineating old age. However, from an ethical point of view, this in itself is problematic. In discussing mental health provision should we focus first on the mental health needs or the assumed needs from being 'old'? Mental health policy certainly in the United Kingdom focuses on young people between 18 and 64. There has been no comprehensive *mental health* policy for the over 65s. Policy governing such services is aimed at *older people* as a generic group although rooting out age discrimination has resulted in health services ensuring an approach that considers need rather than age.[13,14] More recently, the attempt to focus on mental ill health in different age groups in one document as a life span approach is more promising.[15]

The provision of services by age-defined categories ensures an arbitrary focus on chronological age. In working for the good of older people in developing specialist services an inadvertent perpetuation of 'the other' has been established, even though we now can expect to find at least two generations of people in the over 65 age groups. Those clinical issues recognised as relevant for older people do not become significant only on a person's 65th birthday. Research samples regarding older people ranges from 50 years plus. The Geriatric Depression Scale was developed with people aged 55 and over but tends to be used only with the over 65s, highlighting a variation between research and practice, in terms of 'who' older people are. Community services are more and more adopting protocols that enable people with many years of contact with an adult service to remain with that service into old age, instead of being moved into an old age service (unless they develop significant physical health problems or dementing illness, as recommended by the Royal College of Psychiatrists).[16] However, despite these developments, it is indirect age discrimination such as negative attitudes that is of the most concern for older people accessing health care.[17] One of the main problems identified by the MOOTS (Moving Out Of The Shadows) report[18] is the pervasive *care* narratives that accompany services for older people, which should be replaced by narratives that focus on *aspirations*. The Department of Health in the United Kingdom has published two similar documents regarding minimum standards for care homes, one concerning 'adults'[19] and one concerning 'older people'.[20] The one for 'older people' has removed all reference to aspirations, a telling omission.

Mental health care and older people

Most health care for older people takes place in primary care and people over 65 years of age constitute the majority users of health services[21] due to older age being a risk factor for a number of physical illness and also arguably due to the accumulation effects of lifestyle choices over the years. The complexities in relation to older people's mental health are demonstrated, in part, through the relationship between physical and mental health problems. These issues are further compounded by the social context of individuals' lives. The United Kingdom enquiry into mental health and wellbeing in later life[22] identified discrimination, participation in meaningful activity, relationships and poverty as the main areas that influence mental health and wellbeing in later life. Similarly, National Health Service (NHS) Scotland[23] found older people's priorities to be family and friends, positive attitudes, keeping active, maintaining capability and independence and negotiating transitions.

The experience of older people with mental health problems is made more challenging due to the low detection rates of such problems amongst older people.[24] United Kingdom rates for people living in care homes are thought to be underestimated[25] and for older people in general hospital care, over 60 per cent have mental health problems.[26] Further, one survey found that 25 per cent of homeless people in London are over 50 years of age. Half of these have mental health problems, half have alcohol problems and half also have physical health problems.[27] Homeless people are not usually registered with a general practitioner (GP) so this part of the population is largely invisible. Thus, the sophisticated mental health provision discussed in mental health policy excludes people who fall into different special consideration. That is, if you live in a care home your health issues may be served by a GP, although you may have access to some specialist mental health support. If you are homeless, you are likely to access services for homeless people rather than for older people. If you are in prison, you are not likely to have your mental health problems addressed, particularly if you are older,[28] and people over 60 constitute the largest growing population of people in prison.[29] For individuals (of any age) who develop types of dementing illnesses (of which there are several hundred), these are not automatically considered complex health care needs according to the Care Quality Commission criteria for registration for care homes.[30] However, approximately 66 per cent of care home residents have a dementia.[31]

The continued problems faced by older people in health services justify the need for a separate age-classified chapter. We are not, however, focusing exclusively on reduced mental capacity issues, an issue that seems too often assumed to be of primary relevance to older people, whereas it can be relevant to people of all ages. We make reference to this to illustrate where it can be wrongly assumed to be the only mental health issue of concern on the basis of beliefs about older people.

In 1991 Barrowclough and Fleming[32] discussed ethical issues in working with older people focusing on decision making and informed consent. Twenty years later, their discussion is still relevant and the slow change from age discriminatory practices is evidenced by continued debate and policy initiatives that attempt to change such practices. Both Beecham *et al.*[33] and the Royal College of Psychiatrists[34] have recently highlighted continued age discrimination in mental health services. Tools that have been developed since 1991 that aid a more objective approach include the Mental Capacity Act[35] and the Human Rights Act.[36]

Some of the challenges in care provision for older people with mental health problems may result from the continued existence of a paternalistic medical model rather than a humanistic model of care service delivery. Paternalistic approaches to care have been shown to reduce personal control,[37] yet ethical discussions focused around autonomy, beneficence, non-maleficence and justice maintain paternalistic approaches.[38] These traditional ethical values are inadequate to guide day-to-day ethical action[39] (see also Chapter 1). The unique terminology of biomedical ethics can result in it being perceived as a specialist interest subject rather than an everyday accessible issue.

Ethical practice

The starting point for our discourse on ethically based care is grounded in the values of the individual whose life becomes the focus of all care and ethical decisions. This reflects a shift in some aspects of society towards more humanistic approaches to interventions and interactions where the values of the individual concerned are central to decision making. In mental health care this is illustrated through practice development in relation to contemporary recovery values, although this is much less well developed within older peoples services. Alternative approaches to ethics propose a refocus using existential and human advocacy within a relational way of being. These approaches are based on the common humanity of the health care professional and the patient[40] and may reduce the risk of paternalistic ethically based care.

The ethical dilemmas inherent in the context of older people necessitate the ability to balance different ethical demands in situations where a blend of principles, rules, virtues, paradigms and narratives is necessary to achieve practical wisdom.[11] We suggest that these features of ethical decision making must be located within the patient–practitioner relationship. This aspect of practical wisdom should be a continuing professional development aim for practitioners who currently base their ethical practice on Codes of Professional Conduct and legislation. The 'one size fits all' approach (universalism) that could result from only using such resources to guide decision making may not always result in the optimal care for an older person with mental health problems (individualism). To know how to act ethically, health care practitioners must work towards understanding the other's perspective and potential vulnerability.[40]

Professional standards are based on values which reflect those of the society to which care organisations belong. As a result, these values are subject to constant change. Practitioners reflect those values through their personal interpretations. One challenge in current health care services is that, all too often, health care professionals find the paternalistic approach of biomedicine the overarching organisational ethos. Rodney *et al.*[38] found that nurses were working in between their own values and those of their employing organisations, as well as with other competing values and interests. Nordum *et al.*[12] found that nurses regarded the system in which they worked as unethical; not only in its effects on the treatment of older people but also in its dealings with the workforce. It is therefore important to consider the experience of both service users and health care professionals. Austin[13] raises the issue of mental health nurses' moral distress, where nurses gave accounts of lack of resources such as time and staff, lack of respect and absence of recognition for both patients and staff as severely diminishing their ability to provide good quality care.

Health care practitioners have a responsibility to give the best care they can in both non-complex and more challenging situations. In both these situations it is useful to consider ethics as a practical resource to guide decision making. This would necessitate the acquisition of an everyday ethical vocabulary that can also be shared by older people with mental health problems, their families and carers.[11] One starting point may be a definition such as that provided by Hinman[15] who reminds us that at the core, ethics is 'a conscious reflection on our moral beliefs' (p. 5). However, when delivering care, practitioners must take account of patients' moral beliefs alongside professional guidance. Hewitt[16] argued that *relationship-based care* that sets aside self-interest is an ethical practice that places values before research-based evidence.

The type of ethics that can enhance everyday decision making are *practical ethics* – thinking about whether an action is right or wrong; *normative ethics* – using general theories about what is right and good that we can use in practical cases, for example, Codes of Conduct; and *meta-ethics* – the study of the very ideas of right and wrong[17] (see also Chapter 1). These concepts can be applied to practice through reflection on the beliefs and values of the individual and the explicit identification and integration of these into care decisions centred on the person concerned.

Applying practical and normative ethics in an everyday sense can be done in the context of relational ethics which emphasises the contextual features of relationships[39] (see also Chapter 12). This builds on the foundation of previous ethical thinking and focuses on environment, embodiment, mutual respect and relational engagement.[48] Environment explores the organisational system in which care is given and how care relationships are affected by this system. Embodiment recognises that scientific knowledge and human compassion need to be given equal weight and engagement emphasises the development of an emotional connection between nurses and patients, which recognises both nurse and patient as whole beings.[48] Taking a relational ethics perspective means being sensitive to a particular situation through the opening of a dialogue between individuals and an appreciation of the uncertainty inherent in human circumstances.

Hughes[19] relocated his ethical discussion of old age psychiatry away from theorising, firmly from the perspective of the person, emphasising that clinical decisions (such as whether a patient should be told a diagnosis of Alzheimer's disease) are a matter of value of the families and the practitioners involved. In his view, people are situated-embodied-agents, which emphasises the importance of both psychological life and the human body within a context of human social relations, culture and history. His example of a person with a cognitive impairment drinking excessive alcohol explores the dilemma by comparing respecting autonomy, which can mean leaving a person to 'drink himself to death' and the paternalism of compulsory detention in hospital. Traditional ethical principles may clarify the dilemma but do not solve it. Reference to narrative ethics asks us to consider people in the context of their life stories, which may offer different solutions, such as more effective treatment aimed at root causes of drinking behaviours such as trauma in early life.[49]

The World Health Organisation has identified the risk that older people with mental health problems may be seen as 'less than' other members of society, as a global problem.[50] This problem becomes less evident where emotional connections are made between people needing and people delivering care. MacDonald and Mallik[51] found that where practitioners develop a sense of common humanity, between themselves and patients, the resulting emotional connection meant that when nurses perceived violations of patients' dignity or rights, their own emotional responses were a powerful trigger for advocacy. The development of a sense of common humanity may lead to care that contributes to what Aristotle considered human flourishing and practical wisdom; where human flourishing is the ideal goal of human action,[52] an ideal congruent with contemporary recovery values.

Respect for autonomy is a key moral principle in biomedical ethics. It is worth developing this consideration into any discussion of advocacy: the act of informing a person so that they can make the best decisions for themselves.[53] Advocacy not only safeguards but positively contributes to the exercise of self-determination. This is essential if patients are to identify and engage in achieving their aspirations.[54] However, we need to consider how such an emotional connection might be fostered in environments where nurses may be self-protective in stressful circumstances. A 'sliding scale relationship' may be the most practical solution: one that enables not only a recognition of when nurses are more or less emotionally able to move in and out of this connection, but also enables a visualisation of a sliding scale between autonomy and advocacy; where negotiations within relationships recognises each person's strengths and weaknesses on a particular day. A sliding scale relationship between autonomy and advocacy is one of the key features of optimising ethically based care, with recognition of the emotional labour involved on all sides. Where autonomous decisions become more problematic (e.g. in later stages of dementing illness), the ethical challenge should be met by a 'sliding scale' rather than 'all or nothing' approach to decision making; akin to the decision-specific framework utilised by the Mental Capacity Act (2005) but more flexible and reliant on mutual respect (see Chapter 26). This approach necessitates sensitive, ethical assessment of individual's needs.

A life context relational approach is illustrated in Vignette 1.

Vignette 1

Jim, a resident of a care home, is an older man who experiences mental health problems caused by a dementing illness. Staff who had known him for some time concluded that he was a violent, aggressive and difficult man. A health care professional visiting from an external organisation had a meaningful discussion with him (though not using fluent or conventional verbal communication skills) about his current situation; how poor communication between him and the staff resulted in situations deteriorating to conflict. The manager of the home was surprised to hear this and committed to reflect on how they had reached their conclusions and how these had influenced all subsequent interactions with Jim.

Jim's story raises many questions, the most important being the quality of Jim's life and the need for sensitive and self-aware assessments. When attention was focused on his social life and relationship to others, he demonstrated his vulnerability and a willingness to engage in meaningful conversation, provided the listener made the necessary effort. Under pressure to complete their work, staff acquired no insight into the more vulnerable and sensitive aspects of his personality. Care provision was reassessed by the staff following this experience.

This common everyday situation would not necessarily be seen or experienced as an ethical dilemma but can be considered crucial.[55] Randers and Mattiasson[55] point out that issues such as choices of food bear little resemblance to those which are morally dramatic. One interesting example involves the dilemma of whether to lie or be truthful with a resident in hospital who believes they are waiting for a train. The resident is getting into conflict with a carer who insists he is not waiting for a train, he is in hospital. They argue that another carer who provides a 'fanciful' response (i.e. not the truth), by saying 'why don't you sit in the waiting room (pointing towards the dayroom) and wait until your wife comes. I'll go with you. You can have a cup of coffee while you wait.' He responds: 'That sounds very nice' (p. 69), this maintains the patient's dignity. By understanding their perceptions of threatened integrity; the resident was allowed to be themselves. The importance of the role of the patient–practitioner relationship in resolving ethical issues is highlighted by Slettebo and Bunch[56] in the use of strategies of negotiation and explanation to resolve ethically difficult situations, which required discussion with and knowledge of the person.

Unlike the above example, however, Jim was not lacking mental capacity to the same extent. A recent research interview[57] with a staff nurse in a care home ended with the nurse stating that as the unit was not a mental health unit, they did not use the mental capacity legislation.

A working knowledge of this legislation and its application in Jim's case would ensure an understanding of his ability to communicate autonomous decisions.

Reflecting on Jim's care experience, different outcomes could have resulted had a relational ethics approach been used. Jim explained that when he tried to stand up, staff shouted across the communal lounge 'Sit down you are going to fall'; a response possibly guided by risk frameworks, concern for his physical welfare and fear of accusations of neglect. Jim experienced this as a lack of respect, triggering an angry response where he shouted back at the staff, thus reinforcing their perception of him as aggressive. Had an approach based on mutual respect been applied he may have experienced the direction differently, understanding their concerns. Similarly, by using an engagement approach, the emotional connection between Jim and his carers might result in a meaningful understanding of his experience; one that recognised both Jim and the care staff as whole human beings.

Further developments in Jim's care could have been achieved with a sliding scale autonomy/advocacy approach to decisions about his day-to-day care. There was no care assessment or provision that related to Jim's aspirations. Prior to his declining health Jim had been a physical training instructor and in later years had been involved in local football training. Discussion with Jim soon revealed his aspiration to maintain a connection with these interests. This could have been facilitated with minimal time and financial commitment, by ensuring provision of resources and activities related to local football activities. Where Jim was able to make choices on how he spent his considerable 'leisure time', information on the choices available might have resulted in reducing his frustration and an overall improvement in interpersonal relationships.

These approaches could have preserved Jim's human dignity, maximising his physical and psychological safety, as well as preventing and minimising harm. This reflects the moral horizon proposed by Rodney *et al.*[38] 'the good' towards which health care professionals and patients navigate. As a result of not reaching the horizon the resident was left feeling dehumanised, feeling that he was not of value, powerless, unsafe and that he was suffering unnecessarily.[38]

Further complicating issues for decision making are noted in Vignette 2.

Vignette 2

Jack is a 90-year-old man, who is blind. He is admitted to an inpatient ward for assessment following questions about his mental state and psychosis. He appears anxious and afraid in this strange place which he cannot experience visually and this continues over several days. Nurses attempt to develop a relationship with him, serve him meals in his room and reassure him. On one occasion they find his room barricaded, with Jack shouting and sounding distressed inside. They manage to dislodge the barricade, in the process adding to the man's fear. Once inside, he attempts to attack the nurses with a cutlery knife, which he brandishes indiscriminately, as he shouts threats, causing the nurses to retreat. The next few hours are spent trying to talk through the situation to no avail. Eventually, the staff decide, reluctantly, to restrain him, bringing an end to the incident. He is tearful and apologetic. The staff complete an incident form. The following day, the unit manager demands an explanation as to why a 90-year-old blind man was restrained.

It is tempting to view the nurses' action as wrong, as failing to respect Jack's autonomy, in addition to the added physical risks involved in restraining a person of 90, where changes in bone density, could have resulted in more easily fractured bones.[58] It must not be presumed that practitioners and patients hold the same perceptions of ethical issues. For example, in a study across five European countries nurses were found to have more positive perceptions, than patients, of the realisation of autonomy (all five countries) and informed consent (in four of the countries).[28,59] Given Jack's reaction and the violence he was expressing, he may have felt that it was ethically justified for the nurses to intervene as they did. However, the nurses may have been concerned about their decision. Such discussions are rarely if ever conducted in practice settings.

In Jack's case the relational approach did not resolve the crisis. The decision to avoid restraint would allow the situation to continue until he was exhausted; a choice the nurses considered less ethical than physical restraint. The relational framework, however, was reinforced later by the emotional engagement stimulated by the patient's tears and the nurses' acceptance of his apologies, which influenced what happens in the future. Their continued respect for him, rather than making judgements about his behaviour, is the foundation for advocacy–autonomy ethics. From a life context point of view, Jack was known to be a strong, determined person, a former soldier and athlete. Although the nurses may not have known him well, in the short term this information ensured respect for his personal strengths and an understanding of their relationship to someone with such attributes. In the longer term, their relationship could build on further knowledge of the meaning this had for Jack in his life and this connection could contribute to reducing conflict in stressful circumstances.

However, any decision to restrain someone who is 'old' and disabled is necessarily complex. The manager's question implied that it was unacceptable to restrain a 90-year-old blind man, with the implicit assumption that it would be unnecessary due to his frailty and vulnerability. Where some actions are considered unacceptable, on the basis of age and disability, rather than need, a reverse ageism is at work. As a result, staff may be afraid to make clinically sound decisions for fear of criticism based on stereotypes about older people. This might adversely affect good decision making rather than improving protection for the patient and others.

Conclusion

Our approach to ethical care has four key components:

- the values of the person/patient and practitioners;
- the contextual core of the patient–practitioner relationship;
- a sliding autonomy and advocacy scale; and
- a focus on the person/patient's aspirations.

Ethical care decisions made with older people with mental health problems must take into account personal values. This requires development of a vocabulary of ethics that is accessible to the individual and those with a supportive role in their lives. The health care professionals involved in care provision need to be able to reflect on how their values relate to those of the people they are caring for *and* the organisation they work within. These developments could contribute to a more responsive ethical approach to care.

From this foundation a sensitive and flexible, sliding scale of decision making could operate, responsive to the individual's varying needs for autonomy and advocacy. We suggest a greater focus on the aspirations of older people regardless of the setting, rather than services limited to assessing functional care needs. The fundamental component of this ethical framework is the patient–practitioner relationship. This offers an alternative to the paternalism that can result when a purely biomedical ethics approach is used.

The ethical approaches discussed here will be influenced by individual customs and culture. Relational ethics incorporates such differences into its strengths where, rather than worry about whether one is culturally sensitive, the relationship enables a genuine curiosity about such customs and culture and open dialogue about how people live their lives. The relationships that inform ethical practice are well thought out, conscious and reflective, where practitioners can focus their efforts, enabling ethical flexibility in determining care.

Such an approach is applicable to people of any age. We have focused on older people as they experience the greatest challenges; those with mental health problems even more so. A life context relational approach offers a way of breaking down these barriers.

Notes

1 Hilton, C. (2005). The clinical psychiatry of late life in Britain from 1950–1970: an overview. *International Journal of Geriatric Psychiatry* 20:423–8.

2 Collier, E. (2008). Historical development of psychiatric classification and mental illness. *British Journal of Nursing* 17(14):890–4.

3 American Psychiatric Association (APA) (1987). *Diagnostic and Statistical Manual*, 4th edn. Washington, DC: APA.

4 Brothwood, J. (1971). The organisation and development of service of the aged with special reference to the mentally ill. In: Kay, D.W.K. and Walk, A. (Eds.) *Recent Developments in Psychogeriatrics: A Symposium*, London: RMPA, pp. 99–112. Cited in Hilton op. cit.

5 Jolley, D., Kosky, N., and Holloway, F. (2004). Older people with long-standing mental illness: the graduates. *Advances in Psychiatric Treatment* 10:27–36.

6 Beekman, A.T., Copeland, J.R., and Prince, M.J. (1999). Review of community prevalence of depression in later life. *British Journal of Psychiatry* 174:307–11.

7 Baldwin, R.C. (2002). Depressive disorders. In: Jacoby, R. and Oppenheimer, C. (Eds.) *Psychiatry and the Elderly*, 3rd edn. Oxford: Oxford University Press, pp. 627–76 (Chapter 27).

8 World Health Organisation (WHO). http://www.euro.who.int/mentalhealth (accessed 15th Dec 2009).

9 de Mendonça Lima, C.A., Levav, I., Jacobsson, L., and Rutz, W. (2003). Stigma and discrimination against older people with mental disorders in Europe. *International Journal of Geriatric Psychiatry* 18:679–82.

10 Wills, A. and Olivieri, S. (August 1998). Anorexia nervosa in old age. *Aging and Mental Health* 2(3):239–45.

11 Mangweth-Matzek, B., Rupp, C.I., Hausmann, A., Assmayr, K., Mariacher, E., Kemmler, G., Whitworth, A.B., and Wilfred, B. (2006). Never too old for eating disorders or body dissatisfaction: a community study of elderly women. *International Journal of Eating Disorders* 39(7):583–6.

12 Adams, T., and Collier, E. (2009). Services for older people with mental health conditions. In: Barker, P. (Ed.) *Psychiatric and Mental Health Nursing: The Craft of Caring*, 2nd edn. London: Edward Arnold, pp. 486–92 (Chapter 56).

13 Department of Health (2005). *Everybody's Business – Integrated Mental Health Services for Older Adults*. London: Care Services Improvement Partnership (CSIP).

14 Department of Health (2006). *A New Ambition for Old Age: Next Steps in Implementing the National Service Framework for Older People*. London: Department of Health.

15 Department of Health (2009). *New Horizons in Mental Health: Towards a Shared Vision for Mental Health – Consultation*. London: Department of Health.

16 Royal College of Psychiatrists (2009). *Links Not Boundaries: Service Transitions for People Growing Older with Enduring or Relapsing Mental Illness*. London: Royal College of Psychiatrists.

17 Audit Commission (2006). *Living Well in Later Life. A Review of Progress Against the National Service Framework for Older People*. London: Audit Commission, Health Service Commission, and Commission for Social Care Inspection.

18 Bowers, H., Eastman, M., Harris, J., and Macadam, A. (2005). *Moving Out of the Shadows. A Report on Mental Health and Wellbeing in Later Life*. London: Help and Care Development Ltd.

19 Department of Health (2003a). *Care Homes for Older People, National Minimum Standards.* London: The Stationery Office.

20 Department of Health (2003b). *Care Homes for Adults (18–65), National Minimum Standards.* London: The Stationery Office.

21 Age Concern (2008). *Primary Concerns. Older People's Access to Primary Care.* London: Age Concern Reports. http://www.ageconcern.org.uk/AgeConcern/Documents/Primary Concerns report(1).pdf (accessed 15th Dec 2009).

22 Lee, M. (2006). *Promoting Mental Health and Well-Being in Later Life. A First Report from the UK Inquiry into Mental Health and Wellbeing in Later Life.* London: Age Concern/Mental Health Foundation.

23 NHS Scotland (2004). *Mental Health and Well-Being in Later Life: Older People's Perceptions.* Edinburgh: NHS Scotland.

24 Watts, S.C., Bhutani, G., Stout, I.H., Ducker, G.M., Cleator, P.J., McGarry, J., and Day, M. (2002). Mental health in older adult recipients of primary care services: is depression the key issue? Identification, treatment and the general practitioner. *International Journal of Geriatric Psychiatry* 17:427–37.

25 MacDonald, A.J.D. and Carpenter, G.I. (2003). The recognition of dementia in 'non EMI' nursing home residents in South East England. *International Journal of Geriatric Psychiatry* 18:105–8.

26 Royal College of Psychiatrists (2005). *Who Cares Wins. Improving the Outcome for Older People Admitted to the General Hospital: Guidelines for the Development of Mental Health Liaison Services for Older People.* London: Royal College of Psychiatrists.

27 St Mungo's (2004). *Leading London's Services for People Who Are Homeless and Vulnerable. St Mungo's: Biggest Ever Survey into the Problems of Homeless People. 50:50 The Big Stat.* London: St Mungo's.

28 Scott, H. (2003). Older people in prison are not having their health needs met. *British Journal of Nursing* 12(16):944.

29 Prison Reform Trust (2008). *Doing Time: The Experiences and Needs of Older People in Prison. A Prison Reform Trust Briefing.* London: Prison Reform Trust.

30 Care Quality Commission. http://www.cqc.org.uk/guidanceforprofessionals/socialcare/careproviders/guidance.cfm?widCall1=customWidgets.content_view_1&cit_id=2641 (accessed 15th Dec 2009).

31 Dening, T. and Milne, A. (2009). Depression and mental health care homes for older people. *Quality in Ageing, Policy Practice and Research* 10(1):40–6.

32 Barrowclough, C. and Fleming, I. (1991). Ethical issues in work with older people. In: Barker, Philip J. and Baldwin, Steve (Eds.) *Ethical Issues in Mental Health.* London: Chapman and Hall, pp. 68–83.

33 Beecham, J., Knapp, M., Fernandez, J., Huxley, P., Mangalore, R., McCrone, P., Snell, T., Winter, B., and Wittenberg, R. (2008). Age discrimination in mental health services. PSSRU discussion paper 2536. www.pssru.ac.uk.

34 Royal College of Psychiatrists (2008). *Fair Deal for Mental Health.* London: Royal College of Psychiatrists.

35 Mental Capacity Act (2005). Ch. 9. The Stationary Office: London.

36 Human Rights Act (1998). Ch. 42. The Stationary Office: London.

37 Falk, R. and Adeline, R. (December 1995). Advocacy and empowerment: dichotomous or synchronous concepts? *Advances in Nursing Science* 18(2):25–32.

38 Rodney, P., Varcoe, C., Storch, J.L., Mc Pherson, G., Mahoney, K., Brown, H., Pauly, B., Hartrick G., and Starzomski, R. (2002). Towards a moral horizon: a multisite qualitative study of ethical practice in nursing. *Canadian Journal of Nursing Research* 34(3):75–102.

39 MacDonald, H. (2007). Relational ethics and advocacy in nursing: literature review. *Journal of Advanced Nursing* 57(2):119–26.

40 Austin, W. (2001). Relational ethics in forensic psychiatric settings. *Journal of Psychosocial Nursing* 39(9):12–7.

41 Beauchamp, T.L. and Childress, J.F. (2001). *Principles of Biomedical Ethics*, 5th edn. Oxford: Oxford University Press.

42 Nordum, A., Tojuul, K., and Sorlie, V. (2005). Ethical challenges in the care of older people and the risk of being burned out among male nurses. *Journal of Clinical Nursing* 1114:1248–56.

43 Austin, W. (2003). Unable to answer the call of our patients: mental health nurses' experience of moral distress. *Nursing Inquiry* 10(3):177–83.

44 Barnes, M. and Brannelly, T. (2008). Achieving care and social justice for people with dementia. *Nursing Ethics* 15(3):384–94.

45 Hinman, L.M. (2003). *Ethics: A Pluralistic Approach to Moral Theory*, 3rd edn. Belmont, CA: Wadsworth Thomson.

46 Hewitt, J. (2009). Redressing the balance in mental health nursing education: arguments for a values-based approach. *International Journal of Mental Health Nursing* 18:368–79.

47 Law, S. (2007). *Philosophy*. London: Dorling Kindersley.

48 Bergum, V. (2004). Relational ethics in nursing. In: Storch, J.L., Rodney, P., and Starrzomski, R. (Eds.) *Toward a Moral Horizon: Nursing Ethics for Leadership and Practice*. Scarborough, Ontario: Prentice Hall.

49 Hughes, J.C. (2002). Ethics and the psychiatry of old age. In: Jacoby, R. and Oppenheimer, C. (Eds.) *Psychiatry in the Elderly*, 3rd edn. Oxford: Oxford University Press, pp. 863–95 (Chapter 36).

50 World Health Organisation (2002). *Missing Voices: Views of Older Persons on Elder Abuse*. http://whlibdoc.who.int/hq/2002/WHO_NMH_VIP_02.1.pdf (accessed 15th Dec 2009).

51 Macdonald, H. and Mallik, M. (1997). Advocacy in nursing – perceptions of practicing nurses. *Journal of Clinical Nursing* 6:303–13.

52 Van Hooft, S. (1995). *Caring: An Essay in the Philosophy of Ethics*. Boulder, CO: University Press of Colorado.

53 Kohnke, M.F. (1990). The nurse as advocate. In: Pence, T. and Cantrall, J. (Eds.) *Ethics in Nursing: An Anthology*. New York, NY: National League of Nursing.

54 Gadow, S. (1999). Relational narrative: the postmodern turn in nursing ethics. *Scholarly Inquiry for Nursing Practice. An International Journal* 13(1):57–70.

55 Randers, I. and Mattiasson, A. (2004). Autonomy and integrity: upholding older adult patients' dignity. *Journal of Advanced Nursing* 45(1):63–71.

56 Slettebo, A. and Bunch, E.H. (2004). Solving ethically difficult care situations in nursing homes. *Nursing Ethics* 11(6):543–52.

57 Yates-Bolton, N. (2009). Meaning and purpose in the lives of nursing home residents. Paper presented at RCN International Nursing Research Conference, Cardiff, March, 2009.

58 Woodrow, P. (Ed.) (2002). *Ageing Issues for Physical, Psychological and Social Health*. London: Whurr Publications.

59 Leino-Kilpi, H., Valimaki, M., Dassen, T., Gasull, M., Lemonindou, C., Scott, P.A., Ardt, M., Schopp, A., and Kalijonen, A. (2003). Perceptions of autonomy, privacy and informed consent in the care of elderly people in five European countries: comparison and implications for the future. *Nursing Ethics* 10:39–47.

21 'Race' and culture

Suman Fernando

Introduction

The concept of 'race' was evident in sixteenth century English literature when there was a rather vague (racial) awareness of, for example, Jews and Muslims as non-Christians. The concept developed into the modern idea of race during the rise of European power and its conquest of the Americas.[1] Major figures during the (European) 'Enlightenment' of the eighteenth century expounded what are now seen as racist views but then mere wisdom of the times; for example, ideas voiced by David Hume and Immanuel Kant.[2] As Darwinian ideas penetrated European thinking, race was seen as subspecies on the basis of which scientific racism developed.[3] Today, there is some confusion about what is meant by 'race', essentially whether it is a mere illusion, a purely ideological construct or an essence, something fixed and objective. But on the whole 'race' is seen very much as a social concept rather than a biological one.[4]

The term culture applied to an individual originally referred to a mixture of behaviour and cognition arising from 'shared patterns of belief, feeling and adaptation which people carry in their minds'.[5] During the past 40 years cultural studies have widened their scope to such an extent that the word culture has almost lost a specific meaning. Today, we speak of culture in a very loose sense, as a shorthand for explanations of the way people live or work; so we refer to, for example, family cultures, cultures of institutions or occupations/professions and culture of psychiatry or social work. In all these situations, culture means something quite subtle and intangible, underlying people's behaviour, worldviews and so on. Culture is now difficult to define clearly; it is something living, dynamic and changing – a flexible system of values and worldviews that people live by and through which they define identities and negotiate their lives.[6]

Britain has seen waves of immigration over hundreds of years. Until the mid-twentieth century immigrants were mainly from Europe – (racially) 'white' people. But with break-up of European empires after the Second World War, many people from the Caribbean, the Indian subcontinent and Africa have come to settle in the United Kingdom – people seen as racially different, the 'Other',[7] black- and brown-skinned people. It was in this context of migration that the term 'multiculturalism' came to be used to describe, not just *cultural* mixing that the United Kingdom had always experienced, but *racial* mixing. In the popular mind, and even in professional journals, concepts of 'race' and 'culture' became conflated. And to further complicate the field, the term ethnicity, adding a dimension of personal identity, was used to cover both race and culture. The question on ethnicity in the 2001 British Census[8] under the heading 'What is your ethnic group?' asked about *cultural background* not 'race' reflecting this on-going confusion between the three concepts, race, culture and ethnicity. And confusion of terms is an ideal ground on which discriminatory policies and processes can thrive; what is basically racist can be articulated in cultural terms or those of 'ethnicity'. In the 1960s as black- and brown-skinned people came to Britain (initially from former British colonies and therefore 'British' even before migrating), they were called 'coloured people' or immigrants. Then after Enoch Powell's rivers of blood speech[9] in 1968, 'coloured' became a pejorative term and they were known as Black people. But some people, such as those who derived their origins from the Indian subcontinent preferred the term 'Asian'.

From the early 1980s, Black and Asian people were noted to be suffering from disadvantages in the mental health system; and the issues around these problems have remained virtually unchanged until the present day and are generally known as 'ethnic issues'.[10] More recently, as many new immigrants have come to the United Kingdom from Eastern Europe, the categories 'Black' and 'Asian' have been subsumed under the wider umbrella term 'black and minority ethnic' (BME). This term covers anyone seen as not 'white', but leaving room for the inclusion of white people who may sometimes be seen as 'Other' – such as Jewish people and immigrants from Eastern Europe. Even more recently, a 'new' category has appeared in the British Census, namely, the ethnic category 'mixed-race' and about 15 per cent of BME people choose this category for themselves.[11]

As readers will see, it is not always clear who is included within the BME category but many reports, for example, *Inside Outside*[12] and *Delivering Race Equality*,[13] tend to assume that the disadvantages in the mental health system suffered by Black and Asian people are suffered by all BME people. This is far from clear, since there is no evidence that the people who may not fall into the Black and Asian categories are disadvantaged in the same way or to the same degree. For this reason this chapter avoids using the term BME, instead uses the category 'Black' to mean people who have an indigenous African appearance, whatever their backgrounds and 'Asian' to mean people whose backgrounds stem predominantly from the Indian subcontinent (India, Pakistan and Sri Lanka). In fact the former is a 'race' category and the latter largely cultural.

Racism

The doctrine of racism developed in Western culture in conjunction with ideas about race based on visual observations of people, particularly their skin colour. This view is no longer useful or valid. As the book *Not in our Genes* states, 'Human "racial" differentiation is indeed only skin deep. Any use of racial categories must take its justification from some other source than biology'.[14] Scientific findings can be summarized as follows:

1   Differences *within* races are greater than the differences *between* races on important physical characteristics apart from those used to define race.
2   There is no evidence for designating any race(s) as superior or inferior in terms of ability in any particular sphere or in adaptability to environment.
3   There are no 'pure' races that have genetic characteristics that are unique.
4   Finally, physical characteristics often seen as indicative of 'race', such as thin lips, flat nose and straight hair, are found in all races.[15]

Yet racism persists in many walks of life. In the United States, it still draws mainly from its history of slavery[16] and the genocide of Native Americans.[17] The background to British racism is different. Although traditionally welcoming some European refugees fleeing persecution, the British have never held a favourable attitude towards immigrants to Britain. Moreover, immigrants from parts of the world that used to form the British Empire are viewed with the sort of racism that thrived in that empire,[18] but without the imperial paternalism that existed there towards the 'native'. British racism today is seen in the derision implied in the term 'immigrant' or 'migrant', often used to describe all black- or brown-skinned people wherever they were born rather than to describe real immigrants from (say) Ireland or France, and the contempt implied when people are referred to as 'coloureds' or 'Pakis'. Since the strengthening of immigration rules in the 1970s by the British government, most immigrants to Britain in the twenty-first century are refugees and asylum seekers from areas of conflict and disaster. And from the late 1990s into the twenty-first century it is these refugees and asylum seekers who face most overt hostility for their 'alienness', their 'culture' and their 'race'.[19]

What has happened in the mental health field is that the excessive diagnosis of Black people as 'schizophrenic' – with all the images of fear and otherness inherent in this diagnosis – has interacted with myths about degeneracy of Blacks and stereotypes of dangerousness feeding into historic fears of and hostility towards the 'Other' in British society. So, vicious circles have developed over the years with 'facts' of diagnosed psychoses being muddled with fear, distrust and paranoia on both sides of the fence – the 'white establishment' of institutional psychiatry and a constituency of Black and Asian patients.[20]

Why ethical issues have become central

Issues around perceived differences in 'race' and cultural background among people served by mental health services in the United Kingdom have been highlighted in the literature since the early 1980s. These mainly refer to racial and cultural variation in the extent and mode of admission to psychiatric institutes as well as care in the community. The main thrust of these issues is that Black and Asian people, but mainly the former, are disproportionately diagnosed as suffering from schizophrenia, detained compulsorily under the Mental Health Act, labelled as both 'mad' and 'bad', and not referred for talking therapies. The complex background to this state of affairs has been explored extensively elsewhere.[21] Apart from pressures resulting from racism in society at large which give rise to stress on Black and Asian people, the issues reflect the effects of both institutional practices and cultural insensitivity of mental health services underpinned as they are by psychiatry and (Western) psychology.

If we home in on what is wrong with psychiatry, it is likely that the main faults lie in the subjective nature of its diagnosis making, attribution of largely biogenic causation to the illnesses the diagnoses are supposed to signify, its failure as a 'medical' process to allow for cultural differences in the way emotions are expressed and the power of stereotypes and images prevalent in society to influence its practice. The result is that Black and Asian people who access – or are forcibly brought into – mental health services dominated by psychiatry face both racial bias and insensitivity to their cultural background in terms of how health and illness are perceived and analyzed, and the remedies for ill-health are constructed. Thus, since most mental health services are influenced by psychiatry, Black and Asian service users experience services that are institutionally racist. This is mainly implemented through two basic parts of psychiatric practice – risk assessments and diagnosis.

Risk assessments

The domination of risk assessments is particularly dangerous to liberty and human rights because they are based mainly on subjective judgements which, by being set out as clinical opinions, cannot be challenged in a court of law. The contexts in which these risk assessments take place are therefore of supreme importance. What happens at the coal face of every day psychiatric practice is characterized by a mixture of institutional racism[22] and cultural insensitivity. The problems can be summarized as follows:

(a) Failure by most professionals in the mental health field, whatever their ethnicity, to allow for racial bias in their practices.
(b) Racism embedded in institutional practices in the delivery of services is widespread and seldom counteracted in practice.
(c) The intensity of social pressures that impinge on Black and Asian people is not being fully recognized by most practitioners.
(d) Justified anger arising from racism in society is not being taken into account when assessments are made, leading to expression of anger being mistaken for symptoms of illness or deviancy.
(e) Misinterpretation of the sense of alienation felt by many Black and Asian people often goes unchallenged. The net result of all this is that a disease model (reflected in 'symptoms') or criminal model (requiring control and/or exclusion from society) – or both – is seen as the most appropriate response to many Black and Asian people presenting to services or brought into the service compulsorily.

The usual diagnosis in such cases is either 'psychosis' or 'schizophrenia'. For further discussion of these matters readers should consult well-known texts on interplay between mental health, race and culture.[23]

Unfortunately, for those who use mental health services, risk assessments have come to dominate psychiatric practice in many settings in the United Kingdom. This process is promoted by government as good practice and rendered more or less obligatory by the Mental Health Act as revised in 2007 and the corresponding Code of Practice[24] (see Chapter 23). The process of assessing risk used in the United Kingdom depends largely on professionals making judgements about the likelihood that someone designated as a 'patient' may be dangerous or 'at risk', that is, a danger, to others or society at large. It is here that common sense images play their most damaging role in institutionalizing misperceptions; this is because judgements that are largely based on subjective impressions are given professional backing as 'clinical judgements', thereby becoming seen as fact – even as being 'evidence-based' since an opinion given by a professional assumes a status of something objective. The situation has now reached a point where we need to ask whether the practice of psychiatry in the way it is now pursed is ethical.

Diagnosis

The origins of the current diagnostic-illness model of psychiatry for encapsulating human problems are in the emergence of ideas often referred to as the 'Enlightenment'. As European thinking emerged from the dark ages, the main features of the paradigm[25] within which the natural sciences (physics, chemistry, etc.) were pursued in the eighteenth and nineteenth centuries, and within which Western psychology and psychiatry developed, were positivism, causality, objectivism and rationality.[26] Later, psychology, which was initially about the mind, the spirit and the soul, became increasingly biological under the influence of Darwinism.[27] Gradually the importance of heredity (and later genetics) came to the fore. With psychology espousing eugenics founded by Francis Galton,[28] a cousin of Charles Darwin, mental illness was attributed to inborn defects that could not be corrected, tying in with Morel's concept of degeneration of the mid-nineteenth century and the developing science of genetics[29] (see also Chapter 2). By the middle of the twentieth century all mental disorders were firmly set as inborn conditions with medical psychiatrists using an illness model for conceptualizing a vast range of human problems and thereby becoming the arbiters of right and wrong thinking, believing and behaving. This is the background in which diagnosis in psychiatry must be seen.

Psychiatry maintains its status today as a medical specialty by claiming to use scientific methods of study and research, seemingly objective techniques of observation and assessment of 'patients', and an open mind about its information base structured in it a model of medicalizing all problems seemingly located in the mind. Its influence in Western societies and latterly across the globe stems from its recognition, whether rightly or wrongly, as a 'medical science'. In practice, signs and symptoms located in the mind, deduced from an interview between doctor and patient, are assumed to be analogous to physical signs and symptoms obtained by examination of the body; and mental disorders are assumed to be equivalent to disorders of the heart, the lungs or the nervous system. However, this is far from being the case.

First, 'findings' in the so-called examination of 'mental state' that psychiatrists perform are not objective observations but inferences deduced from behaviour, including speech, during a psychiatric interview. Such an interview is essentially an encounter between two or more people and hence affected by all the feelings and tensions that may exist between the participants as well as the attitudes and beliefs of the 'observer', in this case the psychiatrist.

Second, the inferences deduced by the observer are obtained and fashioned by a structure that represents thinking embedded in a cultural tradition that existed at the time psychiatry developed, and more generally ideas about meanings given to various aspects of the 'person' being examined, matters concerning the meaning of 'illness' and the concept of 'health'. In other words ideas about health and illness that inform the examination draw from the culture that the psychiatrist has been trained in – the culture of psychiatry itself.

An important fact to take on board in considering the process of making a diagnosis is that psychiatric diagnoses are not based on objective observations or indeed any kind of 'test'. The question of what is 'abnormal' (pathological) about a belief, behaviour or emotional state is, in the final analysis, one of ethical or moral judgement. Jeff Coulter, a sociologist writing from an ethnomedological perspective states,

> A brief exposure to actual psychiatric work would reveal at once that any determination of insanity or mental illness begins (and usually ends) with judgement about the 'wrongness' of the talk and/or conduct of the person in question, seen against a background of observed and reported social events in his [or her] recent biography, and must also include some assessment of the person's cognition of his [or her] own conduct – or 'knowing its nature'.[30]

Thus, in certain contexts, some beliefs, feelings, conduct or ways of thinking may be deemed pathological if they are 'wrong' or 'bad' in the light of usual psychiatric practice (i.e. what training instils in the psychiatrist) and general common sense (i.e. ethical values of the diagnostician). And signs of illness are identified and labelled (to give just a few labels) as delusions, hallucinations, depression, elation, pathological jealousy, confusion, clinical depression, hypomania, paranoia, schizophrenia or psychopathic disorder. The context is formed by the process of diagnosis in which the psychiatrist is trained, the overall culture in which it is made, and the forces that bear down on the whole process – all of which may harbour various 'isms' including racism and moreover has not room for allowing proper degree of access for cultural diversity.

It is well established that variations in the incidence of diagnosed illness may have a lot to do with social influences and racist influences. For example, overtly racist ideas about Asian and African people held during the first half of the twentieth century tallied with reported paucity of depression and guilt among people of Asia and Africa and Black Americans at that time.[31] Much later in the 1970s, by which time overt racist ideas about Africans and Asians had become unfashionable, a subtle racism was evident in what was reported as underdevelopment of emotional differentiation among people from (industrially) under-developed countries and African-Americans.[32]

In the 1970s there was a campaign in the United Kingdom opposing what was then called the abuse of psychiatry in the (communist) Soviet Union, where political dissidents were being sent to secure hospitals with diagnoses of schizophrenia. One of the problems, although not the only one, was that many Soviet psychiatrists used a very broad definition of mental disor-der where beliefs and behaviours such as 'reformist tendencies' (sometimes designated as 'reformist delusions'), 'inclination to fruitless philosophising' and 'indulging in anti-Soviet agi-tation'[33] were designated as symptoms of schizophrenia – an 'illness' that psychiatry considers is characterized by delusions, bizarre behaviour and so on. In other words, political dissidence was interpreted as an alien way of thinking that fitted easily into the concept of schizophrenia.

About one hundred years earlier, a similar situation was evident in the Southern states of the United States. Samuel Cartwright, a psychiatrist who studied several illnesses allegedly peculiar to African-Americans, described *drapetomania*, a term derived from two Greek words, one meaning 'runaway slave' and the other 'mad' or 'crazy'. The diagnostic symptom of the illness limited to Black people was recurrent running away (absconding) from slavery. Cartwright devised a treatment plan to cure drapetomania of restricting social interaction while ensuring good food and adequate clothing, essentially a form of manipulating the social environment to ensure compliance seen as a cure of the illness.[34] Similar situations have been evident elsewhere, such as apartheid South Africa, when the oppression through the psychiatric system was racially motivated.[35]

The nature of the diagnostic system has been deeply implicated in all the instances noted above. Today, it is likely that institutional racism plays some part in oppressive practices in mental health services in a similar way through the process of diagnosis – the main diagno-sis involved being schizophrenia. It was noted earlier that the high rates at which schizophre-nia is diagnosed among Black people in the United Kingdom is now well established but the meaning of this fact is contentious.[36] The result is that today (December 2009) we have traditional psychiatrists, apparently blind to the limitations of what diagnosis signifies and to institutional racism, claiming that there is an 'epidemic' of schizophrenia among Black people in the United Kingdom attributable, not so much to genetic vulnerability as to 'fac-tors in childhood'.[37] This notion has been taken up by a racist right-wing political party (which the author does not wish to cite) and even the respectable press in blaming family structures of British African-Caribbean people and calling for 'social engineering'.[38] In this context, the ethics of continuing to use the diagnosis of schizophrenia is becoming a matter of human rights – the rights of Black families and individuals to be considered culturally equal to their white counterparts – a political question that needs to be taken up in conjunc-tion with a call for respect of difference – itself an ethical issue.

Respect for difference

British society, like many other parts of the world, is characterized by cultural hybridity and a mixture of cultural forms. Further, the cultural forms, whether of an individual or a society, are not static but ever-changing. We could either see all this as bewildering, frightening and a source of instability, or as a challenge to us all as human beings to put into practice the peren-nial human values of tolerance and understanding. As a psychiatrist and advocate of peace and harmony among people, I have no hesitation in recommending the latter approach. The other one clearly leads us into the arena of conflict and misunderstanding – the pathway to dissension, disharmony and break-up of society. The question of how to meet this challenge hinges around the role of respect. But respect like any other human attitude has to be managed in the context of the here and now – the world as we find it.

What is the practical meaning of respect in actual delivery of mental health services? We have seen how diagnosis, especially the diagnosis of schizophrenia, and the emphasis on risk assessments in practice are identifiable as impediments to proper and fair functioning of mental health services, especially in the case of Black and Asian people. The mental health scene today is far from an ideal place for harmony and peace to thrive, as far as issues of race and cultural difference are concerned. Respect for deviance is in short supply; in fact the rule appears to be *dis*respect for many characteristics of service users that mental health professionals find difficult to understand (because their cultures are unfamiliar); additionally professionals often allow their own prejudiced assumptions to dominate their relationships with service users, especially those who represent to them the 'Other' in terms of skin colour or culture. The result is the unnecessary attribution of pathological labelling, even the diagnosis of illnesses such as schizophrenia.

The issue of incorporating respect while carrying out risk assessment is a difficult matter. There is a responsibility on professionals in mental health care to consider all aspects of a situation before acting – especially when the safety of people other than the service user may be at risk. But risk should never be the main basis for taking action and professionals should never take on a God-like position of judging someone else's behaviour or assuming their intentions to be dangerous, unless there is overwhelming evidence as judged by their state of mind alone. And professionals should be willing to present such evidence to a court of law where they can be challenged. A presumed 'illness' such as schizophrenia should not warp professional judgement of another human being. Respect for others should take precedence.

The cultural insensitivity of the psychiatric system often jars with the needs of people requiring help with their mental health when they are seen as Black or Asian – and that applies even when the professionals concerned in applying the system are themselves Black or Asian. A well-known study – perhaps the only one so far to properly investigate the issues of bias in diagnosis – showed many years ago that it is mostly the system of psychiatry and the context within which it is practiced that give rise to racial and gender biases in diagnosis.[39] Too often the training and power structures of the psychiatric system appear to brainwash professionals into behaving without the respect and understanding that they would otherwise have as ordinary human beings. Clearly, training and governance in the mental health services must address the importance of respect for one another because, whether acting the roles of the professional or the patient, we are all still people in one human race. Training needs to emphasize the fact that mental health services are about human beings helping other human beings – not just professionals treating patients.

In many respects with regard to race and culture, psychiatry as a system has become part of the problem faced by Black and Asian people, rather than being a process that could be used for helping them when they are distressed or trying to find their way through life's problems. However, many professionals in the mental health system do help people who come to them as patients, whatever their colour or cultural background, but they seem to do so *in spite of* rather than because of the system. The system needs to change radically to be more in tune with what all of society has a right to demand of it – a fair and just way of helping people with mental health problems. Although this chapter has highlighted the processes used for risk assessment and diagnosis, it may well be necessary for the whole system (of psychiatry) to be fundamentally overhauled in order to render it fair and ethical.

Conclusions

It was argued earlier in this chapter that the combination of the biased risk assessment process together with flaws in the way diagnoses are made, especially that of 'schizophrenia, leads to a system of psychiatry that is basically unethical in a society where there are people from many different cultural backgrounds and where racism is institutionalized in the mental health system. However, it is noteworthy that the statistics reflected as ethnic inequalities in mental health service delivery, especially at the hard end of compulsory admission and forensic psychiatry, are very similar to ethnic statistics in education and the judicial, criminal justice system. The ethnic statistics that strike one in examining these systems are (a) the high rates at which Black children are excluded from school[10] and (b) the overrepresentation of Black people in the prison population.[11] So we might ask similar questions about ethics in some practices in those systems too. Indeed what is seen as unethical practice in psychiatry may well merely reflect general problems in society. In which case, it is likely to be unrealistic to look for change in psychiatric practice alone without seeking to bring about changes in society in general.

Notes

1   M. Banton, *Racial Theories*, Cambridge: Cambridge University Press, 1987.
2   E. Eze (Ed.), *Race and the Enlightenment. A Reader*, Cambridge, MA: Blackwell, 1997.
3   A. Chase, *The Legacy of Thomas Malthus: The Social Costs of New Scientific Racism*, New York, NY: Alfred Knopf, 1997; L. Graves, *The Emperor's New Clothes. Biological Theories of Race at the Millennium*, New Brunswick, NJ: Rutgers University Press, 2002.
4   M. Omi and H. Winant, *Racial Formation in the United States: From the 1960s to the 1990s*, New York, NY: Routledge, 1994.
5   A. H. Leighton and J. M. Hughes, 'Cultures as Causative of Mental Disorder', *Millbank Memorial Fund Quarterly* 1961, 39(3), 447.
6   Homi Bhabha, *The Location of Culture*, London: Routledge, 1994, emphasises the hybridity of cultural forms and behaviour in today's world; Edward Said, *Culture and Imperialism*, London: Vintage, 1994 discusses culture in the context of power; Suman Fernando, *Mental Health, Race and Culture*, third edition, Basingstoke: Palgrave/Macmillan, 2010 considers culture in the context of mental health.
7   Fernando, *Mental Health, Race and Culture*, op. cit. pp. 3, 154. Western ideas of the 'Other' are explored by Ryszard Kapuscinski, *The Other*, translated by Antonia Lloyd–Jones with an introduction by Neal Acherson, London: Verso, 2008.
8   *Census 2001*, London: Office for National Statistics, available http://www.statistics.gov.uk/census2001/census2001.asp, accessed 20 December 2009.
9   A speech by then Tory Government Minister Enoch Powell to the Annual General Meeting of the West Midlands Area Conservative Political Centre, Birmingham, England on April 20, 1968 had extensive media coverage and is often quoted as a landmark in British race relations history. It is available at http://www.vdare.com/misc/powell_speech.htm, accessed 20 December 2009.
10 An updated table of ethnic issues is given in Suman Fernando and Frank Keating (Eds.), *Mental Health in a Multi-ethnic Society*, second edition, London: Routledge, 2009, p. 7.
11 Ibid.
12 National Institute for Mental Health in England (NIMHE), *Inside Outside: Improving Mental Health Services for Black and Minority Ethnic Communities in England*, London: Department of Health, 2003.
13 Department of Health, *Delivering Race Equality in Mental Health Care: An Action Plan for Reform Inside and Outside Services and The Government's Response to the Independent Inquiry into the Death of David Bennett*, London: Department of Health, 2005.
14 Steven Rose, R. C. Lewontin and Leon Kamin, *Not In Our Genes, Biology, Ideology and Human Nature*, Harmondsworth: Penguin, 1984, p. 127.

15 F. Osborne, 'Races and the Future of Man'. In: R. H. Osborne (Ed.), *The Biological and Social Meaning of Race*, San Francisco, CA: Freeman, 1971, pp. 149–57.

16 The impact of slavery passed down the generations has been documented by J. DeGruy Leary, *Post Traumatic Slave Syndrome. America's Legacy of Enduring Injury and Healing*, Milwaukie, OR: Upton Press, 2005.

17 David Hurst Thomas, *Skull Wars*, New York, NY: Basic Books, 2000, shows how the treatment of indigenous Americans as a subhuman species involved all walks of white American society including the scientific establishment.

18 Well covered by Ann McClintock, *Imperial Leather, Race, Gender and Sexuality in the Colonial Contest*, New York, NY: Routledge, 1995.

19 The nature of racism is explored in many books: Frantz Fanon, *Peau Noire, Masques Blancs*, Editions de Seuil, 1952, translated into English by M. L. Markmann, *Black Skin, White Masks*, New York, NY: Grove Press, 1967, pp. 109–40; J. McCulloch, *Black Soul, White Artefact, Fanon's Clinical Psychology and Social Theory*, Cambridge: Cambridge University Press, 1983, pp. 119–24; D. T. Goldberg, *Racist Culture. Philosophy and the Politics of Meaning*, Oxford: Blackwell, 1993, pp. 117–47; Omi and Winant, op. cit., pp. 69–76; Suman Fernando, *Cultural Diversity, Mental Health and Psychiatry. The Struggle Against Racism*, Hove, East Sussex: Brunner-Routledge, 2003, pp 15–29; Reena Bhavnani, Heidi Safia Mirza and Veena Meeto, *Tackling the Roots of Racism. Lessons for Success*, Bristol: Policy Press, 2005, 149–61.

20 Frank Keating, D. Robertson, A. McCulloch and E. Francis, *Breaking the Circle of Fear, A Review of the Relationship Between Mental Health Services and African and Caribbean Communities*, London: Sainsbury Centre for Mental Health, 2002; Fernando, *Cultural Diversity, Mental Health and Psychiatry*, op. cit., pp. 29–45.

21 Fernando, *Mental Health, Race and Culture*, op. cit., pp.10–45.

22 The notion of institutional racism first appeared in the book by Stokely Carmichael and Charles Hamilton, *Black Power*, Harmondsworth: Penguin Books, 1967. It was quoted as the main problem within the London Metropolitan Police leading to their failure to properly investigate the murder of a black teenager in 1993 in the report by the Home Department, *The Stephen Lawrence Inquiry. Report of an Inquiry by Sir William Macpherson of Cluny*, London: Her Majesty's Stationery Office (HMSO), 1999. Institutional racism in the United Kingdom is defined in that report; and discussed in relation to mental health and psychiatry by Fernando and Keating, op. cit., pp. 13–15; Fernando, *Cultural Diversity, Mental Health and Psychiatry*, op. cit., pp. 162–5.

23 R. Littlewood and M. Lipsedge, *Aliens and Alienists. Ethnic Minorities and Psychiatry*, second edition, London: Unwin Hyman, 1989; S. P. Sashidharan, 'Institutional Racism in British Psychiatry', *Psychiatric Bulletin*, 2001, 25, 244–7; Kamladeep Bhui, *Racism and Mental Health*, London: Jessica Kingsley, 2002; and Fernando, *Cultural Diversity, Mental Health and Psychiatry* op. cit.

24 *Mental Health Act (Chapter 12)*, London: The Stationery Office, 2008; Department of Health, *Code of Practice Mental Health Act 1983*, London: The Stationery Office, 2008. The changes in legislation on compulsory detention enacted in 2007 tightened the Mental Health Act so that practitioners have to pay greater attention since 2008 to risk of harm to other people; and the new Code of Practice followed suit.

25 A paradigm is defined by T. S. Kuhn, *The Structure of Scientific Revolution*, third edition, Chicago, IL: University of Chicago Press, 1962.

26 Some ideas that emerged during the (European) Enlightenment are found in Toni Morrison, *Playing in the Dark: Whiteness and the Literary Imagination*, London: Pan Macmillan, 1993; I. Marin-Baró, 'Towards a liberation psychology'. Translated by A. Aron in A. Aron and S. Come (Eds.) *Writings for a Liberation Psychology*, Cambridge, MA: Harvard University Press, 1994; P. Roger, 'Individuality in French Enlightenment Thought: Exaltation or Denial?' In: S. Bagge (Ed.), *Culture and History: The Individual in European culture*, Cambridge, MA: Scandinavian University Press, 1994, pp. 72–83; D. Outram, *The Enlightenment*, second edition, Cambridge: Cambridge University Press, 2005; G. Smith, *A Short History of Secularism*, Cambridge: Cambridge University Press. Positivism is the belief that reality is rooted only in what can be observed and knowledge limited to events and to empirically verifiable connections to events; this means ignoring everything prohibited by the existing 'reality'. Causality implies a mechanical cause and effect model being universally applicable to all events and that nothing is truly random

and nothing beyond understanding, i.e. supernatural. Objectivity suggests that feelings can be considered as things 'out there' to be studied as objects, and that moral judgements are not valid. And rationality maintains that the final arbiter of truth is reason and all assertions verifiable by logical reasoning. The background to all this is discussed at length in Fernando, *Mental Health, Race and Culture*, op. cit., pp. 48–60.

27 G. Murphy, *An Historical Introduction to Modern Psychology*, fourth edition, London: Routledge and Kegan Paul, 1938.

28 F. Galton, *Hereditary Genius: An Inquiry into Its Laws and Consequences*, London: Macmillan, 1869.

29 B. A. Morel, *Traité des Maladies Mentales* (Treatise on Mental Illness), Paris: Masson, cited by I. I. Gottesman, *Schizophrenia Genesis. The Origins of Madness*, New York, NY: Freeman, 1991.

30 J. Coulter, *The Social Construction of Mind: Studies in Ethnomethodology and Linguistic Philosophy*, London: Macmillan, 1979, pp. 144–5.

31 E. M. Green, 'Psychoses among Negroes – A Comparative Study', *Journal of Nervous and Mental Disorder*, 1920, 41, 697–708; E. Kraepelin, 'Die Erscheinungsformen des Irreseins', *Zeitschrift für die gesamte Neurologie and Psychiatrie*, 1920, 62, 1–29, translated by H. Marshall, reprinted as 'Patterns of Mental Disorder'. In S. Hirsch and M. Shepherd (Eds.), *Themes and Variations in European Psychiatry*, Bristol: John Wright, 1974, pp. 7–30; J. C. Carothers, *The African Mind in Health and Disease: A Study in Ethnopsychiatry*, WHO Monograph Series No. 17, Geneva: World Health Organisation, 1953.

32 J. Leff, 'Culture and the Differentiation of Emotional States', *British Journal of Psychiatry*, 1973, 123, 299–306; J. Leff, *Psychiatry Around the Globe. A Transcultural View*, New York, NY: Marcel Dekker, 1981.

33 H. Fireside, *Soviet Psychoprisons*, New York, NY: Norton, 1979, pp. 4, 10.

34 S. A. Cartwright, 'Report on the Diseases and Physical Peculiarities of the Negro Race', reprinted from the New Orleans *Medical and Surgical Journal*, May 1851, 691–715 in A. C. Caplan, H. T. Engelhardt and J. J. McCartney (Eds.), *Concepts of Health and Disease*, Reading, MA: Addison-Wesley, 1981, pp. 305–25.

35 Psychiatric services for black people in South Africa documented in an official report for the American Psychiatric Association by A. Stone, C. Pinderhughes, J. Spurlock and M. D. Weinberg, 'Report of the Committee to Visit South Africa', *American Journal of Psychiatry*, 1978, 136, 1498–506.

36 The argument centres largely on the nature of psychiatric diagnosis – does it represent merely a bio-genetic condition of personal illness or is it a hypothesis advanced on the basis of a narrow understanding of the human condition and human problems of living and thinking. This question is explored in several books including Fernando, *Mental Health Race and Culture*, op. cit.

37 C. Morgan and G. Hutchinson, 'The Social Determinants of Psychosis in Migrant and Ethnic Minority Populations: A Public Health Tragedy', *Psychological Medicine*, doi10.1017/S0033291709005546. Published online: 1 April 2009; J. P. Selten and E. Cantor-Graae, 'The Denial of a Psychosis Epidemic, *Psychological Medicine*, doi: 1010.1017/S0033291709005546, Published on line 1 April 2009.

38 M. Lewin, 'Causes for Controversy' *Society Guardian*, 9 December 2009, p. 3. reports that a schizophrenia 'epidemic' among African Caribbeans in the United Kingdom has induced the Department of Health to move away from having specialized services for ethnic minorities towards dealing with 'sensitive social issues'. The article quotes a retired professor at the Institute of Psychiatry advocating social engineering to strengthen family structures among African-Caribbean people.

39 M. Loring and B. Powell, 'Gender, Race and DSM-III: A Study of the Objectivity of Psychiatric Diagnostic Behavior', *Journal of Health and Social Behavior*, 1988, 29, 1–22.

40 Social Exclusion Unit, *Minority Ethnic Issues in Social Exclusion and Neighbourhood Renewal*, London: Cabinet Office, 2000; Social Exclusion Unit, *Mental Health and Social Exclusion*, London: Office of the Deputy Prime Minister, 2003.

41 G. Barclay, A. Munley and T. Munton, *Race and the Criminal Justice System. An Overview to the Complete Statistics 2003–4*, London: Criminal Justice System Race Unit, 2005. Available http://www.homeoffice.gov.uk, accessed 20 September 2007 but this and other documents listing the over-representation of Black people in the prison population appears to have been removed from the home office website.

22 Suicide

John Cutcliffe and Paul Links

Introduction

There can be few ethical issues that prompt more passionate and polarized debate than those matters pertaining to end of life decisions.[1] Similarly, a discussion of suicide and care of the suicidal person would be incomplete (and ill-informed) without consideration of ethical issues, informed by a wide range of disciplines as Davidson[2] noted, 'approaching the understanding of suicide exclusively from within one's own discipline is like looking close-up at dots in a pointillist canvas'.

There is currently no unifying ethical discourse pertaining to suicide that achieves consensus; views, beliefs and resultant practices are heavily influenced by numerous ethical stances. Mishara and Weisstub[3] offer a useful categorization of the three predominant positions: the *Moralist*, the *Libertarian* and the *Relativist*. These will serve as underpinning ethical framework(s) for exploring our contemporary issues.

According to Mishara and Weisstub the Moralist position contends that suicide is unacceptable, with the overriding moral obligation to protect life (and prevent suicide). Examples include the notion that it is a sin against God to take one's life[4]; for Plato[5] suicide is an act not only against oneself but against one's society. Moralists utilizing this reasoning (see Chapter 1) regard not engaging in suicide as a categorical imperative; suicide can never be justified as an end in and of itself.

In contrast, Libertarian perspectives include a person's right to die by suicide, especially where suicide is a reasonable and calculated act to avoid pain.[6] Alternatively, a person's decision to die by suicide may simply be a rational, contemplated decision.[7] Libertarian views of suicide do not regard it as a sin against God or against society, viewing the right to suicide as sacrosanct.[8] Relativist ethicists determine the 'rightness or wrongness' of suicide, and any corresponding obligation to intervene (or not), by consideration of the contemporary, situational and cultural variables and the anticipated consequences of action/inaction. Someone adopting the Relativist perspective may in one instance support an individual's right to suicide and in another instance deny the same right.

A brief history of suicide

Prior to the eighteenth century, prevailing views of suicide were framed by theology and philosophy. The first tentative challenge to these orthodox views occurred during the Renaissance; followed, during the 'Age of Enlightenment', by open defiance. During the eighteenth century 'science' began to offer explanations for suicidal behaviour. George Cheyne proposed that a fresh, humid, unstable ocean climate predisposed the mind to suicidal madness. Other early 'scientific' theories included the view that imbalanced and/or irregular circulation of blood and humors through the brain were responsible or that the suicidal person was out of phase with the external world because the 'fibres' were either slack or immobilized by too much tension.[9] However crude or implausible these explanations were, 'science', and with that medicine, had begun to dominate the aetiology (and resultant 'treatment') of suicidal people.

The well documented and significant increase in the number of people interned in so-called insane institutions during the same time period led scholars and intellectuals of the day to link suicide with 'madness'. See, for example, Black's[10] estimates of inmates at Bedlam who had made at least one suicide attempt. During the 'Age of Enlightenment', discourses on suicide were increasingly driven by reasoning rather than religious orthodoxy.[9] It is critical to note that the shift of the 'authoritative voice' on suicide, from religious orthodoxy to 'science' (medicine) occurred as a result of socio-political changes in society rather than as a result of 'scientific discovery'. It was a sociological development; an issue of semantics; of naming things rather than discovering evidence of the aetiology of suicide *per se*.

Whose life is it anyway?

A critical question in suicide is, Who owns our bodies? Within bio-medical ethics increasing emphasis is given to body ownership (see Chapters 8 and 11). The Libertarian perspective predicates, as do most Western (developed) countries, that a person owns his/her body; bodies and body parts may be used *only* with the explicit permission of the person. Yet, the idea of 'body ownership' is relatively new and not unchallenged. Historically, people believed they were 'owned' by God; their bodies were 'on loan'. Theological arguments aside, only recently have vast numbers of the global population (e.g. women, children, slaves, serfs), been able to claim ownership of their own bodies, which were viewed as the 'property' of another. Some cultures believed that people were 'owned' by their ruler, King, Chief, Emperor, etc.

Moreover, there is little evidence to indicate that 'self-ownership' occupies a prominent position in contemporary suicide/mental health policy/practice. Additionally, the power to assume ownership of other people's bodies is enshrined in the mental health law of numerous countries (see Chapters 23–25). Furthermore, in several countries the policy and legal frameworks that surround the provision of mental health care are becoming increasingly coercive (moralist) and less Libertarian[12] (see Chapter 23). Thus, the potential for the suicidal person's body to taken over by another (under mental health law) is becoming more commonplace.

If mental health professionals hold/or respect the contemporary view that a person owns his or her own body,[13] this may generate a major ethical dilemma, possible moral distress and the need to deal with the resultant discomfort or dissonance.[14] While nurses can enact a conscientious objection (e.g. dealing with terminations) in other areas of healthcare, no such facility exists in caring for suicidal people. Further, there is little attention given to how professionals, especially nurses, might deal with their moral distress and any other intra or inter-personal issues arising out of such a situation.

Direct and indirect harming of our bodies

Many activities can result in physical harm to one's body, even though that may not be the original objective or purpose of the activity (e.g. contact sports like rugby). Here, people can risk harm without any public ethical or moral outcry. Other activities carry the risk of serious physical injury, if not death (e.g. extreme sports). Moreover, it is clear that many other activities have a statistically significant effect on shortening a person's life (smoking tobacco, abstaining from physical exercise and eating a high fat/high sugar diet). In all these cases the person clearly owns his/her body and can abuse it to the point of causing his/her death.

Then, in cases where people habitually engage in self-harming behaviour,[1] when one compares the seriousness and extent of the damage caused by people who engage in contact sports, extreme sports, etc., with people who self-harm, almost inevitably the physical damage occurring in the former category is far more serious and extensive. Yet, inversely, the ethical standpoint is most often more Draconian (i.e. excessively harsh and/or severe/Moralistic) and paternalistic in the cases of self-harm than it is in 'sporting' activities. It would be seriously imprudent then to posit a simple positive correlation between the potential seriousness and/or extent of bodily harm and the degree of paternalistic removal of an individual's rights to personal body ownership. One might speculate that the often posited relationship between suicide and self-harming behaviour, particularly given the inappropriate conflation of these behaviours as related in intent, only different in severity, has contributed (and still is contributing) to the transference of paternalistic responses to suicide to self-harming. Such scenarios further highlight the potential for significant moral distress in psychiatric/mental health (P/MH) nurses who hold and/or respect the contemporary view that a person owns his or her own body; wherein such nurses would have to reconcile the above-mentioned incongruity with the overarching mental health policy, and the organization's, physician's and/or family's requirement to keep the person physically safe.

Is suicide ever reasonable?

Contemporary views accept that, in some circumstances, suicide can be reasonable.[15] Nonetheless, there is hardly a consensus. Thomas Szasz[16,17] has readily supported the idea that suicide *can be* the reasonable thing to do and that suicide is not an illness. The absence of a formal diagnosis within the DSM IV TR manual appears to support Szasz's view. Szasz argues that suicide is a fundamental human right; society does not have the moral right to interfere, by force, with a person's decision to engage in this act. Accordingly, the only person responsible is the person him or herself. Since suicide is perceived (by some) as undesirable, the same people insist on holding someone or something responsible for it. Yet for those who believe that suicide can be the right thing to do there is no need to apportion blame.

Others have advanced the position that suicide can be reasonable when specific conditions exists. Speijer and Diekstra[18] and later Werth[19] produced lists of 'conditions', which they believed constituted a legitimate case for when suicide might *NOT* be prevented (see Tables 22.1 and 22.2). Werth's[20] extensive research in this area appears to suggest that there is around a 70–80 per cent acceptability rate for rational suicide across a wide range of disciplines involved in end of life care (e.g. counsellors, psychotherapists, psychologists, members of ethics committees, social workers and members of the American Association of Suicidology). It is worth noting that the views of P/MH nurses are rarely canvassed and published.

---

[1] For the sake of debate, we accept the well established argument that the dynamics of habitual self-harming and suicidal behaviour are *not* the same. While suicide is a death orientated act, individuals who habitually self-harm are sometimes aiming to keep themselves safe from suicide.

Table 22.1 The required conditions

- The choice of ending life by suicide is based on a free-will decision; not made under pressure.
- The person is in unbearable physical or emotional pain with no improvement expected.
- The wish can be identified as an enduring one.
- At the time of decision the person is not mentally disturbed.
- No unnecessary and preventable harm is caused to others by the suicide.
- The helper should be a qualified health professional and a doctor if lethal drugs are prescribed.
- The helper should seek professional consultation from colleagues.
- Every step should be fully documented and the documents given to the proper authorities.

Source: Adapted from Speijer and Diekstra.[18]

Table 22.2 Werth's[19] criteria for rational suicide

The person considering suicide has an unremitting 'hopeless' condition.

Hopeless conditions include, but are not limited to, terminal illness, severe physical and/or psychological pain, physically or mentally debilitating and/or deteriorating conditions or quality of life no longer acceptable to the individual.

The person makes the decision as a free choice.

The person has engaged in sound decision-making, which includes the following:

> consultation with a mental health professional who can make an assessment of mental competence;
> non-impulsive consideration of all alternatives;
> consideration of the congruence of the act with one's personal values;
> consideration of the impact on significant others;
> consultation with objective others (e.g. medical and religious professionals) and with significant others.

Source: Adapted from Werth.[19]

Can rational or appropriate suicide exist?

The prevalent view within the general public is that there can be no such thing as a rational suicide. Indeed, for many in the general population the desire to take one's own life is immediately associated with 'madness'. As a result, rational suicide then would be an oxymoron. Yet, once the assumption that all people who take their own lives must be suffering from a so-called mental illness (and with that, irrational thought) is called into question, then rational suicide becomes a realistic possibility.

Suicide, mental health problems and psychiatric diagnosis

Correlations have been established repeatedly, between certain mental health diagnoses, most notably depression, and increased risk of suicide.[20,21] However, others have cast doubt on the view that *all* people who attempt suicide must have a so-called mental illness. Tanney[23] drew attention to three principal problems in relation to such studies, namely:

1   Difficulties and imperfections in the practice of diagnostics.
2   Insurance-driven health care systems and the necessity for diagnostic categories.
3   Limitations of method and design.

van Praag's[24] life-long work on diagnosis and classification of mental health problems draws attention to the problems in distinguishing between 'real' or 'clinical' depression and sadness/distress/mourning. Diagnosing clinical depression is imperfect and problematic because no clearly demarcated boundaries exist.

> The border then, between sadness/distress and depression is blurred, and psychiatry so far, has failed to study this issue systematically . . . that border, if such a zone exists at all, is *phenomenologically defined* [original emphasis] and poorly studied. Mourning, for instance, may and often does, produce a mental state undistinguishable from major depression. (p. 83)

Moreover, no DSM-IV diagnosis exists for 'being suicidal' yet this state is 'morphed' into a DSM-IV diagnosis: depression. However, Shneidman[25] was critical of the alleged isomorphic (i.e. having the same form/appearance) relationship between depression and suicide.

> Converting suicide into depression is a kind of methodological sleight of hand. The central fact about depression is that one can lead a long happy life with depression ... suicide and depression are not synonymous.

> the biologizing of suicide is an integral part of the medicalization of what is essentially – so I believe – a phenomenological decision of the mind. (p. 73)

Tanney reminded us that the majority of people who complete suicide do not actually access formal mental health care services. For those that do, the standard procedure is that they must be given a psychiatric diagnosis, particularly in insurance-driven health care systems as in the United States. Tanney concluded that this could result in an overestimation of mental health problems among suicide completers. Finally, several methodological limitations have been noted in epidemiological studies that attempt to measure the correlation between rates of suicide in people given a psychiatric diagnosis. These include sampling bias, problems related to definition and conceptualization, the lack of a shared/common nomenclature, and the exclusion of actively suicidal people from controlled trials.

Rational suicide

Under the best of conditions, life is short, periodically painful, fickle, often lonely and anxiety provoking. Frankl[26] argued that life, almost inevitably, is about suffering. Similarly, Maltsberger[27] drew attention to the imperfect nature of life and living and to the pivotal developmental task of accepting the limitations of life: 'Successful adulthood demands that one must passively endure disappointment over and over again. . . . Maturity demands that one must accept passive suffering without flying into rages against life or against one's body' (p. 86).

There is a compelling body of evidence that shows links between mental health problems (so-called mental illness/disorder) and suicide acts, increased suicidality and increased risk. However, the alleged isomorphic relationship has been challenged comprehensively, leading to the more enlightened, contemporary view that suicide does *not* necessarily equate with irrationality *or* mental illness; though it is abundantly clear that it *can*: 'For the majority of suicidal acts, mental disorders may be a necessary but not sufficient element. The suicidal process, pathway or trajectory of suicide, or suicidal career is not, however, synonymous with mental disorder phenomenology.'

Psychiatric/mental health nurses and assisted suicide

Despite the increased focus on assisted suicide during the last 20 years, there is disturbingly little written by nurses or focused on nurses, with some notable exceptions.[28-31] Closer inspection reveals that P/MH nurses' contributions are almost entirely absent; King and Jordan-Welch's[28] cursory inclusion and the 4.5 per cent of the sample of Kowalski's[29] survey sample notwithstanding. The relative absence of the views of P/MH nurses regarding the matter of rational suicide is puzzling. Though suicide is not a mental health problem *per se,* mental health services have a long history of providing services for suicidal people. Within these one can locate the extensive history of P/MH nurses working with suicidal people. Mishara[32] highlighted this common service delivery arrangement: 'In hospital settings, it is the psychiatric or mental health nurses who are most available to engage in more extensive interactions with suicidal people' (p. xiii).

Furthermore, P/MH nurses as front-line carers for suicidal people are by no means limited to hospital settings. While significant international variation in service delivery is evident, P/MH nurses are to be found working with suicidal people in various community settings; emergency rooms, crisis counselling and help lines, general practitioner (GP) surgeries and psychotherapy clinics. Given this level of involvement one would have intuitively expected there to be a corresponding level of input into the debate from P/MH nurses. Silverman[33] offered a persuasive argument regarding the involvement and input into debates around assisted suicide: 'it only seems natural that the development of expertise and experience in these matters should first fall to the health and mental health professionals who more often interact with these (suicidal) patients as part of their daily lives' (pp. 543–4).

In light of Silverman's comments it is all the more difficult to reconcile the limited P/MH nursing contribution to this debate with the amount of time P/MH nurses spend in clinical interactions with suicidal people.

Making a reasonable choice

Decisions about suicide clearly involve affect which may distort judgment. Indeed, people with mental health problems may, at times, experience severe limitations on making fully informed decisions.[34,35] Over the years, this has led to such people being excluded from commenting on their own care and treatment; being unable to decide for themselves what is in their own best interest.

Judging what is (or was) a reasonable choice for the P/MH nurse in these cases of requests for assisted suicide would likely be determined using what the community defines as 'good' and/or appropriate standards of care. In most countries, decisions regarding what is appropriate will, likely, be influenced by case law. However, determining what is a reasonable, ethical or 'right' course of action is always difficult given that there is wide variation in what would constitute 'ethical, good and/or appropriate standards of care' *and* due to the absence of existing case law featuring the actions or inactions of P/MH nurses.

Thus, it is entirely understandable if practitioners err on the side of caution when making such decisions, for fear of criminal prosecution and reprisals from their professional registration body. Furthermore, one would hope and expect that clear and concise directions on such ethically problematic matters would be forthcoming from our professional bodies; sadly this is not the case. In the United Kingdom, for example, the Nursing and Midwifery Council (NMC)[36] stipulates that it is the duty of all registered nurses to protect and support the individual health of clients. Yet in the same document, all nurses are reminded of their duty to respect the individual rights of the person and respect his/her human dignity. Interestingly, these duties have been used as arguments both for and against assisted suicide. As with many other ethical dilemmas in healthcare, in the case of assisted suicide it appears difficult, if not impossible to adhere to all the standards/rules at the same time. Inevitably, one has to adjudicate between two or more, sometimes conflicting standards/rules, and make judicious choices between them.

First considering 'Irrational' suicide; that is, cases where a suicidal person's affect and/or constricted thoughts have ruled out any other options. Or/and cases where intervention from the mental health care services might bring about a change of heart; where there is only a temporary desire to die. In such cases it might be imprudent to respect the suicidal person's right to autonomy since it is quite probable that his/her autonomy is already compromised As a result the person's decision to take his/her own life is not a fully informed choice; it is a 'Hobson's choice' forced upon them by their constricted thoughts, affect and particular world view at that moment in time. In such cases it appears to be reasonable (if not to be required) for professionals to lean towards non-maleficence and beneficence; adopting a paternalistic stance and preventing the person's suicide. While recognizing the breach of the person's individual human rights (right to liberty and freedom of choice and personal dignity), we are comfortable with this course of action in some (many) circumstances (hence our Relativist approach). This means that we temporarily assume 'ownership' of another's body to prevent the suicide. However, although we have the 'evidence' of feedback and thanks from people in these circumstances, at the time that the person's liberty and freedom were temporarily removed, the person may well not have been grateful; the subsequent thanks was offered subsequent to the events.

An alternative response might be indicated if we understand the person's decision to die and regard this as rational. (See the criteria in Tables 22.1 and 22.2.) In these situations, it might be inappropriate to intervene and prolong life, as this would amount to prolonging the person's suffering; thus violating the ethical code of beneficence and non-maleficence. Alternatively, if we agree to assist the person with suicide this could be seen as upholding – even championing – the person's right to autonomy; respecting the person's human rights and, some would argue, the individual's personhood and dignity. As noted above, we are comfortable with temporarily assuming 'ownership' of another's body and preventing suicide, and in support of that, we have the 'evidence' of feedback and thanks from these people – *ex post facto*. However, would we receive the same thanks from those whose suffering was prolonged? Given their contributions to this debate, we leave the last words to Maris[37] and to Werth.[15]

> Sometimes we just need to die, not to be kept alive to suffer pointlessly, and we deserve to be helped in such instances. (Maris *et al.*, 2000)

> We do a disservice to our clients if we do not prepare ourselves to deal with these issues with them, or at least, know to whom we can refer them so they can receive the services they need. (Werth and Holdwick, 2000, p. 533)

Notes

1 Battin, M.P., Rhodes, R., and Silvers, A. (1998) (Eds.). *Physician-Assisted Suicide: Expanding the Debate.* Routledge, London.
2 Davidson, L. (2003). Book reviews: contemporary perspectives on rational suicide. *American Journal of Geriatric Psychiatry* 11, 108–9.
3 Mishara, B.L. and Weisstub, D.N. (2005). Ethical and legal issues in suicide research. *International Journal of Law and Psychiatry* 28, 23–41.
4 Aquinas, T. (1945). *Basic Writings of Saint Thomas Aquinas* (2 vols.). Random House, New York, NY.
5 Plato (1992). *Republic* (Translated by G.M.A. Grube, Revised by CDC Reeve). Hackett Publishing Company, Indianapolis, IN.
6 Humphrey, D. (1991). *Final Exit: The Practicalities of Self-Deliverance and Assisted Suicide for the Dying.* Delta Publishing, New York, NY.
7 Diekstra, R. (1992). Suicide and euthanasia. *Giornale Italiano de Suicidologia* 2, 71–8.
8 Ten Have, H.A.M.J., Weile, J.V.M., and Spicer, S.F. (1998). *Ownership of the Human Body: Philosophical Considerations on the Use of Human Body and its Parts in Health Care.* Kluwer, New York, NY.
9 Minois, G. (2001). *History of Suicide: Voluntary Death in Western Culture* (Translated by G. Lydia Cochrane). Johns Hopkins University Press, New York, NY.
10 Black, W. (1811). *A Dissertation on Insanity* (2nd edn.). MacDonald & Murphy, London.
11 Naverson, J. (1983). Self-ownership and the ethics of suicide. *Suicide and Life-Threatening Behavior* 13(4), 240–53.
12 Hannigan, B. and Cutcliffe, J.R. (2002). Challenging contemporary mental health policy: time to assuage the coercion? *Journal of Advanced Nursing* 35(5), 477–84.
13 Werth, J.L. (1999) (Ed.). *Contemporary Perspectives on Rational Suicide.* Brunner/Mazel, Philadelphia, PA.
14 Corley, M.C., Minick, P., Elswick, R.K., and Jacobs, M. (2005). Nurse moral distress and ethical work environment. *Nursing Ethics* 12, 381–90.
15 Werth, J.L. and Holdwick, D.J. (2000). A primer on rational suicide and other forms of hastened death. *The Counselling Psychologist* 28(4), 511–39.
16 Szasz, T. (1985, February). *Suicide: What is the Physician's Responsibility?* Unpublished paper presented at the Harvard Medical School, Cambridge, MA.
17 Szasz, T. (1990). *The Untamed Tongue.* Open Court Publishing, Chicago, IL.
18 Speijer, N. and Diekstra, R. (1980). *Assisted Suicide: A Study of the Problems Related to Self Chosen Death.* van Loghum Slaterus, Deventer.
19 Werth, J.L. (1996). *Rational Suicide? Implications for Mental Health Professionals.* Taylor & Francis, Washington, DC.
20 Werth, J.L. (1999). *Contemporary Perspectives on Rational Suicide.* Taylor & Francis, Philadelphia, PA.
21 Barraclough, B., Bunch, J., Nelson, P., and Sainsbury, P. (1974). A hundred cases of suicide: clinical aspects. *British Journal of Psychiatry* 125, 35–73.
22 Beautrais, A.L., Joyce, P.R., Mulder, R.T., Fergusson, D.M., Deavoll, B.J., and Nightengale, S.K. (1996). Prevalence and co-morbidity of mental disorders in persons making serious suicide attempts: a case–control study. *American Journal of Psychiatry* 153, 1009–14.
23 Tanney, B. (2000). Psychiatric diagnosis and suicidal acts. In: Maris, R.W., Berman, A.L., and Silverman, M.M. (Eds.). *Comprehensive Textbook of Suicidology.* Guilford Press, New York, NY, pp. 311–41.
24 van Praag, H.M. (2004). Stress and suicide: are we well equipped to study this issue? *Crisis: The Journal of Crisis Intervention and Suicide Prevention* 25(2), 80–5.
25 Shneidman, E. (2000). *Autopsy of a Suicidal Mind.* Oxford University Press, Oxford.
26 Frankl, V. (1959). *Man's Search for Meaning.* Washington Square Press, New York, NY.
27 Maltsberger, J. (2004). Consultation by John T. Maltsberger. In: Shneidman, E. (Ed.). *Autopsy of a Suicidal Mind.* Oxford University Press, Oxford, pp. 85–90.
28 King, P. and Jordan-Welch, M. (2003). Nurse-assisted suicide: not an answer in end-of-life care. *Issues in Mental Health Nursing* 24, 45–57.

29 Kowalski, S.D. (1997). Nevada nurses' attitudes regarding physician-assisted suicide. *Clinical Nurse Specialist* 11(3), 109–15.

30 White, B.C. (1999). Assisted suicide and nursing: possibly compatible? *Journal of Professional Nursing* 15(3), 151–9.

31 White, B.C. and Zimbelman, J. (1999). Why nurses must actively participate in the debate on assisted suicide: a symposium. *Journal of Professional Nursing* 15(3), 139–41.

32 Mishara, B.L. (2007). Foreword. In: Cutcliffe, J.R. and Stevenson, C. (Eds.). *Care of the Suicidal Person.* Churchill Livingstone, Edinburgh, pp. xiii–xiiii.

33 Silverman, M.M. (2000). Rational suicide, hastened death, and self-destructive behaviours. *The Counselling Psychologist* 28(4), 540–50.

34 Cutcliffe, J.R. and Milton, J. (1997). In defense of telling lies to cognitively impaired elderly patients. *International Journal of Geriatric Psychiatry* 11(12), 1117–8.

35 Beauchamp, T.L. and Childress, J.F. (2001). *Principles of Bio-Medical Ethics* (5th edn.). Oxford University Press, Oxford.

36 United Kingdom Central Council (now Nursing and Midwifery Council) (2004). *The NMC Code of Professional Conduct: Standards for Conduct, Performance and Ethics.* NMC, London.

37 Maris, R.W., Berman, A.L., and Silverman, M.M. (2000). *Comprehensive Textbook of Suicidology.* Guilford Press, New York, NY.

Section 4 – Ethical dilemmas

Phil Barker

The 300-year-old history of psychiatry has been a colourful and dramatic affair, often embellished with grandiose, self-serving ambition and not a little care and compassion. Sadly, compassion and carefulness do not win Nobel prizes and have usually been displaced in favour of the latest 'ground-breaking discovery'. We need to remember that we remain steeped in history, which is being written as we speak. The names of the characters may change but the perennial story remains fairly constant. Person falls down in the stream of life. Who will pick him or her up? Why should they bother?

1   *What is the point of mental health care?* If interplanetary beings colonised the Earth, and discovered 'people with mental health problems', would they establish 'acute psychiatric units' in 'district general hospitals' to address their needs? Most 'mental health care' is a tired revision of the asylum mentality. Perhaps, the colonising aliens would consider 'what kind of help do these people need – and where might be the best place to provide it?'

> How do we ensure that *persons* and their individual problems are not drowned by the rising tide of bureaucracy, competing professional demands and the pressure to 'patch' people up in preparation for 'discharge'?
> How do we ensure that the various members of the team are focused on the needs of the person and not on their own, professional, self-interest?

2   *Mad, bad or dangerous to know?* The people who are to be found in any forensic service represent every section of society and evoke every sentiment from pity to disgust. Some would say that they are 'all god's children' and should be treated as such. Others, especially the popular press, would disagree with such a soft-hearted attitude. Given the nature of their offences many will find it difficult to excuse them – even allowing for some 'abnormality' of mind.

> How do you maintain a principle of beneficence, in the face of your own prejudices?

3   *Addicted to life?* When multi-millionaire golfers and film stars enter 'therapy' for their 'sex addiction' we might be forgiven for treating this as a face-saving publicity exercise. Who is not addicted to some 'thing' in these needy times?

> How are you 'helping' someone by encouraging the view that their problems are a function (either wholly or in part) of some abstract notion of 'addiction'?

If people believe that they 'have' an 'addiction', what right have you to disagree with them, whatever the evidence to the contrary?

4   *The innocent, abused and tormented: an everyday story of childhood?* Few people today have had anything less than an 'awful' experience of childhood. However, many young people experience losses, trials and tribulations as part of their growing up. Only some of them end up in mental health care. For those who do, we might ask:

What do young people 'need' when they are in 'distress'?
Where is the 'problem': in the young person, their family, or the world at large?

5   *Dignity, respect and old age: mutually incompatible?* If we are fortunate, we may live to become *old.* It is largely a state of mind, in any case. Some people *feel* old, despite their age. The problem, if there is one, lies not so much in years, as in the extent to which people are still 'living' – doing something that they consider 'useful'.

How do you feel about people you consider to be old and 'useless'?
Leaving aside the diktats of some Code of Ethics, why *should* you treat me (an older person) in a dignified and respectful manner?

6   *Lost in translation?* I may know a lot about the pyramids, the Pharaohs and the Suez Canal, but what do I know about 'being' an Egyptian?

If everyone is as unique as their fingerprint, why would you assume that 'race' or 'culture' defined a person?
How does 'race' or 'culture' influence your personal identity?
What is the 'difference' present in people from other 'cultures' that inspires so much fear or suspicion?

7   *Whose life is it anyway?* People might regret killing themselves – but how would we ever know? Suicide can be unpleasant for those left to mourn or clean up. However, if people do not own their own lives, what can they own?

Is suicide ever reasonable?
How can we begin to talk, reasonably, about suicide, without acknowledging that we all have a right to kill ourselves?
When people ask, 'should I kill myself?' are they asking 'why should I live?' Do we have any right to answer either question?

Section 5

The legal context

Section preface

Phil Barker

Throughout recorded history, all societies have developed and modified laws, aimed at the government of the populace. The idea that 'ignorance of the law is no excuse' originated with the Romans, although today few people could claim 'knowledge' of every law that might pertain to them. Every government passes a wealth of legislation, much of which we only become aware of, when it affects us directly.

Dickens first coined the phrase 'the law is an ass', but it has proven to be a popular complaint down the years, as people discover, to their cost, that the rules of law do not always make for 'common sense'. However, simply because it might displease us, does not mean that it is wrong, far less *unethical*: or does it?

Section 5 provides some examples of mental health legislation. The 'law' and 'ethics' can often appear to share some common ground. Hopefully, legislators draw upon ideas of what is 'right' and 'proper', and especially what is 'fair' and 'just', when framing laws that set limits on our freedom, or define penalties to be levied in the case of some 'wrongdoing'. However, laws are developed to enable the government of society and its members. Few such laws are universally popular. People are bound to disagree with some law, if only because it does not meet their needs. In and deed, some might argue that 'law' and 'ethics' are potentially incompatible.

For much of its early history, the conditions governing the 'care' and 'custody' of people in asylums were the responsibility of local authorities. Only in the mid-nineteenth century were moves made to begin to establish more general forms of legislation, aimed at addressing the country as a whole. In Section 5 I have chosen examples of aspects of mental health legislation which, although very different, serve as good examples of the moral reasoning behind their creation, if not also the ethical dilemmas that have led to revisions, over time.

I have chosen the current *Mental Health Laws* in *England and Wales*, *Ireland* and *Scotland*, since these will be relevant to a substantial proportion of readers. However, given the international influence of British legal philosophy, over many centuries, these pieces of legislation may find echoes in the mental health laws of many other countries.

Arguably, the most radical legal proposal made in the whole history of psychiatry was Thomas Szasz's proposal of the 'psychiatric will', whereby people might make a legal provision regarding how they would wish to be treated, should they find themselves in psychiatric hands. Although still unpopular in many circles, Szasz's proposal found support in the contemporary notion of the *advance directive*, which provides people with the legal means to control their future care and treatment – at least in principle.

Finally, arguably the most contentious issue in the history of psychiatry has been the idea of *diminished responsibility*, whereby people may be found unfit to stand trial, by virtue of some form of 'insanity'. Where people stand accused of a crime, they may seek to use the *insanity defence*, as a means of avoiding the full punishment of the law. This issue is not only legally complex but also fraught with ethical dilemmas.

23 Mental health law in England and Wales

Tony Warne, Joanne Keeling and Sue McAndrew

Introduction: taking control

In 1785, the philosopher and social theorist Jeremy Bentham developed the epitome of social control, the *Panopticon*. Designed as a prison it allowed an observer to observe '*all*' without the prisoners knowing. It was described as having the sentiment of invisible omniscience.[1] Whilst it did not come to fruition during Bentham's life, his design and the intentions behind it became a metaphor for the way in which modern societies continue to want both to observe and modify behaviour. Michel Foucault, in *Discipline and Punish*, provided the most coherent explication of this metaphor and its application to the social institutions such as psychiatry, medicine and their physical manifestations as prison and hospitals. Not only prisons, but all hierarchical structures in society like the army, the school, the hospital and the factory evolved throughout history to resemble Bentham's Panopticon. The notoriety of the design today (although not its lasting influence in architectural realities) stems from Foucault's famous analysis. This chapter explores the way such thinking can be seen in the legislation governing contemporary mental health services in England and Wales. The lessons, however, have international appeal.

Like many other countries, over the past two decades in the United Kingdom there has been a sustained and purposeful shift from institutional to community care. There has been no corresponding shift in public perception around the safety of others who live close to places providing mental health services. Stigma and misinformation combine to perpetuate new urban myths describing the level of dangerousness and risk associated with those with a mental illness. Despite evidence to the contrary, there has been a growing pre-occupation with public safety; in particular protection from those who might have a mental illness. One consequence of this concern has been the consideration of ways in which those deemed to be mentally ill and presenting a 'risk' might be better controlled, thus offering greater public protection. Establishing better methods of control has centred on amendments to existing mental health legislation.

The *1959 Mental Health Act* in England and Wales marked a transition from the '*legalism*' of the *1890 Lunacy Act*, with its nineteenth century libertarian concerns, to a welfare statute in which decisions about the involuntary treatment for people with a mental illness became primarily a medical responsibility. Many iterations of this Act have occurred since, and this chapter employs the latest changes to this legislation as a starting point. A brief look at the reform of the current legalisation allows for an exploration of some of the drivers for these changes. This chapter discusses the intention of these reforms, the inconsistencies and unintended outcomes and explores the issues that result for mental health nurses and other professionals as they learn to work within this new legislative framework for practice.

The torturous process of reform

Changing this legislation for mental health reform proved to be a tortuous task[2] going through several incarnations before emerging as the Mental Health Act of 2007.[3] It was not the anticipated root and branch review of legislation but a series of amendments to the 1983 Mental Health Act,[4] the main purpose of which was and remains

> to ensure that people with serious mental disorders which threaten their health or safety or the safety of the public can be treated irrespective of their consent where it is necessary to prevent them from harming themselves or others.

Whilst the desire to better control 'risk' permeates the current legislation, paradoxically, the initial changes were made in response to what came to be known as the 'Bournewood judgment': a case brought before the European Court of Human Rights (ECHR) in 2004. A man diagnosed with autism was kept at Bournewood Hospital against the wishes of his carers. The ECHR found that man's admission to and detention in hospital under the 'common law of necessity' amounted to a breach of Article 5(1), deprivation of liberty; and of Article 5(4), the right to have lawfulness of detention reviewed by a court.

However, the intention to reform mental health legislation formed part of the newly elected Labour Government's programme of health care modernisation.[5,6] For mental health services emphasis was on community services as opposed to the hospital treatment model embraced by the 1959 and 1983 Mental Health Acts. These policy initiatives gave a clear signal from the Government that mental health legislation needed to reflect an agenda of ensuring patient *compliance*.[7]

Several reasons have been advanced as to why reform was necessary; legal, medical, political and policy considerations have all been espoused as drivers for reform. According to Hewitt[8] the resulting change is attributable to political and pragmatic considerations rather than legal or medical ones. For example, a number of high-profile homicides, associated with failures in mental health services to treat the perpetrators,[9] prompted a long-standing Government concern about the small number of people deemed to be dangerous.

An Expert Committee was charged with considering a root and branch review of the legislation that would reflect contemporary patterns of care; promote the rights of the individual and promote public safety.[9] The two important principles underlying this work were (1) non-discrimination and (2) patient autonomy.[10]

The committee proposed significant proposals for reform in 1999.[11] But, whilst some of these were incorporated many of the original recommendations were omitted.[8,9] Unsurprisingly, the overwhelming response was of an opportunity missed.[2]

A Draft Mental Health Bill was published in June 2002. The main areas of concern focused on the very broad definition of mental disorder, the concept of treatment within the community and the changed role of the tribunal system.[9,12] The Draft Bill was controversial and evoked an almost unprecedented response from all interested parties.[6,8,10,13] This led, in part, to the formation of the *Mental Health Alliance*, an umbrella organisation of 77 groups which opposed the Government's plans for mental health reform. Membership of the Alliance included The Law Society, Royal College of Psychiatrists, The British Association of Social Workers, MIND, Rethink, Mencap and The Sainsbury Centre for Mental Health.

The Alliance's concerns centred on the Government's overemphasis on risk and the potential threat posed by people with mental health problems. It was believed that the

Government had used the legislation to further emphasise control. Whilst psychiatry was being used as an instrument of social control,[14] psychiatrists were losing autonomy.[15] (See also Chapters 2 and 3, 23 and 29.)

In the face of such criticisms the Government took a further 2 years to revise and publish a new Mental Health Bill.[5] The Joint Parliamentary Committee, appointed to scrutinise the 2004 Bill, found it to be flawed fundamentally.[8] The Joint Committee made 127 recommendations which broadly mirrored those made previously by the Mental Health Alliance.[2] The Government responded with a further Bill.[16] Although this did not appear to address the original concerns, it was introduced to the House of Lords, transferred to the Commons on 7th March 2007 and received Royal Assent on 19th July 2007.[3] The Mental Health Act is the Act of Parliament of the United Kingdom that sets out the responsibilities of those providing services for people requiring care and treatment for a mental illness. In particular this legislation sets out the legal arrangements under which individuals might be detained in hospital and/or treated against their wishes. This Act significantly amended the previous legislation The Mental Health Act 1983. The Act applies only to the people of England and Wales. In Scotland, only those parts of the Act set out in Section 146 apply, the rest is covered by the Mental Health (Care and Treatment – Scotland Act, 2003), and in Northern Ireland, only those parts set out in Section 147 apply, the other aspects are covered by the Mental Health Order (Amendment – Northern Ireland 2004).

It has been suggested that the new Act[3] is now in line with the Human Rights Act.[17] Careful examination of the new Act, however, gives rise to important moral and ethical questions both for those delivering and those in receipt of mental health care.

A brief overview of the changes

The Mental Health Act (2007)[3] includes the following amendments to the previous 1983 Act:

- *Definition of mental disorder*: All references to categories of disorder have been abolished so that a single definition applies throughout.
- *Criteria for detention*: The 'treatability test' has been replaced by a new 'appropriate medical treatment' test which will apply to all the longer-term powers of detention. As a result, it will not be possible for patients to be compulsorily detained, or their detention continued, unless medical treatment – appropriate to the patient's mental disorder and all other circumstances of the case – is available to that patient. According to the 'New Horizons'[18] consultation policy document this is particularly pertinent to those deemed to have *a personality disorder*. These people can now be treated under the Act *if appropriate therapies are available*.
- *Professional roles*: Functions previously performed by the approved social worker (ASW) and responsible medical officer (RMO) can now be taken on by a broader range of professionals qualified in mental health care.
- *Supervised community treatment (SCT)*: SCT for patients can be exercised following a period of detention in hospital. *Practitioners will have the power* to require patients who are in the community and deemed to present a risk, to receive treatment and/or be recalled to hospital.
- *Nearest relative*: Patients have the right to make an application to the county court to displace their nearest relative. Likewise, the Act enables county courts to displace a nearest relative who it thinks is not suitable to act as such. In addition civil partners are now included in the list of nearest relatives.

- *Electro-convulsive therapy (ECT)*: New safeguards for patients have been introduced. For example, the *abolition of power to impose ECT where the patient is detained but has the capacity to make a decision in a non-emergency situation*. Where this is not the case a *nurse as well as a doctor* is required to make an informed decision regarding this treatment.
- *Tribunal*: The periods after which hospital managers must refer certain patients' cases to the Tribunal, if they do not apply themselves, have been reduced. Separate changes to the Tribunal system also came into effect in November 2008 (see *Tribunals Service: Rules and Legislation* for further information).
- *Advocacy*: There will be a duty placed on Mental Health Trusts to provide specialist advocacy support for people detained under the Act. Such support will be provided by independent mental health advocates.
- *Age-appropriate services*: Hospital managers are required to ensure that patients aged under 18 admitted to hospital for mental disorder are accommodated in an environment that is suitable for their age (subject to their needs). It is envisaged that this will be implemented in April 2010.

In addition, the Act has also extended the rights of victims by amending the *Domestic Violence, Crime and Victims Act*,[19] introducing new rights for individuals who become victims of those recognised as mentally disordered offenders and who are not subject to restrictions. Likewise, the *'deprivation of liberty safeguards'* was introduced in a revision of the *Mental Capacity Act* (MCA)[20] and implemented in April 2009 (see Chapter 26). These changes to the MCA provide procedures whereby a person in a hospital or care home, who lacks capacity to consent to being there, can have the deprivation of their liberty authorised. This legislation sought to address the 'Bournewood Gap', providing a framework that would allow a person 'detained', by way of 'best interest', as opposed to being sectioned, to be able to challenge his/her detention. The notion of 'best interest' raises a number of moral and ethical questions which will be discussed later. However, suffice to say here is that the MCA principles of supporting a person to make a decision when possible, and acting at all times in the person's best interests and in the least restrictive manner, must apply to *all* decision-making regarding the deprivation of a person's liberty.[21]

These changes could suggest, seductively perhaps, that the amendments take account of public safety whilst at the same time safeguarding those deemed to be in need of mental health care. However, it is easy to spot inconsistencies: The Act *'abolished categories of disorder'*, but mentions treating those people diagnosed as having a personality disorder; reference is made to the *'abolition of power to impose ECT'* yet practitioners are empowered, *if they believe it is necessary*, to implement supervised community treatment. Likewise, there are several grey areas. For example, a nurse is now also required to give information regarding what is predominately a medical intervention (ECT), yet the inequity of power often inherent in the nurse–doctor relationship makes this largely a rhetorical discussion. The making of decisions in situations where there is perceived to be a *'lack of capacity to consent'* or the issue of *'best interest'* likewise raises the question of who is making the decisions and whose best interest might this refer to.[22]

In trying to find a path through these numerous contradictions various moral and ethical dilemmas are created for mental health care professionals. Clearly, greater care, thought and consideration is required before decisions are made and enacted in clinical practice.[23] In aspiring to achieve a balance between good mental health care and providing a safe space for the person and public alike, we need to tread carefully though what could prove to be a legal mind field.

Navigating the legal mind field

The areas that are particularly problematic for practitioners are the abolition of diagnostic categories; the 'new' appropriate medical treatment test; ECT; new professional roles and SCT. The first three areas are, in many ways, interrelated, whilst new roles and SCT have major implications for mental health nurses working in the community.

For some, the abolition of the four legal categories of mental disorder might be welcome. From a Government perspective abolishing the four legal categories will ensure that people who '*need*' compulsory treatment are not excluded on the basis of a legal classification. In future '*decisions will be based on the needs of patients and the degree of risk posed by their disorder, not on their diagnostic label*'. Professionals need to prove that detention is required on the basis of individually assessed need and risk, as opposed to relying on a diagnosis.[24]

Closely linked to the abolition of diagnostic categories are the '*criteria for detention*' and the new '*appropriate medical treatment test*'. The interrelatedness of these two additions centres on the criteria for detention being predicated upon the 'treatability' of the person detained. Whilst there is some debate around what legally constitutes medical treatment[25,26] the underpinning philosophy of the new test is that it is applicable to all groups of patients liable to detention, regardless of their diagnosis and that it is more '*holistic*' in nature. Hence, clinicians need to base their decisions about treatability, not only on clinical factors, but also on whether treatment is culturally appropriate, the proximity of the treatment to the patient's home and consequently, the effect the treatment will have on the patient's ability to sustain relationships with family and friends. However, this is not always an easy task to achieve, and factoring in these considerations will also need to be undertaken against other aspects of interpersonal therapeutic relationships.[27]

There is now an explicit requirement for treatment to have a therapeutic purpose as long as such treatment is practically available and appropriate for a specific person. But, caution does need to be exercised here if we consider caveats such as evidence-based practice and what that has meant politically for those with mental illness.[27,28] For example, brief therapy, cognitive behaviour therapy and short-term psychopharmacology have been said to provide the evidence base for treating a vast range of mental health problems.[29] This has led to the demise of longer-term therapeutic approaches, such as psychoanalysis and psychodynamic and person-centred counselling.[30] As many of those who experience severe and enduring mental health problems do so as a result of historical trauma, the efficacy of brief interventions focusing on the here and now are often ineffective in the long term.[30] We suggest that the consequence of such emphasis on the 'quicker fix treatments' has resulted in a restricted menu of available and/or appropriate treatments that can be accessed by those experiencing mental distress.

Similarly, what is seen as being the '*appropriateness*' of treatment, and who makes that decision, provides an opportunity to revisit the professional versus patient debate.[31] There is a growing recognition by service providers that many users of mental health services are best able to articulate how they experience their mental health problem. Such patient experience knowledge can often challenge the assumptions made of an individual's experience that arise through the application of a diagnostic category.[32] If '*treatment which is appropriate to the patient's mental disorder and all other circumstances of the case is made available to that patient*' the expectation would be that services will be required to engage with service user needs, as opposed to the more common situation of service users being constrained to engaging only with those services available to them.[10]

Working in such a way that reliance on diagnosis is not paramount could be beneficial. However, the proviso in the 1983 Act that treatment might alleviate or prevent deterioration in the patient's condition has been removed. The Government's rationale is that previously test of 'treatability' focused too much on treatment outcome. This is the legal stipulation that arises in case law when patients win their discharge because the treatment they are receiving is not '*working*'.

The Government believes that the new test strengthens both the criteria for detention and its clinical purpose. Conversely, by removing the need for a favourable treatment outcome, some patients can be detained just because treatment is available, whether or not it is effective or even that they want such treatment. Far from ensuring that people are not detained inappropriately, and ensuring that their fundamental right to liberty remains intact, this change could allow mental health law to be used to justify detention on the grounds of paternalism and public safety: the professional 'knows best' and 'appropriate' treatment is available.[33]

Human Rights issues are equally difficult: '*whose rights*' are at issue when depriving people of their liberty is concerned. As noted, '*practitioner power*', '*best interest*' and '*capacity to make decisions*' are all concepts that need to be exposed to ongoing thoughtful debate before being embedded within professional practice.[10] Given that 'empowerment' is a key concept of contemporary mental health practice, such paradoxes reflect the confusing nature of current professional discourse surrounding the amendments to the criteria for detention.[34]

Laws regulating mental health work can lead to ethical, moral and political dilemmas. Changes to the MCA[20] ensure that a person in a hospital or care home, who lacks 'capacity', can be legally deprived of their liberty. Capacity refers to the person's 'capacity' to understand the nature and purpose of a recommended treatment, the consequences of accepting or rejecting it and the ability to make an informed decision, which he or she can then communicate.[34,35] The principles of the MCA aim to support a person in making a decision, acting at all times in the person's best interests, in the least restrictive manner. That said, mental health professionals risk adopting a paternalistic stance whereby capacity, or the lack of it, is assumed and treatment is imposed as being in the person's '*best interest*'.[10]

For some, the prescribing of involuntary treatment is primarily predicated on social ideology rather than epidemiology and/or clinical evidence.[36] Mental health professionals acting on little more than society's wisdom and values will result in mental health care that fails to contextualise the experience of the person seeking help.[37] Whilst the Mental Health Act[3] allows mental health practitioners the right to make decisions on behalf of the patient and against the patient's will when necessary, this will only reinforce the notion of 'the professional knows best'. This view has long been evident in and continues to pervade mental health care with the patients' opinions regarding care planning and decision-making appearing less valued.[38] Such powerlessness will only re-establish the existing hierarchy within healthcare professions; those left in the care of professionals becoming acutely aware of their lack of control over being able to change anything. The consequences for many individual is the surrendering of personal choice; becoming a passive recipient, unable and afraid to challenge professionals. One way to ensure that a person's '*best interests*' are addressed is through advance directives[20] (see Chapter 26). Advance directives provide the practitioner with an ethically authentic statement clarifying what treatment the person would '*not*' have chosen under the present circumstances.[39] Patients cannot refuse 'care'-only treatment; leading to both a personal and professional debate as to what constitutes care as opposed to treatment, particularly as there is no definition of 'care' within the MCA[20] (for further discussion see Chapter 26).

Far from strengthening the criteria to detain, the amendment may enable practitioners to use the Mental Health Act to detain people where treatment is available *despite* a lack of a clinical diagnosis. The Mental Health Act[3] can be viewed as a law that could potentially satisfy public pressure to deal with '*dangerous*' individuals with the propensity to offend, but who may have never committed any crime. The new legislation is said to be in keeping with Human Rights legislation. However, detention to remedy public protection issues – turning perceived 'dangerous individuals' into 'patients', whether intentionally or under the guise of Human Rights reform – could prove costly, both legally and practically.[27] If legislation is to be used to reduce risk of public harm, this needs to be generic, rather than singling out those with a 'mental illness'. This risks further discrimination and stigmatisation of those with mental illness and possible avoidance of services by those needing them most.[27,36]

Everybody's business

Perhaps one of the most far-reaching changes to the Mental Health Act[3] involves the role and responsibilities of mental health professionals. The new Act sees the replacement of the RMO and ASW with two new roles: the 'Responsible Clinician' (RC) and 'Approved Mental Health Professional' (AMHP). Development of these roles was predicated on the need to abandon the tradition of restricting roles to a specific professional group; encouraging qualified mental health practitioners, with the '*right skills*' and '*expertise*' and who are likely to be familiar with the person experiencing distress, to extend their role. The RC, in effect, replaces the role of RMO, in taking responsibility for deciding when a person can be granted leave of absence and/or be discharged from hospital. The practitioner needs to complete a formal programme of training before being approved. The challenge to medical hegemony is interesting. By drawing from the broader mental health team it is anticipated that opportunities will be created whereby the person's needs are matched to appropriately skilled professionals.[6] This might result in ensuring that the person's difficulties are recognised and addressed in keeping with their wishes and that non-medical professionals will have more opportunity to extend their role in a variety of ways; for example, through therapeutic endeavour.

The main argument for the change to the role of AMHP is that it will speed up the process of mental health assessment. The training remains based around the existing ASW training and remains under the jurisdiction of the Local Authority, both for approval purposes and for fulfilment of duties under the Act. One obvious concern is the potential conflict involved in serving two masters.[6] If a person is detained against their will at the request of a mental health professional, who *then* has an active role in their treatment and care, regardless of familiarity, trust in the relationship might well be compromised.

Other concerns include a threat to existing roles; blurring of role boundaries; no financial compensation (diluting quality by doing it on the cheap); and no power at the practitioner level, as not able to enforce the provision of appropriate services. With both roles there is further ambiguity relating to how the RC can decide to continue detention but is not competent to say it should commence.[10] Such anomalies may undermine professional integrity, in turn having a detrimental effect on the person considered in need of detention.

The amendments to the Act[3] are particularly pertinent for those receiving treatment within the community where compliance may falter. This is particularly relevant to Community Mental Health Nurses (CMHNs), the largest group delivering community mental health care. Under the new Act, CMHNs, with others, have the power to require those receiving care *and* deemed a risk, to receive treatment and/or be recalled to hospital through SCT.

The professional discourse around SCT is vast and international in nature.[6,41–43] A central concept is that of balancing patients' rights with that of community protection.[6] Those subject to this new power need to meet criteria similar to *Section 3 (admission for treatment)*, the prerequisite for SCT being that they have been assessed and treated in hospital *previously*. The similarity in legal status between those subject to SCT and people detained in hospital begs the question: Is the community a new virtual psychiatric institution?

Politically, SCT is considered to be an answer to the '*revolving door*' scenario, where those who do not comply with community treatment need readmission. It is hoped that it will also reduce the risk of social exclusion that can result from detention under the Act. However, people will still be legally '*subject*' to SCT. Therefore, it is unclear as to how SCT will reduce social exclusion. Conversely, it could be argued that this creates an exclusion clause for people who have not been subject to previous treatment in hospital but nevertheless could be offered SCT as an alternative to formal in-patient treatment from the outset.[6]

Although people are under no legal obligation to accept treatment under SCT, *or* to keep in contact with services, they can be recalled to hospital for treatment '*where clinically necessary*'. Similar situations have emerged in past case law, where patients detained under Section 3 of the Act, might spend most of their time in the community on Section 17 leave, as long as a treatment plan was still '*clinically necessary*'. So what makes the SCT any more palatable than detaining patients on a treatment section? The only obvious benefit is that the person may remain in the community, with SCT representing a 'community Section 3'.[8]

Indeed, SCT might only be useful for monitoring patients in the community, fast tracking them back into hospital when 'necessary'. This raises the question why the Government did not embed the Care Programme Approach (CPA) more in statute, as opposed to introducing a new provision for '*community detention*'. This would have maintained a degree of autonomy for patients discharged from hospital, with healthcare professionals expected to ensure adequate monitoring rather than expecting the patient to comply with professional wisdom.[14,15] People would not have the stigma of being '*detained*' in the community, retaining the same rights and freedoms as others without a diagnosed mental illness. Of course not everyone with such a diagnosis would want to be (or could be) managed in the community in this way. For some, hospital admission might be appropriate, providing that they had some control over their discharge as they improved. This is illustrated by the case of *R* v. *Kearney* where a patient was detained under Section 37 and a further restriction order Section 41 in the community.[1] The appellant did not object to the hospital order being in place, but appealed against the restriction order that would restrict his subsequent leave and discharge. This suggests that people may recognise the need to be detained in hospital for a period of treatment but do not wish this to diminish their freedoms in the community.

Additionally, the concept of ensuring community safety has come under heavy criticism in professional debate. Mental health professionals have been given the extended role of '*community supervisors*',[16] which has the potential for a conflict of interests. Whilst '*a clear separation of the therapeutic from the supervisory*' has been advocated,[16] there are concerns that this has become eroded due to the introduction of '*excessive legalism*' within the mental health system. Whilst not advocating the abolition of clinical judgement it is interesting that other European countries allow courts to make decisions on treatment, avoiding the '*dualism*' that may occur where professionals operate SCT.[15] In the absence of this provision, attention needs to be given to professional training for the role of '*community supervisor*'. The central prerequisite for any meaningful intervention is the therapeutic relationship. This could become secondary to community supervision, emphasising compliance as a condition of SCT. For interventions to be therapeutic both mental health professional and the patient need to hold a similar interpretation of its value and necessity. Account needs to be taken of how these two distinct roles might be managed or how the mental health professional might reconcile their therapeutic role with their statutory responsibility inherent in the SCT.[17]

There could also be a tendency to use coercive methods to foster treatment compliance within SCT, especially given audit and clinical governance factors. Professionals may highlight the benefits of SCT as opposed to informing patients of the restrictions SCT may place on their home lives. However, any restrictive measures, in this case SCT, must be justified clinically and legally. Failure to justify coercive treatment can be challenged in the courts.[48] Although the European Convention on Human Rights exempts people with mental disorder from its protection against detention,[17] this must not be seen as justification to act unethically; under the guise of promoting the organisational good at the expense of the patient's right to informed consent.

Contemporary health policy aimed at modernising nursing careers clearly proposes greater involvement of service users at all stages of the nurses' development.[16,49] Service user involvement, within mental health services and nurse education, is largely advocated, encouraged and accepted, with the service users having an increasing effect on the planning, delivery and evaluation of services and programmes of learning.[50,51] Despite such initiatives, the Mental Health Act[3] appears to perpetuate the gross imbalance of power between those who *deliver* and those who *use* services.[11] The professional continues, for the most part, to set the agenda, determine treatment and define its parameters. To promote public safety, the amended Act aims to ensure a more positive experience for those experiencing mental ill-health, whilst empowering mental health professionals to use their expertise as 'custodians of those who are at, or present, risk'.[52] However, the notion of expert custodian needs careful consideration, Nurses, in particular, might have concerns over such 'reductionism' and its possible impact on professional identity. Such notions limit further the influence of service users in a protectionist policy context, which seeks to ensure public safety at all costs.[53] Such paternalism filters into the direct care relationships between providers of community services (often the mental health nurse) and service users. All too often the service provider defines the service users' problems and determines solutions based on professional models, with little regard for the experiences, expertise and unique life circumstances of the individual.[54]

Conclusion

Despite the evidence, the past two decades has witnessed a growing pre-occupation with public safety, particularly related to those who might have a mental illness. One consequence has been a series of legal reforms related to the control of those deemed to be mentally ill and a 'risk' to public safety. Although many factors contributed to these reforms, a few high-profile homicides associated with failures in the mental health system became important catalysts. The new legislation can be a minefield of ethical and moral dilemmas for all professionals involved. Far from ensuring that people are not detained inappropriately and that their fundamental rights remain intact, mental health law could be used to justify detention on the grounds of paternalism and public safety. If legislation is to be used to reduce risk of public harm, this should be generic, rather than focused on people with a mental illness.

Bentham saw his Panopticon as a new way of '*obtaining power of mind over mind*'[55]: the opposite of therapeutic endeavour that seeks to offer a meaningful experience to people seeking mental health care. The new legislation has the potential to evoke a conflict of interest for professionals, not least in terms of reconciling their therapeutic role with that of their new statutory responsibilities of containment. Instead of a Panopticon what is called for is a *panorama*: greater clarity, over a much wider area of information, is needed before decisions are made and enacted under the name of mental health care.

Notes

1 Lang, S.B. (2004). The impact of video system on architecture. Unpublished dissertation. Lausanne: Swiss Federal Institute of Technology.

2 Daw, R. (2007). The Mental Health Act 2007: the defeat of an ideal. *Journal of Mental Health Law* 16: 131–48.

3 *Mental Health Act 2007* London: HMSO.

4 *Mental Health Act 1983* London: HMSO.

5 Department of Health (2004). *Draft Mental Health Bill.* London: The Stationery Office.

6 Fawcett, B. (2007). Consistencies and inconsistencies: mental health, compulsory treatment and community capacity building in England, Wales and Australia. *British Journal of Social Work* 37(6):1027–42.

7 Salize, H. and Dressing, H. (2004). Epidemiology of involuntary placement of mentally ill people across the European Union. *British Psychiatry* 184:163–8.

8 Hewitt, D. (2006). Incapable patients and the law. *British Medical Journal* 332:237.

9 Bowen, P. (2007). *Blackstone's Guide to the Mental Health Act 2007.* Oxford: Oxford University Press.

10 Richardson, G. (2007). Balancing autonomy and risk: a failure of nerve in England and Wales. *International Journal of Law and Psychiatry* 30(1):71–80.

11 Department of Health (1999). *Review of the Mental Health Act 1983. Report of the Expert Committee.* London: Department of Health.

12 Bracken, P. and Thomas, P. (2004). Out of the clinic and into the community. *OpenMind*, March/April 2004.

13 Eldergill, A. (2002). Is anyone safe? Civil compulsion under the Draft Mental Health Bill. *Journal of Mental Health Law* 8:331–59.

14 Bean, P. (1996). *Mental Disorder and Community Control.* Cambridge: Cambridge University Press.

15 Moncrieff, J. (2003). The politics of a new Mental Health Act. *British Journal of Psychiatry* 183:8–9.

16 Department of Health (2006). *Modernising Nursing Careers: Setting the Direction.* London: Department of Health.

17 *Human Rights Act 1998* London: HMSO.

18 Department of Health (2009). *New Horizons: Consultation Document.* London: Department of Health.

19 *Domestic Violence, Crimes and Victims Act 2004* London: HMSO.

20 *Mental Capacity Act 2005* London: HMSO.

21 Rapaport, J. and Manthorpe, J. (2008). Family matters: developments concerning the role of the nearest relative and social worker under mental health law in England and Wales. *British Journal of Social Work* 38(6):1115–31.

22 Singhal, A., Kumar, A., Belgamwar, R. and Hodgson, R. (2008). Assessment of mental capacity: who can do it? *Psychiatric Bulletin* 32(1):17–20.

23 Smith, H. and White, T. (2007). Before and after: introduction of the Mental Health (Care and Treatment) (Scotland) Act 2003. *Psychiatric Bulletin* 31(10):374–7.

24 Davidson, G. and Campbell, J. (2010). An audit of assessment and reporting by approved social workers (ASWs). *British Journal of Social Work* 40(5): 1609–27.

25 Craw, J. and Compton, M. (2006). Characteristics associated with involuntary versus voluntary legal status at admission and discharge among psychiatric inpatients. *Social Psychiatry and Psychiatric Epidemiology* 41(12):981–8.

26 Bolton, D. (2007). *What is Mental Disorder? An Essay in Philosophy, Science and Values.* Oxford: Oxford University Press.

27 Szmukler, G. and Appelbaum, P. (2008). Treatment pressures, leverage, coercion and compulsion in mental health care. *Journal of Mental Health* 17:233–44.

28 Lawton-Smith, S., Dawson, J. and Burns, T. (2008). Community treatment orders are not a good thing. *The British Journal of Psychiatry* 193(2):96–100.

29 Richardson, G. (1999). *Review of the Mental Health Act 1983: Report of the Expert Committee.* London: Department of Health.

30 Slade, M. and Priebe, S. (2001). Are randomised controlled trials the only gold that glitters? *British Journal of Psychiatry* 179:286–7.

31 Dawson, J. and Szmukler, G. (2006). Fusion of mental health and incapacity legislation. *British Journal of Psychiatry* 88:505–9.

32 Applebaum, P. (2007). Assessment of patient's competence to consent to treatment. *New England Journal of Medicine* 357:1834–40.

33 Eastman, N. (1999). Public health psychiatry or crime prevention? *British Medical Journal* 318:549–51.

34 Staden, C. and Kruger, C. (2003). Incapacity to give informed consent owing to mental disorder. *Journal of Medical Ethics* 29:41–3.

35 Law Commission (1995). *Mental Incapacity*. Law Commission Report no. 231. London: HMSO.

36 Szmukler, G. and Holloway, F. (2000). Reform of the Mental Health Act. *British Journal of Psychiatry* 177:196–200.

37 Owen, G., Richardson, G., David, A., Szmukler, G., Hayward, P., and Hotopf, M. (2008). Mental capacity to make decisions on treatment in people admitted to psychiatric hospitals: cross sectional study. *British Medical Journal* 337:448–59.

38 Hui, A. and Stickley, T. (2007). Mental health policy and mental health service user perspectives on involvement: a discourse analysis. *Journal of Advanced Nursing* 59(4):416–26.

39 Halpern, A. and Szmukler, G. (1997). Psychiatric advance directives: reconciling autonomy and non-consensual treatment. *Psychiatric Bulletin* 21:323–7.

40 Merchant, C. (2004). 'Roles' from mental health. *Today Paper*, April 2007.

41 Romans, S., Dawson, J., Mullen, R., and Gibbs, A. (2004). How mental health clinicians view community treatment orders: a national New Zealand survey. *Australasian and New Zealand Journal of Psychiatry* 38:836–41.

42 Mullen, R., Dawson, J., and Gibbs, A. (2006). Dilemmas for clinicians in use of community treatment orders. *International Journal of Law and Psychiatry* 29:535–50.

43 Dawson, J. (2006). Fault-lines in community treatment order legislation. *International Journal of Law and Psychiatry* 29:482–94.

44 Campbell, P. (2001). The role of users of psychiatric services in service development: influence not power. *Psychiatric Bulletin – Royal College of Psychiatrists* 25(3):87–8.

45 Campbell, J. (2010). Deciding to detain: the use of compulsory mental health laws by UK social workers. *British Journal of Social Work*: 40(1):328–34.

46 Turner, T., Salter, M., and Deahl, M. (1999). Mental Health Act reform: should psychiatrists go on being responsible? *Psychiatric Bulletin* 23:580.

47 Hurley, J. and Linsley, P. (2006). Proposed changes to the Mental Health Act of England and Wales: research indicating future educational and training needs for mental health nurses. *Journal of Psychiatric and Mental Health Nursing* 13:48–54.

48 Bindman, J., Maingay, S., and Szmukler, G. (2003). The Human Rights Act and mental health legislation. *British Journal of Psychiatry* 182:91–4.

49 Department of Health (2008). *NHS Next Stage Review: A High Quality Workforce*. London: Department of Health.

50 Pilgrim, D. and Waldron, L. (1998). User involvement in mental health service development: how far can it go? *Journal of Mental Health* 7(1):95–104.

51 Warne, T. and McAndrew, S. (2006). Transferring anonymity for a few choice words. *Nurse Education in Practice* 6:63–8.

52 Sarkar, S.P. (2002). A British psychiatrist objects to the dangerous and severe personality disorder proposals. *Journal of the American Academy of Psychiatry and the Law* 30:6–9.

53 Perkins, R. and Repper, J. (2003). *Social Inclusion and Recovery: A Model for Mental Health Practice*. London: Bailliere-Tindall.

54 Warne, T. and McAndrew, S. (2007). Passive patient or engaged expert? Using a Ptolemic approach to enhance mental health nurse education and practice. *International Journal of Mental Health Nursing* 16:224–9.

55 Bozovic, M. (1995). *The Panopticon Writings*. London: Verso.

24 Mental health law in Ireland

Denis Ryan and Agnes Higgins

Background

The treatment of the insane has a long history in Ireland. Henry and Deady[1] as cited by Deady[2] argued that the evolution of Irish mental health services has traversed a continuum from being community based, through institutionalised care, returning in the second half of the twentieth century to a community-based focus. In his account of the history of institutionalised mental health services at Grangegorman in Dublin, Reynolds[3] suggested that the first formal provision of care for the insane can be traced to 1708, when William Fownes is credited with constructing special cells within the Dublin City Workhouse for the care of the most disturbed lunatics.[3] Following that, St Patrick's Hospital, which continues as a hospital today, was founded on monies bequeathed for the purpose of building a hospital for the 'fools' and 'mad' by Jonathan Swift, Dean of St Patrick's hospital (author of Gulliver's Travels).[4]

Nearly 100 years later the Richmond Hospital opened in 1815 as the first of a suite of public psychiatric hospitals. A further 21 asylums were built and opened during the remaining part of the nineteenth century.[5] Descriptions of these developments are interesting at a number of levels, but principally because they describe the historical context for the treatment and care of those who now would be described as having 'mental health problems or difficulties'.

Evolution of mental health legislation in Ireland

Across the period of institutionalised care arrangements, mental health care in Ireland has been managed under legislation. Irish mental health legislation has a long and staggered history. Robins[1] noted that there were systems in place in pre-Christian times which gave societal guidance on managing the insane. From the nineteenth century, Irish mental health legislation broadly mirrored legislation applied in England, Scotland and Wales until after Irish independence in the early part of the twentieth century. Finnane[5] described in great detail the process by which legislation was passed as early as 1817 in Ireland to allow for the provision of public asylums for the entire country. Subsequent to this, a significant number of mental health acts were implemented, including the Lunacy (Ireland) Act 1821; the Criminal Lunatics (Ireland) Act 1838; the Private Lunatic Asylums (Amendment) Act 1842; the Central Criminal Lunatics Asylum Act 1845; the Lunacy Act 1867; and the 1945 Mental Treatments Act.[6] Throughout the nineteenth century, committal abuses were frequent and persistent.[7] Indeed by the year after the Mental Treatment Act was introduced, there were some 17,708 individuals resident in asylums in the Republic of Ireland[8] from a population of 2,955,107 in 1946.[9] Until the enactment of the 1945 legislation, as with other jurisdictions, social exclusion was the preferred societal response to the management of people who experienced 'mental disorders'.[10] Prior to the enactment of the 1945 legislation, compulsory detention was permissible, but there was no obligation on families to take patients home following a period of incarceration or when they were deemed to be well enough to leave the hospital system. This among other social issues may have been largely responsible for the inordinately high levels of residency in the Irish mental hospital system which peaked in the late 1950s.

While various amendments were added to the 1945 legislation up to 1961, by the end of the twentieth century there was general consensus that the Irish psychiatric legislation had become outdated, and attracted both national and international criticism, for the inadequate level of protection afforded to persons subjected to involuntary psychiatric detention.

In response, the *Oireachtas* (Irish Parliament) attempted to reform the 1945–61 legislation and passed the Health (Mental Services) Act in 1981. However, this legislation was never implemented because it became apparent that if implemented, it would be in breach of European guidance; specifically the *Council of Europe's* 'Recommendation for the Legal Protection of Persons Suffering from Mental Disorders Placed as Involuntary Patients' (1983),[11] in preparation at this time. Consequently, the 1945 Mental Treatment Act remained the core legislation governing psychiatric care in Ireland for over 50 years. A White Paper published by the Department of Health in 1995 did acknowledge that the 1945 Mental Treatment Act was not in keeping with the terms of the European Convention on Human Rights and Fundamental Freedoms; the Council of Europe Recommendation 83(2) for the Legal Protection of Persons Suffering from Mental Disorders Placed as Involuntary Patients (1983) and the UN Principles on the Protection of Persons with Mental Illness and for the Improvement of Mental Health Care (1991). However, it was not until the summer of 2001 that new legislation, *The Mental Health Act 2001*, was enacted.

Ireland lagged behind international trends in the latter period of the twentieth century in relation to the move towards deinstitutionalisation.[12] Similar trends of being a 'follower' rather than 'leader' may also be true in terms of legislative reform. Mental health or treatment legislation has largely been directed at protecting the rights of citizens. In that sense the law is a mechanism for setting out society's obligations as well as those of individual citizens. The law has been described as the most powerful instrument for both the articulation and imposition of duties – partly because failure to meet duties may be responded to in a range of ways where individuals can seek legal remedies.[13]

Any consideration of the current legal framework for mental health care in Ireland needs to acknowledge that the current situation is neither context free nor can it be considered in isolation from the historical evolution of mental health legislation or policy. Legislation cannot, and should not, be considered outside the societal norms, the legal context and the function of the law as a means of assuring the rights of citizens or society as a whole. However, any legal framework is also likely to result in ethical challenges as the assurance of rights for one party may negatively impact on the rights or actions of others.

Current mental health/treatment legislation

The *Mental Health Act* (2001) is currently the principal piece of legislation governing mental health service provision in Ireland. The Act was formally enacted by the *Houses of the Irish of*

Oireachtas (Parliament) in 2001; however, to allow for the necessary preparatory work to be undertaken to facilitate its full implementation and statutory regulations to be crafted to support the legislation, it was introduced on a phased basis and was not implemented in full until 2006. The Act replaced all older pieces of legislation and owes much to the influence of international policy and legislative trends.

The 2001 *Mental Health Act* is chiefly concerned with two aspects of mental health care:

1   involuntary detention of persons with 'mental disorders' in approved centres;
2   mechanisms for assuring standards of mental health care.[11]

The previous legislation contained some provision for service users to have a right to second opinions and other such protections against inappropriate involuntary detention. Current legislation has significantly strengthened those processes through a range of measures; including the automatic and independent review of involuntary admission and renewal orders by a Mental Health Tribunal. It has also enshrined explicit rights to second opinion, and the provision for a 'Mental Health Commission', responsible for ensuring mandatory legal representation at tribunal hearings and for commissioning an independent psychiatric medical opinion.[15] It is also presumed to be evidence of a commitment to a 'quality assured' service. The principal function of the Commission, as specified in the Act, is, 'to promote, encourage and foster the establishment and maintenance of high standards of good practice in the delivery of mental health services and to take all reasonable steps to protect the interests of persons detained in approved centres'. While a previous Inspectorate system was in place, its remit was constrained to inspections of mental hospitals and its membership limited to a consultant psychiatrist supported by an experienced nurse (normally at Director of Nursing level). That has now been considerably expanded to incorporate other aspects of the mental health care system – including community residential services – and its membership expanded to reflect a more multidisciplinary input.

In a comprehensive review of the Irish legislation, Eldergill[16] argues that the primary principles upon which the 1945 legislation was based were paternalistic and the 2001 legislation is based on similar statutory principles. Section 4 of the 2001 Act sets out the principle of 'best interest' of the individual, where decisions regarding involuntary or compulsory admission to hospital are made. However, it also identifies the need to give 'due regard' to the interests of other persons, who may be at risk of harm *if* the decision to detain someone were not made. The concept of 'best interests' is not clearly defined and, as a result, practitioners have little legislative guidance on how to protect these 'best interests'. In essence, a third-party makes an 'objective', decision on what would be 'best' for a person, irrespective of their present wishes or past opinions. Carney[17] cites Peay[18] who suggested that 'best interests', on its own, is little more than an 'empty vessel into which adult perceptions and prejudices are poured' (p. 7). As the 2001 Act is concerned with issues relating to compulsory detention of those deemed to have a 'mental disorder', as well as the protection of the rights of those citizens who require compulsory admission,[16] it can be argued that referring to it as a *Mental Health Act* is in itself a misnomer.

This *dual* mandate of 'purposeful protection' provides not only a backdrop to the legislation but also poses two fundamental dilemmas for those charged with making decisions around involuntary detention and containment, namely, the dilemma associated with *excluding* people from the protection afforded by this legislation and the dilemmas associated with caring for those offered care within the context of the legislation. Some of these issues will be dealt with in the following sections.

The dilemma of exclusion

The legislation is intended to afford greater protection to citizens *against* inappropriate detention, but Section 3(1) stipulates that a person *can* be involuntarily admitted to an 'approved
centre' if he/she is suffering from a mental disorder, mental illness, severe dementia or significant intellectual disability, *where there is*

(a)   A serious likelihood of the person concerned causing immediate and serious harm to
      himself or herself or to other persons, or

    1   because of the severity of the illness, disability or dementia, the judgment of the
        person concerned is so impaired that failure to admit the person to an approved
        centre would be likely to lead to a serious deterioration in his or her condition or
        would prevent the administration of appropriate treatment that could be given only
        by such admission, and
    2   the reception, detention and treatment of the person concerned in an approved
        centre would be likely to benefit or alleviate the condition of that person to a material
        extent.

There are, however, some interesting exclusions. Subsection 8(2) specifically stipulates that
those suffering 'solely' from addiction to drugs or intoxicants, personality disorder *or* those
who are considered 'socially deviant', may not be detained on an involuntary basis, however
much it might be in their best interest. Interestingly, the concept of being 'socially deviant'
is not defined.[19]

The *Declaration of Human Rights* (1948) specifically includes health as a fundamental right
and Ireland is a signatory to that declaration. While the declaration may well be aspirational, it is arguable that the state owes a duty of care to vindicate such rights where an
individual's capacity to ensure their own rights is diminished. The anomalies, with regard
to reconciling the competing demands already referred to, become apparent when these
specific exclusion criteria are considered: from a legal perspective; from the perspective of
the moral imperative related to the presumed *duty of care*; and from the ethical principle of
fidelity (outlined later).

Arguably, the state has an obligation to intervene in *all* circumstances, *on an equitable
basis*, where diminished capacity exists. In that sense, exclusion from the protection
afforded to those with other forms of diminished capacity can be seen as inequitable: failing to respond to the individuals' 'best interest'. It could also undermine the ethical obligation of practitioners – who work in services managed by the state – to abide by the
principle of *fidelity*.

Healthcare practitioners are ethically obliged to operate in the best interests of the 'sick'.
While this legislation is directed at protecting individuals against inappropriate detention
and mistreatment, ironically, this concern for the best interests of the individual may lead to
ethical dilemmas for those empowered (by the state) to make detention decisions. In a recent
survey, over 55 per cent of Irish consultant psychiatrists[20] expressed concern that people
requiring admission would *not* be admitted because of this legal stipulation. The issue of
capacity and the fact that the new legislation is deficient in relation to this criterion has been
acknowledged by the Mental Health Commission,[15] which has called for legislative reform
to address this deficiency.

Whether or not someone is 'solely' suffering from an addiction or also has some other
'co-morbid condition' has been identified as an area of potential difficulty. This may lead

to situations where clinicians may diagnose 'other conditions' in an effort to ensure the 'best interests' of the individual. O'Donoghue and Moran[20] hypothesised that when involuntary admission is deemed to be the safest course of action, psychiatrists may admit people with a diagnosis of psychiatric illness of an acute nature, such as 'adjustment disorder' or 'brief depressive episode' (p. 26), in an attempt to circumvent the exclusion criterion. The ethical dilemmas associated with such a practice are considerable. However, it should be remembered that clinicians in different settings in Ireland have engaged in such practices in the past – in the 'best interest' of others and in many ways contrary to existing policy. Prior to the decriminalisation of suicide anecdotal evidence suggests that deaths by suicide were often recorded in other ways – to serve the best interests of families.[21]

Self-reported ethical concerns of mental health nurses

Recently, we canvassed the views of members of the Irish Institute of Mental Health Nursing on issues of ethical concern relating to the new legislation. (The following quotes are all taken from this consultation.)

The principal areas of concern related to the difficulties of having someone admitted to care where admission was warranted. For example, in the case of those aged under 18, except where they were married (permitted at 16 under Irish law), the capacity to voluntarily seek hospitalisation has been withdrawn:

> Now sixteen and seventeen year olds cannot choose to go into psychiatric care under their own steam as they are deemed to be children. Therefore their parents can effectively sign them in against their will and they will be deemed an involuntary admission, because their parents deemed to do so possibly without their permission.

With regard to persons with significant mood disorders, either family doctors or psychiatrists may be reluctant to engage with compulsory detention because of fear of litigation:

> An area I am concerned with in the new mental health act is around having people admitted involuntarily or rather the difficulty with this process. I have twice been approached by families of mentally ill clients where the clients in question have clearly been very Manic and despite the consultants have been unwilling to admit them against their will. In one of these cases the young gentleman in question ran up bills for over 10,000 Euros. His family were very distraught with the situation and in fact the young man had placed himself in significant danger before finally being admitted. It feels now like Consultants and indeed GP's are afraid to admit some of these clients in case of legal throwbacks.

These concerns relate to the person's (presumed) right to appropriate services which appeared to be obstructed by the stringency of the admission criteria.

Overall, the effect of the Act in reducing the involuntary admission rates is interesting. *The Report of the Inspector of Mental Hospitals* in 2008[22] reveals that in the first few years since its full implementation, the involuntary admission rates (per 100,000 of total population) had fallen to a rate of 47.29 compared with a rate of 50.14 in 2007. While these figures indicate a clear improvement in terms of involuntary detention, concerns remain that this reduction has possibly been achieved at the potential cost of denying treatment where it was needed *and* warranted. If true, this would point to further ethical dilemmas for practitioners.

Fidelity and a flawed healthcare system

The concept of 'fidelity' is a central ethical principle in mental health care practice: the commitment of the practitioner to serve the well-being of the person 'faithfully'; to keep their interests first above all others and to maintain their trust and confidence. It requires practitioners to fulfil their promise to care for people with faithful attention.[23] In our view, all patients and their carers have a right to expect the highest standard of care possible. Given the fact that those who are involuntarily detained have their liberty removed with the authority of the state, there is a greater requirement to provide them with comprehensive, competent care and treatments in an environment that affords them dignity and is sensitive and responsive to their needs.

Green and Bloch[24] argued that working within 'flawed' health care systems poses significant challenges for healthcare professionals in terms of the principle of *fidelity*. Being or remaining faithful to the needs of an individual within services which might be described as not being 'fit for purpose' poses one of the most fundamental of challenges for those who work within such systems and who are aware of the limitations of the services. This does not suggest that services must in all instances be perfect or ideal, but they should be considered sufficient to meet the legitimate needs of those who utilise them.

In 2006, the expert group on mental health stressed the need for Irish mental health services to move beyond the current biological and illness focus towards a more 'biopsychosocial model of practice'.[18,25] More recently, in 2008 the Inspector of Mental Health Services in Ireland published a report, the second appraisal of the Irish mental health services since the full implementation of the 2001 Act. While acknowledging that there is an evolving tangible shift in ethos towards a commitment to excellence, nationwide, services were still seen as organisationally problematic. Service users remained in inappropriate settings; services often lacked comprehensive or coherent structures; resources and practices were often inadequate or restrictive; all in all the report was seen as a 'damning indictment' of Irish mental health services.

Such views, expressed by an independent statutory Inspectorate, hardly inspires trust among the citizens who may need to use such a service. Moreover, it hardly describes a service which is 'fit for purpose'. This is especially worrying in light of the fact that the findings of these reports of the Inspectorate broadly echo the findings of previous reports from the mid-1980s onwards. The surprise is not that the findings are new, but that such inadequecies have continued for so long and have not been resolved by service providers – invariably the state itself. Involuntary detention of people in a system which is neither fit for purpose *nor* adequate poses ethical challenges for all healthcare professionals involved in depriving people of their liberty in 'their best interests'. Mental health services almost universally formally suggest that they are committed to the provision of services that are 'evidence based' and underpinned by principles of 'best practice'. Providing care in settings which are found by an independent Inspectorate to be unfit for purpose is arguably both impossible and unethical and could be interpreted as condoning the inadequate standards.

Providing care in such circumstances challenges practitioners who are professionally mandated to operate within professional codes of conduct and to adhere to ethical principles, which collectively emphasise that it is not sufficient to *do no harm*. One needs to contribute to society by *preventing* harm.

The principles of beneficence and non-maleficence are arguably the longest standing ethical principles associated with caring practices and are perhaps the most frequently associated with the Hippocratic oath and medicine (see also Chapter 1). The mandate imposed upon practitioners – to do good and avoid causing harm – is welcomed by most practitioners. Wells *et al.* (2000)[26] reported that the desire to do good and make a positive impact on the lives of those who experience mental distress featured strongly in relation to choosing a career in mental health nursing in Ireland. However, it is not only important in terms of influencing career choice. Higgins *et al.*[27] noted that many actions of psychiatric nurses in Ireland were driven by a sense of paternalistic protectionism and a strong sense of beneficence. This extended, at times, to nurses making decisions to withhold information about side effects of prescribed medication, which was needed by service users to inform autonomous decision-making, and justifying their actions by appealing to the principle of beneficence and 'best interests'.

Indeed, Shanley *et al.*[28] portrayed many nurses and mental health professionals (at least in the past) as people who have failed to demonstrate adequate concern for the basic human rights of patients, citing a series of reports in Australia that were critical of both the attitudes and practices of mental health workers, which ironically lead to greater stigmatisation, as well as an increased sense of inferiority and shame experienced by people with a mental illness.

The dissonance between excellence and minimal standards

Attempts to provide 'quality' care, within accepted guidelines, also warrant comment as there can be dissonance between the espoused views and/or wishes of healthcare professionals and reports on practice by independent evaluators. A fundamental flaw of the 2001 Act is that it fails to clearly establish a minimum standard of care to which people are entitled.[29,30] Despite this criticism, the statutory regulations supporting the Act are quite prescriptive within a number of areas. Consequently, in 2008, the Inspectorate drew attention to the rights of individuals to have care plans, as set out and defined in the regulations (Regulations 2006 (S.I. no. 551 of 2006)). The 2007 Report noted that there was only an 18 per cent compliance level with this particular regulation. However, in a self-assessment exercise, 83.6 per cent of approved centres for the care and treatment of individuals with mental disorder indicated, in advance of inspection, that in their view, the service was fully compliant with this care requirement.

As discussed, the current legislation in Ireland is built on principles of both beneficence and non-maleficence. Ironically, its core thrust is to protect citizens from the system, which is populated by professionals who claim to base their practice on the very same principles.

White[31] argued that 'modern medical practice is founded on the concept of respecting patient autonomy' (p. 525). The veracity of such a claim needs particular attention when considering mental health services. It would seem reasonable to suggest that many service users might well disagree, especially where various forms of paternalistic, as well as coercive practices, are a normative feature of the care environment. Blackhall *et al.*[32] suggested that in many ways this ethical principle, as operated within healthcare practice, reflects broader trends within Western societies, where the issues of *independence, autonomy* and *choice* are seen as fundamental and virtually inalienable rights. The legislation, as well as many of the practices associated with mental health care, is grounded in principles of protectionism, paternalism and coercion. Autonomy and/or independence are not assumed to be absolute rights in the Irish legislation. Eldergill[16] noted that the concept of individual rights to freedom and the requirement to operate in someone's best interests become secondary considerations where there is a serious risk of harm to other persons. This legitimises and institutionalises forced detention and similar coercive acts within mental health systems. However, simply because such acts are legitimate or permissible does not mean that they are palatable or that they do not generate ethical dilemmas for practitioners.

Coercion and the ethos of care within mental health services

Forced admission to hospital in Ireland is, fundamentally, coercive. Admission to hospital has often been described as not being the desired first option for service users. However, of overall concern is the fact that the Mental Health Commission's[22] report referred to its 'damning indictments' of the system. The need for both a strong legislative framework and appropriate advocacy structures, firmly grounded in civil liberties, finds a strong resonance in international reviews of practice.

So far our examples have concentrated on the impact of the new legislation on the *admission* of patients and concerns with the *rights to treatment* where capacity is a concern (see Chapter 26). Compulsory detention is, by nature, coercive. However, coercion equally applies to treatment processes when individuals are detained. Notably, the 2001 Act provides quite detailed guidance in relation to informed consent to treatment. Consent to treatment must be freely given. Coercion, in various forms, is prohibited or some protections allowed for (see Chapter 13). For example, in the case of psychosurgery or electroconvulsive therapy (ECT), protections involve tribunal approval or need for a second opinion. In ECT if the person is unable or unwilling to consent, a second opinion must be sought from another consultant psychiatrist following 'referral of the matter to him or her' by the treating consultant. The fact that the patient's consultant *nominates* the doctor from whom the second opinion is sought is an obvious weakness, which may give rise to ethical issues.

Coercion and concern for the protection of patient rights lie at the heart of the new legislation. The 2001 Act also specifies that patients may not be restrained or placed in seclusion unless it is necessary for treatment or to prevent persons injuring themselves or others. This improves the situation that pertained under previous legislation, which allowed for ambiguous interpretation. For the first time in law, the rules stipulated the situations where seclusion was *not* to be used, removing the ambiguity which previously existed. The regulations set out in 1961 stipulated that seclusion of a patient in a mental institution meant 'the placing of a patient (except during the hours fixed generally for the patients in the institution to retire for sleep) in any room alone and with the door of exit locked or fastened or held in such a way as to prevent the egress of the patient'.[33] Some relatively recent research in this area noted that the use of such coercive practices was marked by wide variation in Ireland.[34]

Moreover, the 2001 Act does not concern itself with *voluntary* admission. Kelly[6] noted that neither does it contain provision for involuntary treatment (including but not limited to community orders) outside of approved centres; nor does it allow for shorter periods of detention for assessment purposes. In addition, the Act does not give due recognition to situations where detained people no longer meet the criteria for detention, but lack capacity to make decisions about their care. When detention, as set out in the legislation, is no longer warranted, the person must be discharged. Wrigley[35] highlighted some anomalies in that regard, citing a person detained in an approved centre because of severe dementia and *not because of* lack of capacity. However, over time they no longer meet the criteria for detention, but, due to deterioration, now lack the capacity to make decisions about care or to self-care. As the person does not have assets they would not come under Ward of Court legislation. Wrigley argued that moving the person out of the approved centre, in the final weeks or months of their lives, to another care environment would, in the care team's view, be damaging to the person's emotional and psychological well-being. However, to keep them in the approved centre with no status contravenes the legislation. She highlighted the urgent need for this anomaly to be addressed and the need for the enactment of appropriate mental capacity legislation in Ireland (see Chapter 26).

Ironically, a concern has been expressed by medical practitioners that, while the initial effect of the Act has been to improve the care environment for those detained, the resource (time and financial) implications related to engagement with the tribunals and other protective structures mean that resources are being diminished in other contexts. The lack of resources for voluntary patients may affect care negatively, again highlighting the challenges to practitioners complying with the principles of *fidelity*, beneficence and non-maleficence (see also Chapter 1).

Conclusion

Many aspects of the Irish Mental Health Act have been welcomed, such as the automatic review of involuntary detentions, the inclusion of explicit rights to information and the formation of the Mental Health Commission. While little research on the Act is available, anecdotal evidence suggests that Irish mental health care and treatment has improved overall, through its enactment. Its intention to protect the rights of citizens against unjust or unwarranted detention is praiseworthy. However, as the implications of the legislation emerge and following several legal challenges to its application it becomes clear that some of the intended effects have generated dilemmas for the services. The Act also has generated anomalies for the civil liberties and rights to protection of the law of Irish citizens in general. Some aspects of the legislation, which are correctly embedded in an intent to protect citizens, may lack flexibility, which may not be beneficial in individual circumstances. The emergent commentary and analysis in the literature, while limited, suggests a strong desire among practitioners to successfully navigate the stormy waters between assuring rights and ensuring ethical conduct. The anomalies which clearly exist need to be addressed to guarantee a confluence between intent and effect. In addition, there is a need for research into service users' experience of the Mental Health Act and Mental Health Tribunals, before one can comment with confidence on whose best interests are being served or to what extent.

Notes

1 Henry, H. and Deady, R., *Mental Health Nursing in Ireland.* 2001, Red Lion Press: Kilkenny, Ireland.
2 Deady, R., Psychiatric nursing in Ireland: a phenomenological study of the attitudes, values, and beliefs of Irish trained psychiatric nurses. *Archives of Psychiatric Nursing,* 2005, 19(5):210–16.
3 Reynolds, J., *Grangegorman. Psychiatric Care in Dublin since 1815.* 1992, Institute of Public Administration in Association with Eastern Health Board: Dublin, Ireland.
4 Robins, J., *Fools and Mad: A History of the Insane in Ireland.* 1986, Institute of Public Administration: Dublin, Ireland.
5 Finnane, M., *Insanity and the Insane in Post-famine Ireland.* 1981, Croom Helm and University of Michigan Library, Scholarly Publishing Office: London and Ann Arbour, MI.
6 Kelly, B., The Mental Treatment Act 1945 in Ireland: an historical enquiry. *History of Psychiatry,* 2008, 19:47–67.
7 Prior, P., Dangerous lunacy: the misuse of mental health law in nineteenth-century Ireland. *Journal of Forensic Psychiatry and Psychology,* 2003, 14:525–41.
8 Walsh, D. and Daly, A., *Mental Illness in Ireland, 1750–2002: Reflections on the Rise and Fall of Institutional Care.* 2004, Health Research Board: Dublin, Ireland.
9 Central Statistics Office, *Population Statistics 1901–2006.* 2010, Central Statistics Office: Dublin, Ireland.

10 Feldman, D., The contribution of human rights to improving public health. *Public Health*, 2006, 120:61–70.
11 McClelland, R., Webb, M., and Mock, G., Mental health services in Ireland. *International Journal of Law and Psychiatry*, 2000, 23(3–4):309–28.
12 Sheridan, A.J., Psychiatric nursing. In: J. Robins (Ed.) *Nursing and Midwifery in Ireland in the Twentieth Century*. 2000, An Bord Altranais: Dublin, Ireland.
13 Martin, R., The limits of law in the protection of public health and the role of public health ethics. *Public Health*, 2006, 120:71–80.
14 Kelly, B., The Irish Mental Health Act 2001. *Psychiatric Bulletin*, 2007, 31:21–4.
15 Mental Health Commission, *Report on the Operation of Part 2 of the Mental Health Act 2001*. 2008, Mental Health Commission: Dublin, Ireland.
16 Eldergill, A., The best is the enemy of the good: the Mental Health Act 2001. *Journal of Mental Health Law*, 2008:21–37.
17 Carney, T., Best interests or legal rectitude?: Australian Mental Health Tribunal stakeholder & case-flow implications. In: *Mental Health Commission Conference: Promoting Best Interests. Mental Health Act 2001*. 2009, Irish Mental Health Commission: Dublin.
18 Peay, J., *Tribunals on Trial: A Study of Decision-making Under the Mental Health Act 1983*. 1989, Clarendon Press: Oxford.
19 Kelly, B., The Irish Mental Health Act 2001. *Psychiatric Bulletin*, 2007, 31:21–4.
20 O'Donoghue, B.M. and Moran, P., Consultant psychiatrists' experiences and attitudes following the introduction of the Mental Health Act 2001: a national survey. *Irish Journal of Psychological Medicine*, 2009, 26(1):23–6.
21 Smyth, C., MacLachlan, M., and Clare, A., *Cultivating Suicide? Destruction of Self in a Changing Ireland*. 2003, The Liffey Press: Dublin, Ireland.
22 Mental Health Commission, *Annual Report*. 2009, Mental Health Commission: Dublin, Ireland.
23 Roberts, L., Ethical principles and skills in the care of mental illness. *Focus* 2003, 1(4):339–44.
24 Green, S.A. and Bloch, S., Working in a flawed mental health care system: an ethical challenge. *American Journal of Psychiatry*, 2001, 158:1378–83.
25 Government of Ireland, *A Vision for Change: Report of the Expert Group on Mental Health Policy*. 2006, Stationery Office: Dublin, Ireland.
26 Wells, J.S.G., Ryan, D. and McElwee, C.N. 'I don't want to be a psychiatric nurse': an exploration of factors inhibiting recruitment to psychiatric nursing in Ireland. *Journal of Psychiatric and Mental Health Nursing*, 2000, 7(1):79–87.
27 Higgins, A., Barker, P., and Begley, C.M., Iatrogenic sexual dysfunction and the protective withholding of information: in whose best interest? *Journal of Psychiatric and Mental Health Nursing*, 2006, 13(4):437–46.
28 Shanley, E., Jubb, M., and Latter, P., Partnership in coping: an Australian system of mental health nursing. *Journal of Psychiatric and Mental Health Nursing*, 2003, 10(4):431–41.
29 Kelly, B.D., The Mental Health Act 2001. *Irish Medical Journal*, 2002, 95(5):151–2.
30 O'Shea, B., The Mental Health Act 2001: a brief summary. *Irish Medical Journal*, 2002, 95(5):153.
31 White, S.M., Confidentiality, 'No blame culture' and whistleblowing, non-physician practice and accountability. *Best Practice and Research Clinical Anaesthesiology*, 2006, 20(4):525–43.
32 Blackhall, L.T., Murphy, S.T., Frank, G., Michel, V. and Azen, S., Ethnicity and attitudes toward patient autonomy. In: K.W.M. Fulford, *et al.* (Ed.) *Healthcare Ethics and Human Values*. 2002, Blackwell: Oxford, pp. 187–96.
33 Government of Ireland, *Mental Treatment Regulations*. Statutory Instrument, 1961. 261/1961.
34 Maguire, J., *Seclusion Usage in Psychiatric Institutions in the Republic of Ireland and an Analysis of Nursing Attitudes, Knowledge and Experiences Regarding Seclusion*. 2002, Royal College of Surgeons in Ireland, Faculty of Nursing: Dublin, Ireland.
35 Wrigley, M., Capacity: clinical decisions and dilemmas. Paper presented at *Mental Health Commission Conference: Promoting Best Interests: Mental Health Act 2001*. 2009, Dublin.

25 Mental health law in Scotland

Robert Davidson

Introduction

The Scottish Government's *Renewing Mental Health Law* policy statement[1] set out the proposals for a Mental Health Bill and gave consideration to the recommendations made by the Millan Committee in their report *New Directions, Report on the Review of the Mental Health (Scotland) Act 1984.*[2] Consequently, the Mental Health (Care and Treatment) (Scotland) (MH(CT)(S)) Bill[3] was introduced to the Scottish Parliament on 16 September 2002.

The passage of the Bill marked the first major overhaul of mental health law in Scotland for 40 years. It demonstrated a commitment on the part of the Scottish Government to enhance mental health law and to engineer a step-change towards forms of service provision founded in human rights legislation and based on agreed values and principles. The new Act came into effect in October 2005.

To act as a set of 'standards' or 'touchstones', a suite of reasoned principles were put in place to be considered by practitioners, organisations and other parties with responsibilities under the MH(CT)(S)A.[4] These principles seek to ensure that fundamental human rights, such as meaningful participation, intolerance of inequalities and intervening in people's lives with as light a hand as possible, are central to the implementation and interpretation of the legislation.

The principles

Reference is made, frequently, to the '*Millan Principles*'[5] which define the underpinning philosophy of the MH(CT)(S)A[4] and the intentions of its architects. They function as a guide not only to those seeking to interpret the Act coherently and consistently, but also to act as protection for people who use mental health services. Generally speaking, anyone proposing to take any action under the Act must carefully consider the principles prior to proceeding.

The Principles underpinning the MH(CT)(S)A[4] are as follows:

- non-discrimination
- equality
- respect for diversity
- reciprocity
- informal care
- participation
- respect for carers

- least restrictive alternative
- benefit
- child welfare.

The use of compulsory powers

Compulsory orders

The MH(CT)(S)A[1] makes provision for people to be placed on different kinds of compulsory order according to their prevailing needs, vulnerabilities and circumstances. The use of such measures is a matter of enormous consequence. It means that the person is relieved of the right to make autonomous decisions about his/her medical treatment. In this regard it is sobering to reflect, as Patrick (2006)[6] noted that 'compulsory measures are a fundamental attack on the person's autonomy'.

There are three main types of compulsion or civil orders:

1   *Emergency detention*: Allows the person to be detained in hospital for up to 72 hours in situations where hospital admission is required urgently to allow the person's condition to be assessed.
2   *Short-term detention*: Allows the person to be detained in hospital for up to 28 days.
3   *Compulsory treatment order (CTO)*: Authorises either detention in hospital or, if appropriate, care and treatment in the community. Lasts for up to 6 months in the first instance but can, if appropriate, be extended for a further 6 months, thereafter it can be extended for further periods each of up to 12 months duration.

A significant difference in the MH(CT)(S)A,[1] from the previous legislation,[7] is that it is possible for the Tribunal to authorise a CTO that is entirely based outside a hospital setting. Thereby the MH(CT)(S)A[1] separates compulsion from detention, which was not previously possible. This permits the person to be the subject of compulsory measures without the necessity to initially detain him or her in hospital.

The introduction of Community-based CTOs could be seen as offering comfort to those practitioners who have been alarmed by media publicity concerning 'service lapses' prior to homicides viewed as 'preventable'. However, their introduction is not that straightforward with clear benefits all round. CTOs bring ethical and professional dilemmas for practitioners. Not least that increased use of compulsion might result in people being deterred from contacting or using the services put in place to provide care and support, thus making a deterioration of their condition more likely.

Issues related to community-based CTOs

A Community-based CTO might include a range of measures; for example, that the person take medication, live at a certain address, attend certain services at particular times or attend a particular place for treatment. In setting these conditions strict observance of the principle of 'least restrictive alternative' is paramount.

A Community CTO may initially come into force when a person is in the community – to avert the need for admission to hospital – and many will feel that this is a less stigmatising approach. Alternatively, the Community CTO may follow detention and treatment in hospital as a means of ensuring future compliance with treatment – usually medication compliance.

One view might be that treatment on the basis of need should be what drives healthcare intervention. This principle pervades the National Health Service (NHS). The problem in mental health is that not everyone is able to identify their own needs or where they can for a variety of reasons may be unable to voluntarily exercise their right to treatment. As a colleague once remarked:

> Compulsory admission is essential in some circumstances, even though it can be a frightening and demeaning experience for the individual. In many ways it is an act of kindness and a useful and important option in ensuring the person's right to treatment, as long as there are safeguards in place to prevent its misuse.

Alternatively, a situation might exist where a person has made a significant recovery following hospital or community treatment; nevertheless a community order is either granted or continued. This is not done because of concerns regarding their current mental state, but due to a past history of defaulting from agreed treatment. The decision is based on the view that the person's capacity to make sound judgements about future treatment is significantly impaired. Similarly, after granting a community order, should a person's (mental health-related) problems-of-living remain manageable over time, a clinical team might feel that the CTO is working and should therefore be continued. At the same time the person, their carer or advocate, might voice the view that the objectives of the order have been achieved and therefore it should be revoked. The question is at what point will the team deem the order to be unnecessary for the person's continued safety and wellbeing or that of others? Or will defensive practice mean that it will be continued *ad infinitum* or until it is revoked by a Tribunal.

There is the potential for the introduction of Community CTOs to result in a tendency towards defensive practice on the part of those charged with the responsibility for making such decisions. A perceived blame culture (real or imagined), national targets to reduce re-admission rates and the current media attitude towards mental health care are such that if a person is discharged from detention in hospital only to require readmission shortly thereafter, questions are likely to be asked as to why the Responsible Medical Officer (RMO) did not use a Community CTO. Furthermore, forcing compliance is a less problematic option for the defensive clinician than choosing to trust the person (patient).

It may well be that previous failure to follow through with prescribed treatment has had more to do with a person's disorganised lifestyle and forgetfulness rather than refusal to comply. Alternatively, he/she may have been uncomfortable with the unwanted side effects produced by medication, which although dampening down 'the voices' may cause various other problems.

This raises the ethical question of whether Community CTOs are intrinsically fair. Should a person who is not significantly and actively 'unwell' be forced to accept medical treatment they do not want, solely to benefit their health? We do not compel people with heart disease to take medication and make compulsory lifestyle changes – even where it would clearly be in their best interests, prolonging their lives and making economic sense by reducing their future use of essential services. Why then compel people with, for example, depression to do so?

Treatment should aim to improve the quality of life for the individual concerned, not simply remove symptoms. Stopping medication can be a rational decision and people often choose not to comply with aspects of their care plan for justifiable reasons, such as medication side effects. One might reasonably ask whether a person deemed fit to live in the community should not be trusted to make such decisions with the aid of support. Should the approach therefore be to provide that support within the context of a trusting relationship rather than relying on coercive and compulsory measures? Does the development of a trusting relationship not lie at the very heart of mental health care and mental health nursing in particular?

Inquiries into suicides and homicides[8] frequently point to issues such as poor risk management, communication problems, inadequate care planning, service gaps and ineffective interagency working as the most common contributing factors. It might be argued therefore that the introduction of Community CTOs, rather than addressing these issues, fails to tackle the root causes of the problem. Many people, and their carers, will say that the principal reason why they required readmission to hospital was that they were unable to access the range of supports and interventions in the community that they felt they required. Practitioners must ask themselves if they should be forcing people, under a threat of readmission, to engage with a limited choice of service options many (most) of which they find unappealing or irrelevant to their needs.

Community CTOs, medication and the role of the CPN

It is the responsibility of the Mental Health Officer (MHO) to apply to the Mental Health Tribunal for a Community CTO to be granted. This is done on the basis of two medical reports detailing the clinical rationale for the application.

It is likely, however, that the Community Psychiatric Nurse (CPN) will have the major part to play in ensuring that the person complies with the measures specified in the order. This has significant implications for the therapeutic alliance between the person and the CPN. The nurse must strive to ensure that his/her role does not shift from one of therapeutic partner to one of 'mental health act enforcer' where reluctance on the person's part to comply is met with the warning of a possible enforced return to hospital. In such circumstances the hope-inspiring, trusting relationship and therapeutic alliance necessary to support and promote the person's recovery would be impossible to achieve.

Medication is the easiest treatment to deliver on a compulsory basis. It is readily available and requires little effort or thought for overstretched practitioners. It is much more difficult to compel people who require services such as counselling, cognitive behavioural therapy (CBT) or other talking treatments, which many CPNs see as their core function. These non-pharmaceutical interventions require voluntary participation. Medication is not always desirable or helpful and some may argue that it is only justifiable if it brings about a better life for the individual – matched with past or current wishes and aspirations. If it does not, the ethical question is whether we are only compelling the person to take the medication to appease a society which otherwise ignores, denies or stigmatises them.

Where medication brings benefits, these are likely to be limited unless the drug(s) are combined with access to a range of other interventions and services, such as practical support to overcome problems-of-living, adequate housing, education, training and employment. If Community CTOs focus only on medication they are likely to be, at best, only partially effective, and in some cases potentially harmful if they precipitate a person's complete disengagement from essential support. Treatment perhaps should be more clearly defined in legislative terms in relation to detailing access to a wider range of non-pharmaceutical therapeutic interventions.

Delivering key principles in practice

Mental health nurses and other practitioners must always practice ethically and work within the law. This means that in striving to meet people's needs, their practice must be underpinned by core values and principles which acknowledge people's rights as valued members of society. Nurses are the predominant mental health professionals in terms of numbers and as such they have a key role in bringing about cultural change. They and other practitioners must:

- explore, respect and learn from people's personal experience of mental health problems;
- seek to determine people's personal wishes, aspirations, concerns and fears;
- involve people in their care in a manner which is meaningful to the person and bring tangible benefit.

They must also practice within the parameters set out in:

- practitioner codes of conduct;
- good practice guidelines/statements;
- national legislation – including the principles and spirit underpinning that legislation.

The emphasis is no longer about doing things *to* people or doing things *for* them. Neither is it about protecting them from all possible harm. It is about working with and alongside people: positively managing risks rather than vainly trying to eliminate them altogether. It is about promoting people's recovery, sense of self-determination, self-worth, self-respect and dignity and supporting them to live lives that are meaningful to them.

Respecting diversity, challenging inequalities and non-discriminatory practice

These principles require the practitioner to practice in a manner which respects the person's background, 'differences', 'preferences' and 'uniqueness'. Understanding, and demonstrating that these factors have been taken into account when working with people to build their care plan, is of vital importance. The practitioner must also seek to ensure that people with mental health problems are afforded the same rights and respect as other members of society when they engage with services.

To challenge inequalities, the practitioner needs to have an understanding of the actual and potential consequences of stigma, discrimination and social exclusion. It is their duty to do everything within their power to challenge negative attitudes, discriminatory behaviours and language that is disrespectful; to question value-laden judgements and opinions held by other Mental Health Practitioners and to combat unfairness and injustice towards people with mental health problems.

Reciprocity

This principle is probably the least well understood. If a person is subject to compulsory measures under mental health legislation, it is essential for practitioners to ensure that the services provided are appropriate. If statutory services are overriding the person's civil liberties for the purposes of providing care and treatment, the MH(CT)(S)A[1] places a duty upon the health and social care authorities – and by inference the health and social care practitioners practicing within a clinical or local authority setting – to provide care of a standard and quality that is *adequate* to meet the person's needs and safe and proportionate to the degree of vulnerability the person presents. Interventions should bring benefit and they should be matched to need. In short the services should *'make a difference'*. Whilst working within organisational policy and towards organisational aims, some of which might be resource and efficiency focused, the practitioner is duty bound to ensure that services are safe, effective and person-centred and to speak up and challenge service managers and others on behalf of people when they feel that these factors are being compromised.

The provision of meaningful, person-centred care requires practitioners to be comfortable with relinquishing control. The lived experience of mental health problems and the journey of recovery are factors unique to each person. That is a fact of life. To respect and work with this 'fact of life' means practitioners having to operate in a manner that moves away from the outdated notion that they are the (so-called) *experts* who will proffer guidance and advice that must be followed at all times.

New ways of working, being led and promoted by nurses, acknowledge and respect the knowledge and wisdom that comes from a 'lived experience'. They seek to build upon people's strengths and abilities. They turn the old ways on their head and view the person and their carers as the experts and the practitioners as their apprentices. They focus less on obstacles and more on what is positive and possible.

This requires practitioners to develop and hone new skills that are founded in values, which promote autonomy, self-direction, social inclusion and a shared responsibility for positive risk-taking.

They must work in a way that both recognises and tackles the – sometimes obvious/sometimes latent – power imbalances which exist between practitioners and people in receipt of care. This is especially true in the case of people subject to compulsory measures under mental health legislation.

Resorting to compulsion is not the only choice. Practitioners must develop skills in communication and rapport building which enable them to establish and maintain helping relationships that respect peoples' rights, maintain their dignity and help them to make sense of their world. They must also support them to recognise and evaluate the advantages and disadvantages of specific therapeutic interventions and make informed choices which help them regain control of their lives.

To paraphrase NHS Education Scotland's 10 Essential Shared Capabilities for Mental Health Practice.[9]

> The provision of meaningful person-centred care means agreeing on goals that fit with the achievable wants and aspirations of the person, their carers and family, rather than focusing on the interventions which Mental Health Practitioners might think that the person needs. It then focuses on what needs to be done now, who will do what and how progress and success will be identified.

Participation

The principle of *'participation'* is focused on the person being enabled and empowered to participate in his/her care as fully as possible. It is fundamental to the concept of *'working in partnership'* with the person. It decrees that people, and others important to them, should be partners in their care rather than passive recipients of treatment prescribed by 'experts'.

This presents a quandary for the practitioner who is accustomed to working within a traditional, practitioner-led culture which allows them to feel safe and in-control. The ethical question is how do practitioners accommodate the requirement to empower people and offer meaningful choice within a system which can be overly focused on risk and process and which has the legal power to infringe upon people's rights and freedoms? In the course of professional practice, we must never forget that the best strategy for risk minimisation is the engagement of the person in a trusting therapeutic alliance.

Participation means establishing positive helping relationships, giving due regard to people's stories, experiences, aspirations and past and current feelings. In the course of accurately determining a person's past and current views, the principle of *'participation'* is likely to also mean that the practitioner has to consult other people important to the person, such as carers, relatives or perhaps independent advocates, who effectively become members of 'the wider partnership' along with the person and the multidisciplinary team.

Effective communication is essential if participation is to be meaningful. This might include the use or involvement of communication aids, interpreters, signers or as previously mentioned independent advocates. Communication can be further enhanced by people's stories and wishes being recorded in their own words rather than in practitioner language. This allows the person to validate the practitioner's interpretation and understanding of their unique situation.

For people to participate in a meaningful way they must be given information about services and service options, interventions and treatment strategies and the advantages and disadvantages of taking any mooted course of action. This information must be presented in a form and at a pace that is comprehensible to the person. Importantly, they must be supported to understand it.

The giving of verbal information should always be the first option. This allows the person to pause, reflect, ask questions, seek clarification and slow things down when they feel the need. Written information should only be viewed as a back-up to face-to-face communication, not a substitute. The person's understanding should be gauged and the subject matter revisited again later if it is felt that he/she does not fully understand all or part of what is being explained.

Respect for carers

This principle is closely linked to the principle of 'participation' as it involves respecting the experiences that people have had, or are having, as carers.

As far as it is practicable to do so, it means giving due regard to their stories and views. It enables them to become part of 'the partnership' as far as their abilities and wishes, the wishes of the person being cared for and considerations for confidentiality allow.

It is not uncommon for the carer to also be the person's Named Person, chosen by the person to provide support when he/she is engaged in any proceedings under the Act.

Named Persons, carers and families need to be given appropriate information to enable them to participate in care and in supporting the person. Once again some good practice rules apply in that written information should be provided to support verbal explanation. All information should be provided in ordinary (not practitioner) language. Written information should be provided in a format that the carer can readily understand with due regard given to overcoming communication obstacles.

Where carers have health and social care needs of their own they should be given relevant information and 'signposted' to appropriate services.

Least restrictive alternative

This principle brings most angst to Mental Health Practitioners as they struggle with the ethical dilemma of balancing people's vulnerabilities with their freedoms as members of a just society.

It compels practitioners to adopt an approach which places the minimum restriction on people's lives commensurate with the provision of safe and effective care.

Many deliberate and unwitting actions taken by Mental Health Practitioners have the effect of unnecessarily limiting the freedom of people in their care. Sometimes these actions are meant in the person's best interests but often they can be more about the best interests of the practitioners themselves or their employing organisations.

We all have the right to take risks in our personal lives and these risks can be variable depending upon our capabilities. So if people have the right to take risks, how do Mental Health Practitioners strike the correct balance between risk of harm and giving people freedom to act? At what point should they get involved? It can be a difficult dilemma when one is trying to fulfil a duty of care and the person being cared for is ignoring their advice or rejecting their support. Practitioners should not feel compelled to protect people from every potential mishap and disappointment. Indeed evidence of responsible risk-taking is an indicator of good mental health practice.

Living a meaningful life involves taking measured risks and living with the possibility of failure. Sometimes the courses of action we take are unsuccessful – we live and learn from that. If practitioners seek to shelter people from failure they are basically communicating to them that they are too vulnerable and that it is too unsafe and too risky for them to make decisions for themselves. Ultimately they stifle the individual's personal growth.

This response to risk is disempowering in the extreme. It erodes any sense of control and self-responsibility the person might previously have felt. It corrodes their self-esteem and self-confidence. It leaves them with a sense of not being listened to. It results in overly restrictive clinical practices that lead to feelings of frustration, resentment and anger. In the end it can completely fracture the therapeutic partnership and give rise to the person taking reckless risks which have more serious and longer-term consequences.

People's recovery can only flourish in a climate where they feel valued and that their rights are respected. In this regard the right to autonomy and self-determination is important and must be promoted in all circumstances where it is safe to do so. In a team culture which is risk-averse, care and treatment strategies are likely to be well meaning but overly parental, overly restrictive and perhaps custodial in nature, thereby stifling the development of the team and the development of the person who is being cared for. In such a culture it is likely that all the significant decisions will rest with the practitioners and the person will be a passive onlooker who is told by the 'authorities' what will be happening to them. The ethically minded practitioner must guard against this.

In a culture that embraces risk and works with it, it can provide opportunities to promote self-direction, self-responsibility and self-esteem – people will 'grow' as individuals and assume greater control over their lives and their behaviours. Having a clear and measured approach to *positive risk-taking* is critical in engendering this type of team culture.

Under the principle of '*least restrictive alternative*' the promotion of safety and positive risk-taking involves sharing decision-making *with* the person being cared for *and* those important to him/her. It acknowledges the potential conflict between considerations for safety and the person's right to autonomy and grasps this nettle by involving the whole team. It concedes that no single individual has all of the knowledge and experience to make all of the decisions unilaterally and safely. It recognises that no single person should be burdened with such a huge sense of responsibility.

The importance of careful and measured assessment cannot be overemphasised. Such an assessment should strive to support the clinical team's understanding of why the person is behaving in the way(s) that they are. The identification of risks and vulnerabilities and the required interventions must be carried out in an open and transparent way.

Benefit

The principle of '*benefit*' involves the core imperative that no one should intervene in a person's life without being confident that the intervention will benefit the person and that the proposed intervention is the only safe and equitable means of achieving this benefit.

Benefit can be difficult to define and in terms of identifying the potential impact on practitioner practice it is therefore probably best to view this principle in the context of all of the others in the set. This effectively means that in trying to deliver 'benefit' the person must

- be supported to participate;
- have their carers/family involved;
- receive all information relative to their care and treatment;
- be supported to tell their own unique story;
- have their culture, lifestyle, choices, values and beliefs respected;
- have equal access to all potential services and supports as others;
- be enabled to speak about their problems of living and their hopes and aspirations for the future;
- be supported in the least restrictive way possible;
- receive care that is effective;
- be supported to recognise their personal progress and derive hope from this.

Conclusion

The Scottish legislation's underpinning principles seek to promote rights and values-based practice. The separation of detention from compulsion strives to support the principle of least restrictive alternative and the concept of care in the community.

If practitioners are to ensure that they are promoting recovery and not simply 'controlling a problematic section of the population', there are a number of professional challenges, ethical dilemmas inherent in the new framework which they must be alive to and which they must endeavour to surmount. There are also a number of changes to traditional, often well-intended, practices which they will have to implement.

In researching the outcomes and effects of the legislation as it becomes established, we must look beyond issues like the number of hospital admissions, length of stay, number of untoward events, suicide rates and size of caseloads to outcomes which are person-centred.

The things that are important to people are: being able to make their own decisions; being able to establish and maintain meaningful personal relationships; being respected; having valued roles in their communities; and having opportunities for personal growth and development. They are looking for services which are appealing, offer real choice and are relevant to their needs. They also want consistent services, of a high standard. They will avoid services of variable quality that seem more concerned with constantly re-inventing themselves under the guise of progress. Person-centred services and service benchmarks will give us a sense of whether or not the legislation is improving the mental health of the people of Scotland.

Notes

1 Scottish Executive Public Health Division. *Renewing Mental Health Law: Policy Statement.* Edinburgh: SEHD, 2001.
2 Scottish Executive Public Health Division. *Millan Committee Final Report. New Directions: Report on the Review of the Mental Health (Scotland) Act 1984.* Edinburgh: SEHD, 2001.
3 Scottish Executive. *Mental Health (Scotland) Bill.* Edinburgh: HMSO, September 2002.
4 Scottish Executive. *Mental Health (Care and Treatment) (Scotland) Act 2003.* Edinburgh: Office of Public Sector Information, 2003.
5 Scottish Executive Public Health Division. *Millan Committee Final Report. New Directions: Report on the Review of the Mental Health (Scotland) Act 1984.* Edinburgh: SEHD, 2001, pp. 16–22 (Chapter 3).
6 Patrick, Hilary. *Mental Health, Incapacity and the Law in Scotland.* Edinburgh: Tottel Publishing, 2006.
7 Scottish Office. *Mental Health (Scotland) Act 1984: An Act to Consolidate the Mental Health (Scotland) Act 1960.* Edinburgh: Office of Public Sector Information, 1984.
8 Parker, C. and McCulloch, A *Key Issues from Homicide Inquiries*, London: Mind, 1999.
9 NHS Education for Scotland. *The 10 Essential Shared Capabilities for Mental Health Practice: Learning Materials (Scotland).* Edinburgh: NHS Education for Scotland, 2007.

26 Advance directives

Jacqueline Atkinson

Introduction

Advance directives seem at first glance to be both simple and straightforward. When well (or 'capable') a person writes down how they want to be treated when they become too unwell (or 'incapable') to make that decision for themselves. This would seem to be the epitome of respecting a person's wishes (autonomy) and also having them involved in decision-making about their treatment, which may improve communication and collaboration with staff. In most people's minds it is probably associated with refusal of treatment in end-of-life situations and may be used synonymously with 'living wills' or 'do not resuscitate' (DNR) orders.[1] They have been discussed and promoted in the media, particularly following the death of the popular Labour politician Mo Mowlam who died in 2005 and who had one in place following her diagnosis with a brain tumour.

It is not surprising that there has been interest expressed by people with mental illness in advance directives.[2] They have been adopted by parts of the user movement as a way of promoting patient choice and autonomy and may be seen as part of a wider involvement of patients in their treatment. The reality of using advance directives is not so straightforward, however, particularly when they are applied to mental illness. This chapter will explore some of these issues.

Advance directives and mental illness

There is no one single definition of an advance directive which suits all situations, apart from the general statement made at the start of this chapter, as different legal jurisdictions have different legal requirements. Added to this, different terms are used to describe them. Thus in Scotland, where they are, unusually, incorporated into the Mental Health (Care and Treatment) (Scotland) Act 2003 they are referred to as advance statements (see Chapter 25). In England and Wales there is general provision made for the making of advance decisions to refuse treatment in the Mental Capacity Act 2005, but nothing specific for mental illness (see Chapter 23). In much of the United States they are referred to as psychiatric advance directives (PADs) and the majority of states have legislation covering them.[3] In this chapter *advance directive* will be used as the generic term.

The idea of advance directives in mental health came to the fore in 1982, when Thomas Szasz suggested a 'psychiatric will' (corresponding to a living will),[1] Howell *et al.* suggested a 'precommitment contract',[5] and following Culver and Gert's use of the term 'Odysseus pact'[6] both Winston *et al.* and Dresser[7] presented ideas for 'Ulysses contracts'. A decade later service users Rogers and Centifanti promoted the 'Mill's will'[8] as they had concerns about the presumption in Ulysses contracts towards accepting treatment. Over time the emphasis has varied between those wanting a person to be able to refuse either all, or certain kinds of treatment and others who saw an advance directive as a way of entering into a dialogue with their doctor or treating team to negotiate an acceptable treatment plan.[9] Indeed, for some people the main objective of having advance directives seems to be to open up channels of communication between staff and patients. This has led some groups, for whom the autonomy of the patient's wishes is primary, to withdraw support for advance directives, although there is support for making them legally enforceable.[10-12]

These different approaches have led to a number of different models of advance directives in mental health being drawn up.[13-15] This takes account of whether the directive is drawn up independently, with an independent staff member, or in collaboration with the patient's doctor; whether it allows for the person to request particular treatments or only to refuse them; and whether it covers wider issues than just clinical treatment. Some may even indicate when the directive is to come into force, and this is the first problematic area in their use in mental illness. In England and Wales, and many states in the United States, it may also incorporate the appointment of a surrogate or proxy decision-maker.

Advance directives, mental illness and capacity

There are some circumstances where it is clear that the person does not have capacity to make a decision about his/her treatment, and these are situations where an advance directive may be useful. Such situations would include the person being unconscious or in a coma and being legally judged to lack capacity under (in)capacity legislation. People may not be able to make capacitous medical decisions in other situations, such as during an emergency, and the law allows for emergency treatment to be given without informed consent in such circumstances, although if an advance directive is in place this should be followed. Even in such circumstances, an advance directive may not be followed if it refuses treatment and, at the time, the patient indicates that he/she wishes to have treatment. Where a decision is in favour of prolonging life, even if the person lacks capacity, most people will be happy to go with that decision. In conditions such as dementia a person may make an advance statement when first diagnosed to cover what will happen to him/her as he/she loses capacity. They may also choose to appoint a proxy or surrogate decision-maker (such as a welfare attorney) under (in)capacity legislation to deal with financial and other practical circumstances.

With a mental illness the situation of when to use an advance directive is even less clear-cut. Mental illness is a fluctuating condition and it is possible to have an acute psychotic episode but still retain capacity. The crucial question is probably whether the person has the capacity to make a decision about his/her medical treatment and is thus a more narrow definition of capacity than that found in (in)capacity legislation. This is the approach taken in Scotland in the Mental Health (Care and Treatment) (Scotland) Act 2003 (see Chapter 27), which introduced a modified capacity criterion for compulsory treatment; that is, 'significantly impaired decision-making ability' (SIDMA) in relation to making medical decisions about treatment. This means that unlike many legal jurisdictions, including England and Wales, a person with mental illness who has capacity to make a medical decision *cannot* be detained and treated against his/her will. Although the law itself and the Code of Practice for its use[16] do not specify how this impaired ability is to be determined, it is, nevertheless, a helpful approach to considering capacity in relation to mental illness. Patrick[17] describes it as 'a more flexible concept than incapacity'. The mental disorder itself is responsible for the impaired decision-making and may mean that decisions about some treatments are capacitous but not others. The Mental Welfare Commission for Scotland[18] advises that capacity to consent to treatment should be assessed for each separate treatment.

If a global assessment of capacity is not appropriate what are the issues in mental illness which mean that a person may be handicapped in making a competent decision? Possibly the most common situation is going to be that of lack of insight. This interferes with the person making competent decisions about his/her treatment because it means that the person has no real understanding that he/she is ill. They may well realize that they are not in agreement with people around them as to what is happening, but may attribute this to problems other than to something in themselves. In other aspects of their life their capacity to make decisions may not be affected. The only issue is that they do not believe they need treatment or they do not believe it will make any difference. In many cases lack of insight will mean that a person refuses treatment when he/she most needs it. For some people this will be a persistent symptom; for others it will be something that happens as they become ill again. It could be argued that advance directives are made for such circumstances. The persons, when they have insight, can specify what treatment they agree to, or want to refuse, when they lose insight. From a clinical and legal perspective the question then arises at what point can a clinician invoke the advance directive and treat the person against his/her current wishes, but following the advance directive, and without the use of mental health or capacity legislation. Although it might be possible to write into the advance directive when it should be used it will always be open to interpretation.

Lack of insight is not the only time a person's mental illness interferes with his/her decision-making ability. A feature of depression is that the person may experience hopelessness and helplessness in his/her thinking, along with a low value of his/her self. In such a circumstance they may believe that there is no point in having treatment, either because it will not work, or because they are not worth receiving treatment. Again, an advance directive may allow the person to specify what treatments he/she will accept or refuse, and when the directive should come into force.

Anorexia nervosa is yet another different scenario. The condition is such that it may always interfere with the person's ability to make a judgement about the need for treatment,[19] but he/she may also recognize that there is a problem and may be willing to make an advance directive to come into effect, for example, when he/she reaches a certain lower weight.

Sometimes a person refuses treatment *as* they become unwell, not for reasons connected with the illness, but for reasons connected to the treatment. Antipsychotic medication has extremely unpleasant side effects and some people may decide that they would rather have a period of illness than take the medication. Similarly some people experience electroconvulsive therapy (ECT) and its consequences as so distressing that they do not want to receive it. Decisions of this type should carry some weight, although some clinicians will argue it helps if they are made in conjunction with the treatment team so alternatives can be agreed. Other considerations may be how long someone may be prepared to be unwell before considering treatment, or if the situation becomes life-threatening.[20]

If someone has to be declared *legally incapable* (or, as in Scotland, subject to a Mental Health Act order) before an advance directive comes into play this will severely limit its use. It does, however, give a clear trigger for its use. Most people with a major mental illness do not become subject to legal conditions; nevertheless their thinking can be impaired and their decisions different from those made when well. Different legal jurisdictions will deal with this differently (see later) but it is in these circumstances where advance directives may be best seen as integrating with other forms of future planning, including joint crisis plans and the care programme approach (CPA).[21]

In making an advance directive a person states his/her (capacitous) wishes at the time, but people may change their minds according to circumstances or the passage of time. If they are well, they can change their advance directive. Indeed, it would be seen as good practice to regularly update an advance directive or at least indicate that it still represents the person's wishes. The problem arises in mental health when someone has written an advance directive agreeing to certain treatment, but he/she becomes unwell and subsequently refuses this treatment. If the law is not invoked then, what status does it have to overrule the person's current decisions? Dunlap[22] puts it well when she describes the situation of someone with an acute psychotic situation as a 'netherworld of quasi competence'.

Advance directives and the law

An advance directive is only worthwhile if it has mandatory power to be used when a person is incapable of making a decision. In many legal jurisdictions, including the United Kingdom, this is the case in physical illness for advance refusals of treatment. The position differs, however, in mental illness. In most legal jurisdictions an advance directive is 'trumped' by the use of a 'Mental Health Act' which allows for compulsory treatment, even if the person objects and has so stated in an advance directive. This is particularly the case where only advance refusals of treatment are allowed. Clinicians, however, may choose to at least consider the person's wishes as set out in the advance statement.

In Scotland the position is somewhat different. When the Mental Health Act 1984 was being reviewed considerable attention was given to the possible role of advance directives.[23,24] There was support from user groups and their representatives although less support from psychiatrists.[25] Advance statements were introduced in the Mental Health (Care and Treatment)(Scotland) Act 2003 along with personal statements. An advance statement allows a person to state both how he/she wishes to be treated for a mental disorder and also how he/she does not wish to be treated, when unwell and unable to make a decision. It is a written, witnessed statement which ideally should be kept in a patient's records and be available to clinicians at the time of making a compulsory treatment order (including a short-term order), who are required to 'have regard' for its contents. It is presented to the Mental Health Tribunal which considers the application for a compulsory treatment order and which also has to 'have regard' for the contents of the advance statement. It is not binding in law and can be overturned. Any treatment given in conflict with an advance statement has to have the reasons for this noted. The patient must be told this and a record of the decision and reasons placed in the patient's medical records. It must also be reported to the Mental Welfare Commission for Scotland, which has produced figures on the overturning of advance directives.[26]

When advance statements were introduced it was intended that 'treatment' referred to medical treatment for the condition. It was also recognized that people might want to give instructions, or state wishes, which were wider than this. For this reason, 'personal statements' were introduced which allow the person to cover a wider set of conditions, including: care of children; care of pets or their home; financial matters; or who they want to visit or restrict visits from. The personal statement does not carry the same weight as the advance statement. For this reason, or perhaps because of lack of clarity in the guidelines, the contents of advance statements vary widely.[27] They have been used less than some people had hoped, for various reasons including: lack of knowledge about them; that they are not legally binding; people being unwilling, when they are well, to think about becoming ill again and planning for this; or people seeing no need as they trust their clinical team to do what is best.[28] For these reasons advance statements have been included in the mini review of the Act which will report on its consultation paper in 2010.[29]

In England and Wales, Sections 24–6 of the Mental Capacity Act introduced advance decisions to refuse treatment. If these are written, signed and witnessed then they are legally enforceable (given certain other considerations) under the Act. This is not the case where someone is subject to the Mental Health Act when a person with capacity can still receive compulsory treatment *for a mental disorder*, although the advance refusal should be considered. If a person has an advance refusal for treatment for a physical condition this should still be enforceable even if the person is subject to the Mental Health Act. This separation of mental disorder and physical illness has been described by some people as discriminatory.

> … the Government is allowing advance refusals in the Mental Capacity Act which would allow people to exercise some dignity and control at the end of their lives, yet is not allowing similar dignity or control over treatment for people in non-life threatening situations, by virtue of them having a mental disorder.[30]

There is also growing interest in more widely defined advance statements (or advance directives, both terms are used), which could include acceptable treatment and the circumstances which make it acceptable for treatment to be refused no matter how ill; treatment the person would rather not receive and the circumstances and the names of someone to be consulted.[31] Although there are similarities with the advance statement in Scottish law, care must be taken in understanding which legal jurisdiction is being referred to and thus the detail of what is required and how it will be used. The National Institute for Clinical Excellence (NICE) Guidelines on schizophrenia[32] include advance decisions and agreements as a standard of care, as does the Guidance on the short-term management of disturbed and violent behaviour in inpatient settings and emergency departments.[33] Audits of the guidelines suggest low usage ranging from no patients having them[34] to a meta-analysis suggesting a compliance rate of 29 per cent.[35]

The law in Northern Ireland is currently being reviewed and it is expected that this will clarify the position of advance statements there. In the United States, Canada and Australia each state, province or territory has a different law governing the use of advance directives.[36]

Problems in the legal status of advance directives

Some service users have either withdrawn support for advance directives or have refused to make them because they are not legally enforceable, and some groups argue for this. Is this a reasonable position to take? This requires consideration of the range of situations in which an advance directive might be made and what it might contain.

Perhaps the arguments for why advance acceptance of treatment is not legally enforceable is the easiest place to start. Nowhere can a patient legally demand and receive a treatment they want. Probably the most commonly given reason for this is that it is for a doctor – as expert – to decide what a treatment should be and not a patient. There are concerns that patients might want inappropriate or contra-indicated treatment. This is not the same as a patient who lists treatments which he/she has received in the past and which he/she is willing to receive again. Similarly, a patient may refuse older medications but may say he/she is willing to try new medications as they become available. Other concerns include patients opting for more expensive treatments and this having an impact on resources and patients with an advance directive having more or more expensive treatments than those who do not.

In some parts of the United States there exists provision for making what is called a Ulysses contract. This is named after the ancient Greek explorer who asked his crew to bind him tightly to the mast so he could hear the song of the Sirens (whilst they had their ears stopped up with wax) but not be lured onto the rocks. A Ulysses contract is seen as a 'self-binding' directive to accept treatment when necessary, and although some people have argued that patients should be able to agree to accept treatment in this way, rather than, for example, be subject to compulsory treatment, others still see it as coercive treatment.[37] As well as concerns that people might be put under pressure to make such a contract, there is also concern that such a contract negates the contemporaneous wishes of the person when ill. It could be argued that, at least in mental health, this is the point of an advance acceptance of treatment and the individual would only make it with this knowledge. It does, however, raise the issue of the 'rights' of the ill person to have his/her wishes heard and respected, even against the wishes of his/her 'well' self.[38]

Another issue that arises with advance statements which are very widely written, such as some of those made in Scotland,[39] is the question of what should count legally as 'treatment'. A person may find meditating with candles helpful in managing agitation but this might require finding a special, secure place (both in terms of fire regulations and freedom from interruption from other patients) and possibly supervision (for fire regulations). It may be that the person's symptoms or behaviour improves, but does this constitute 'treatment'? The resource implications of this, along with other similar requests, may make staff want to have the option to dismiss them. Given that a number of the requests referred to the boredom of inpatient wards it may be that generic changes to the environment might negate the necessity for some of the requests.

In almost all jurisdictions advance refusal for treatment for a mental illness is not binding. The Mental Health Alliance's position (noted in the earlier section)[30] is that it is discriminatory when advance refusal for physical illness is legally binding. What are the reasons for this difference? The first reason is the mental status of the patient, particularly regarding insight into their condition. If someone refuses treatment because he/she does not believe he/she is ill then his/her competence to make an advance directive may be challenged, and clinicians will usually argue that he/she has a duty of care and it is in the person's best interests to be treated. If, however, they refuse treatment because they do not want to experience its potentially negative side effects, it could be argued that it is their decision to make. It does, however, lead to another concern that of how the person is to be managed, or treated, whilst acutely ill and refusing treatment.

This leads to a reason for not wanting to allow patients to refuse treatment which may not be palatable to many and that is resources. Put baldly, if someone with a terminal illness refuses treatment this is likely to hasten their death and management of their condition will be for a limited time. Someone with a recurrent mental illness who refuses treatment when acutely ill is still likely to require care and management. If they pose a risk to themselves or others they will probably be subject to detention under the Mental Health Act. Even if they are not then compulsorily treated they will still require a bed, nursing care and other support. This is likely to last longer than if they received treatment. There are concerns that if a number of patients acted in this way there would be excessive demand on resources.[40]

Research indicates that very few patients refuse all treatment, instead preferring to refuse some, but indicate what is acceptable.[11-46] The 'worse case' scenarios which have received publicity, however, are in jurisdictions where refusal of treatment was upheld in court, thus disallowing treatment under a Mental Health Act. Two involved advance directives. These were the cases of Nancy Hargrave in Vermont[47] and Edwin Sevels in Ontario.[48] Having refused treatment Mr Sevels spent 404 days in seclusion. Another celebrated case in Ontario was that of Scott Starson, who, although not having an advance directive, refused treatment and was found by the Supreme Court to be competent to make that decision and then spent a number of years hospitalized but not receiving treatment.[49,50] A total of six such cases have been found in Ontario, with patients spending more than 20 years in hospital.[51]

There is one aspect, however, where there may be an advantage in making an advance directive for a recurrent illness. The less experience a person has with the situation he/she is trying to predict and plan for the more difficult it will be, and the greater the likelihood there will be problems with his/her planning. For people with mental illness they are likely to be writing an advance directive with some considerable experience of the situations in which they are unable to make decisions and their advance directive will reflect this experience. This is offset, however, by the fact that when the directive comes into force their contemporaneous decisions may not accord with the advance directive (particularly one agreeing to treatment). They will probably want to engage in the decision-making process (even if such engagement is of the order 'everyone go away and leave me alone'), and they certainly should not be excluded. Whereas in many end-of-life situations there is not the possibility for the person to engage in any way, or often to even be aware that such decisions are being taken.

Invoking an advance directive

If an advance directive is only to be used when a person is not capable of making a decision does this mean that a formal or legal test of capacity is necessary before an advance directive can be used? In England and Wales, being subject to the Capacity Act, and in Scotland the Mental Health (Care and Treatment) (Scotland) Act will automatically invoke any advance directive which is in place. But some people may see a use for them before reaching this stage or may prefer to use an advance directive than be subject to such Acts. Some templates for advance directives have a section which suggests when it should be used.[52–54] These give, however, little information on when they are actually invoked. Even if a person outlines the signs of them becoming ill and thus unlikely to make the decision they are putting in their advance directive, there is always the possibility that both at the time and after the event they may have different views about whether it should have been used.

The practicalities of advance directives

Although in some legal jurisdictions a verbal advance refusal of treatment is valid, when it comes to advance directives in mental health they need to be in writing and usually witnessed. Some places have a preferred template which should be used, and many organizations, including hospital authorities and user groups, also have templates which can be used. There may also be regulations about who is eligible to be a witness to an advance directive, as well as what they are witnessing to. This may be no more than a witness to a signature or may range from saying that they believe the person made the directive voluntarily to making a judgement about the person's capacity. An advance directive also needs to be kept up to date and it is generally suggested that it should be renewed at least every 5 years.

An advance directive is only useful if it is available when it is needed. For this reason a copy should be given to the person's psychiatrist and placed in their medical record. It may also be useful for their general practitioner (GP) to have a copy. If it has not been drawn up with the clinical team then it might prove an opportunity for discussing future plans for management should another crisis occur. It is probably also helpful if someone close to the person – a part-ner, parent or close friend – at least knows of the advance directive's existence and where it can be found (if they do not have a copy), so that in an emergency they can remind staff of its existence. Easy access to the advance directive must be balanced with privacy and confidential-ity about its contents where multiple copies are held by family or friends. The need for family to know of its existence is important. One study, where a form of advance directive was placed at the front of the patient's medical record it was still overlooked by many staff.[55]

The ethics of advance directives in practice

Patient autonomy is a guiding principle in health care ethics and for many is the underlying foundation for the use of advance directives. They are a form of substituted judgement where the 'well person' is making a decision which they want treated as a contemporaneous decision when they are unable to make a decision regarding treatment. This automatically gives the 'well' person rights over the 'ill' person, who now has no rights to refuse consent to treatment. If the person consents then the issue of their capacity may not even be raised. It becomes of particular importance if the person wants to revoke the advance directive.

There are differences of opinion about when a person can revoke an advance directive. Many believe that the same conditions should apply as to make one, that is, the person must be competent. Others, however, think that someone should be able to revoke it at any time. Whilst this clearly gives the greatest autonomy to the person it also negates the purpose of an advance acceptance of treatment which a person makes when competent, knowing that when they become ill they will refuse treatment. The question of the 'rights' of the person when unwell to make decisions as to what should happen is complex and includes a consid-eration of which 'decision-making entity' – the well or ill self – should take precedence and involves a consideration not only of autonomy but also what it means to be a person (see Chapter 2) and the role of rationality in our concept of a person.[56]

There is also a question of whether people have a responsibility to accept treatment and thus prevent or at least delay or minimize their use of finite services as well as limit other damage as a consequence of treatment refusal. Most Mental Health Acts require a person to be a risk to either themselves or others before they can be compulsorily treated. Is it rea-sonable to allow a person to refuse treatment if they continue to be a danger to others? Even if detained in hospital such patients may still present a risk and require either seclusion or restraint. A person making an advance directive needs to be aware of these possibilities and in making choices understand that they may need to choose the least worst option. It is unlikely that many people would agree to a person refusing treatment and being allowed to harm others in the name of autonomy. However, whether or not a person could refuse treat-ment and harm themselves is open to debate.

In some cases refusal of treatment may mean that a person dies, not just through suicide but possibly as an end stage consequence of depression, mania or anorexia nervosa.[57,58] This is quite different from someone refusing treatment with a terminal illness. Again some people feel that this is an individual's choice, where, for example, death might be seen as preferable to ECT. Other people will be uncomfortable in allowing someone to die from a condition which could be treated. And it is for this reason Mental Health Acts exist which allow for the compulsory treatment of people at risk who refuse treatment.

Putting advance directives into practice means confronting the ethical dilemmas as well as the practical ones. Since in most places advance directives in mental health can be overruled by the use of a Mental Health Act the dilemmas are usually addressed at an individual clinical level rather than through the law.

Notes

1 Department for Constitutional Affairs. *Making Decisions: Helping People Who Have Difficulty in Deciding for Themselves: Planning Ahead. A Guide for People Who Wish to Prepare for Possible Future Incapacity*, London: Department for Constitutional Affairs, 2003.
2 The term mental illness will be used rather than mental health problems, as to make use of an advance directive requires someone to lack capacity, and this is not a feature of most mental health problems, but may apply at times with people with major mental illness.
3 Atkinson, J. *Advance Directives in Mental Health. Theory Practice and Ethics*, London: Jessica Kingsley Publishers, 2007.
4 Szasz, T. 'The psychiatric will. A new mechanism for protecting persons against "psychosis" and psychiatry', *American Psychologist* 1982, 37: 762–70.
5 Howell, T., Diamond, R. and Winkler, D. 'Is there a case for voluntary commitment?', In: Beauchamp, T. and Wlater, L. (Eds.) *Contemporary Issues in Bioethics*, Belmont, CA: Wadsworth, 1982.
6 Culver, C. and Gert, B. 'The morality of involuntary hospitalization', In: Spicker, J.M., Healy, J.R. and Engelhart, J.R. (Eds.) *The Law Medicine Relations: A Philosophical Exploration*, Boston, MA: Riedel, 1981.
7 Winston, M., Winston, S., Appelbaum, P. and Rhoden, N. 'Can a subject consent to a Ulysses contract? Commentary', *Hastings Centre Report* 1982, 12: 27–80; Dresser, R. 'Ulysses and the psychiatrists: a legal policy analysis of the voluntary commitment contract', *Harvard Civil Rights-Civil Liberties Law Review* 1982, 16: 833–5.
8 Rogers, J.A. and Centifanti, J.B. 'Beyond "self-paternalism": response to Rosenson and Kasten', *Schizophrenia Bulletin* 1991, 17: 1–7
9 Atkinson 2007, op. cit.
10 Atkinson, J., Garner, H.C., Patrick, H. and Stuart, S. 'Issues in the development of potential models of advance directives in mental health care', *Journal of Mental Health* 2003, 12: 463–74.
11 Atkinson, J.M. *Private and Public Protection: The New Mental Health Regime*, Edinburgh: Dunedin Academic Press, 2006.
12 Campbell, P. 'Written in advance', *OpenMind*, September/October 1999: p. 24.
13 Atkinson, J.M., Garner, H.C., Stuart, S. and Patrick, H. 'The development of potential models of advance directives in mental health', *Journal of Mental Health* 2002, 12: 575–84.
14 Atkinson, J.M., Garner, H. and Gilmour, W.H. 'Models of advance directives in mental health care: stakeholder views', *Social Psychiatry and Psychiatric Epidemiology* 2004, 39: 673–80.
15 Henderson, C., Swanson, J.W., Szmukler G., Thornicroft, G. and Zinkler, M. 'A typology of advance statements in mental health care', *Psychiatric Services* 2008, 59: 63–71.
16 Scottish Executive. *Mental Health (Care and Treatment) (Scotland) Act 2003 Code of Practice* (Vols 1,2,3), Edinburgh: Scottish Executive, 2005.
17 Patrick, H. *Mental Health, Incapacity and the Law in Scotland*, Edinburgh: Tottel, 2006.
18 Mental Welfare Commission for Scotland. *Consent to Treatment*, Edinburgh: MWC, 2006.
19 Tan, J., Hope, A. and Stewart, A. 'Competence to refuse treatment in anorexia nervosa', *International Journal of Law and Psychiatry* 2003, 26: 697–707.
20 Atkinson 2007, op. cit.
21 Atkinson 2007, op. cit.
22 Dunlap, J.A. 'Mental health advance directives: having one's say?', *Kentucky Law Journal* 2001, 39: 327–86.
23 Atkinson 2006, op. cit.
24 Atkinson 2007, op. cit.
25 Atkinson *et al.*, 2004 op. cit.
26 Mental Welfare Commission for Scotland. *Overview of Mental Welfare in Scotland 2006–2007*, Edinburgh: MWC, 2007.

27 Reilly, J. and Atkinson, J.M. 'The content of mental health advance directives: advance statements in Scotland', *International Journal of Law and Psychiatry* 2010, 33: 116–21.

28 Atkinson, J., Lorgelly, P., Reilly, J. and Stewart, A. *The Early Impact of the Administration of All New Compulsory Powers Under the Mental Health (Care and Treatment) (Scotland) Act 2003*, Edinburgh: Scottish Executive, 2007.

29 Scottish Government. *Limited Review of the Mental Health (Care and Treatment) (Scotland) Act 2003: Report*, Edinburgh: Scottish Government, 2009.

30 Mental Health Alliance. 'Advance Directives and Advance Statements', www.mental health alliance.org.uk/polic/11AdvanceDirectives.pdf (accessed 7 December 2009).

31 Net Lawman. 'Living Wills and Advance Directives Under the Mental Capacity Act', www.net lawman.co.uk/nfo/living-wills-advance-directives.php (accessed on 7 December 2009).

32 National Institute for Clinical Excellence. *Schizophrenia Core Interventions in the Treatment and Management of Schizophrenia in Adults in Primary and Secondary Care*, London: NICE, 2009.

33 National Institute for Clinical Excellence. *Violence the Short-Term Management of Disturbed/Violent Behaviour in In-Patient Psychiatric Settings and Emergency Departments*, London: NICE, 2005.

34 Macpherson, R., Hovey N., Ranagarth, K., Uppal, A. and Thompson, A. 'An audit of clinical practice in an ACT teams against NICE guidelines in schizophrenia', *Journal Psychiatric Intensive Care* 2007, 3: 113–7.

35 Mears, A., Kendall, T., Strathdee, G., Sinfield, R. and Aldridge, I. 'Progress on NICE guidelines in mental health trusts: meta analysis', *Psychiatric Bulletin* 2008, 32: 383–7.

36 Atkinson 2007, op. cit.

37 Monahan, J., Bonnie, R.J., Appelbaum, P.S., Hyde, P.S., Steadman, H.J. and Swartz, M.S. 'Mandated community treatment', *Psychiatric Services* 2001, 52: 1192–205.

38 Atkinson 2007, op. cit.

39 Reilly and Atkinson 2010, op. cit.

40 Halpern, A. and Szmukler, G. 'Psychiatric advance directives: recognizing autonomy and non-consensual treatment', *Psychiatric Bulletin* 1997, 21: 7–9.

41 Amering, M., Stastny, P. and Hopper, P. 'Psychiatric advance directives: qualitative study of informed deliberations by mental health service users', *British Journal of Psychiatry* 2005, 186: 247–52.

42 Backlar, P., McFarland, B.H., Swanson, J.W. and Mahler, J. 'Consumer, providers and informal caregiver opinions on psychiatric advance directives', *Administration and Policy in Mental Health* 2001, 28: 427–41.

43 Reilly and Atkinson 2010, op. cit.

44 Sherman, P.S. 'Computer assisted creation of psychiatric advance directives', *Community Mental Health Journal* 1998, 34: 351–62.

45 Srebnik, D.S., Rutherford, L.T., Peto, T., Russo, J., Zich, B.E., Jaffe, C. and Holtzeimer, P. 'The content and clinical utility of psychiatric advance directives', *Psychiatric Services* 2005, 56: 592–8.

46 Swanson, J.W., Swartz, M.S., Hannon, M.J. and Elbogen, E.B. 'Psychiatric advance directives: a survey of persons with schizophrenia, family members, and treatment providers', *International Journal of Forensic Mental Health* 2003, 2: 73–86.

47 Appelbaum, P. 'Psychiatric advance directives and the treatment of committed patients', *Psychiatric Services* 2004, 55: 751–3.

48 Ambrosini, D.L. and Crocker, A.G. 'Psychiatric advance directives and the right to refuse treatment in Canada', *Canadian Journal of Psychiatry* 2007, 52: 397–402.

49 Gray, J.E. and O'Reilly R.L. 'The Supreme Court of Canada's "beautiful mind" case', *International Journal of Law and Psychiatry* 2009, 32: 315–22.

50 Sklar, R., 'Starson v. Swayze: The Supreme Court speaks out (not all that clearly) on the question of capacity', *Canadian Journal of Psychiatry* 2007, 52: 390–6.

51 Solomon, R., O'Reilly, R., Gray, J. and Nikolic, M. 'Treatment delayed – liberty denied', *Canadian Bar Review* 2008, 78: 679–719.

52 Papageoriou, A., King, M., Janmohamed, A. and Davidson, O. 'Advance directives for patients compulsorily admitted to hospital with serious mental illness', *British Journal of Psychiatry* 2002, 181: 513–19.

53 Papageoriou, A., Janmohamed, A., King, M. and Davidson, O. 'Advance directives for patients compulsorily admitted to hospital with serious mental illness: directive content and feedback from professionals and patients', *Journal of Mental Health* 2004, 13: 379–88.
54 Srebnik *et al.*, 2005, op. cit.
55 Papageoriou *et al.*, 2004, op. cit.
56 Atkinson 2007, op. cit.
57 Saks, R. *Refusing Care: Forced Treatment and the Rights of the Mentally Ill*, Chicago, IL: University of Chicago Press, 2002.
58 Tan, J., Hope, A. and Stewart, A. 'Competence to refuse treatment in anorexia nervosa', *International Journal of Law and Psychiatry* 2003, 26: 697–707.

27 The insanity defence and diminished responsibility

Tom Mason

Introduction

The one constant theme that will underpin this chapter is that since records began, and written accounts passed on, people considered to be insane (a legal term and not a psychiatric one) who have committed an offence should be treated differently from those offenders who are not considered to be insane. However, throughout history and across countries differences in interpretation, as well as in thinking, have ensured that a complex picture has emerged in contemporary times. Furthermore, the semantics of definition and terminology has subtly developed and altered both the usage and the operations of such terms. Influences from law, psychiatry, penology, legal philosophy and the public have served to constantly review the way in which the mentally disordered offender is treated, managed and contained. All these 'forces' that are brought together ensure that the disposal of such mentally disordered offenders is a dynamic and complex issue that is difficult to unravel, as there is little agreement on philosophical issues, the status of human rights and the role of medical jurisprudence. Medical jurisprudence is concerned with the application of law to medicine and the application of medical science to legal concerns.

Throughout this chapter the reader is asked to be aware of these numerous influences on mentally disordered offenders and the choice of disposal routes and to see the struggle with semantics not as pedantry but as a labour with philosophy and reason. However, it should also be noted that the two disciplines of psychiatry and law have their own language. Eastman[1] refers to these as 'mentaland' and 'legaland' and they sometimes do not speak to each other or, when they do, understand each other. In an attempt at clarity the chapter is divided into four main parts: (a) historical background, (b) insanity defence, (c) incompetence to stand trial and (d) diminished responsibility.

Historical background

As far back as the early Greco-Roman writers there were calls for the insane not to be punished for the crimes that they committed as the insanity itself was perceived as a divine punishment from God.[2] However, the Anglo-Saxon laws up to the Conquest did not view insanity as an excuse, nor a mitigation, for the crime committed.[3] In contrast, the Canon law of the English church insisted that moral guilt (*mens rea*) should establish the culpability of the offender and clearly saw young children and the insane as falling outside of this. *Mens rea* is contrasted with *Actus Reus*, which is concerned with the 'guilty act', and external elements, such as epilepsy or somnambulism, are dealt with in this principle. In the thirteenth century the English judge and ecclesiastic, Henry of Bracton, employed this principle in the legal courts as well as pontificating it in religious doctrine, 'but it was not until the sixteenth century that the recognition of "furious madness" as an excuse led to an acquittal'.[3] This form of insanity defence was offered to the courts over the next two centuries but rarely succeeded. In those that did they were released from criminal proceedings but could be detained under the Vagrancy Act 1744[4] or various Poor Laws, and held in gaols, madhouses or houses of correction. No specific provision was made until 1816 at Bethlem Hospital and the opening of Criminal Lunatic Asylums in Dundrum, Ireland in 1852 and Broadmoor, Berkshire in 1863 (see also Chapters 23 and 24).

A tipping point was the trial of James Hadfield in 1800. Hadfield had been a soldier and had received a head wound during the course of his service. Following discharge from the army Hadfield shot at King George III and at his trial his defence lawyer argued that his attempt on the King's life was due to his having paranoid delusions. This claim was accepted and led to a verdict of 'not guilty' as 'he being under the influence of insanity at the time the act was committed'.[3] Although 'not guilty' Hadfield was remanded to prison amidst great concern that the criminal law had no jurisdiction over him. The Government of the day hastily passed the 1800 Act for the Safe Custody of Insane Persons Charged with Offences, which allowed a court to order the detention of an insane person acquitted of an offence until 'His Majesty's Pleasure be Known'. Of note here is the apparent tension between an offence being committed and how to deal with the offender who is considered insane, this difficulty pivoting on the criminal law of the time and what may be considered a foray into mental health law in relation to the 1800 act. As Blackburn[3] notes 'this Act, then, laid the foundation for all subsequent legislation permitting the preventive and indeterminate detention of mentally disordered offenders'. Also of interest here are the words 'not guilty' as this appears to focus on culpability for the act rather than a question of whether he did indeed shoot at the King. A final note worth considering is the fact that it was the sensational act of an assassination attempt on a highly significant person in society (Royalty) that appears to have provoked such public and political interest in the mentally disordered offender. This would be repeated over the next 200 years.

According to Michel Foucault[5] it is at this point in time, and over the next 35 years (1800–1835) that nineteenth century psychiatry became increasingly important because it initiated a new technological treatment of mental disorder, which empowered a policing of public hygiene through the judicial system. Foucault argues that expansion was clearly evident in a number of psychiatric domains at this point in our history, including the identification of risk, dangerousness and punishment (Table 27.1). Through the creation of *Homicidal Monomania*, a fictitious condition, psychiatrists convinced the courts throughout Europe that they had an expertise in the identification, treatment, prevention and prognosis of this condition.[6] Setting out a series of serious cases coming before the courts over this 35-year period Foucault argues that this was the birth of forensic psychiatry, which he referred to as 'first and foremost a pathology of the monstrous'.[5] What is 'monstrous' is the criminal act and not the mental disorder. There is in Foucault's thesis a clear tension, or vacillation of forces, between public outrage, political and professional power relations and philosophical arguments pertaining to liberalism and humanitarianism over this period.

Insanity defence

In 1843 Daniel McNaughtan attempted to assassinate the Prime Minister, Sir Robert Peel, but in a case of mistaken identity shot and killed his private secretary, Edward Drummond. At his trial it was agreed that McNaughtan suffered from persecutory delusions and a defence of 'partial insanity' was put forward. After due consideration the judge adjudicated confirming a verdict of 'not guilty on the grounds of insanity'. The public were indignant and Queen Victoria, who had witnessed the shooting, was outraged claiming that 'insane he

Table 27.1   Some landmarks in the insanity defence laws

England	USA
Early Roman writers – e.g. Plato, Caelius Aurelianus, Aulus Cornelius Celsus, Augustus, Justinian	
Eleventh century – prior to conquest tenth and eleventh centuries	
Thirteenth century – Bracton – legal and ecclesiastical writer	
Sixteenth century – furious madness	
1744 – Vagrancy Act	
1800 – James Hadfield – ex-soldier with head wound shot at George III. Considered to have paranoid delusions. 'Not guilty due to insanity'. Act for the Safe Custody of Insane Persons Charged with Offences	
1836 – King v. Pritchard[25] – court instructed the jury to consider whether defendant was mute of malice or not, can plead or not and can comprehend the proceedings	
1843 – Daniel McNaughtan – attempted to assassinate the Prime Minister. NGRI.* McNaughtan rules developed	
1852 – Dundrum, Dublin, Ireland opens	
1863 – Broadmoor, Berkshire, England opens	
	1887 – 'irresistible impulse', Alabama – test for volitional control developed
	1870 – 'product of mental illness', New Hampshire
1912 – Rampton, Nottingham, England opens	
	1938 – defective delinquent, sexual psychopath
	1954 – Durham v. US[26] – Durham rule states that an accused person is not criminally responsible if his unlawful act was the product of mental illness. Jury decides on causal relationship between mental state and act
1957 – Homicide Act[19] – insane persons could be charged with manslaughter rather than murder	
1959 – Mental Health Act[27] – became special hospitals	
1964 – Criminal Procedures (Insanity) Act[7]	
1965 – Capital punishment abolished	
	1975 – Drope v. Missouri[28] – Drope indicted for rape of wife. Guilty verdict and sentenced to life. Second day of trial Drope attempted suicide. Reports from wife of 'strange behaviour' and psychiatric report rejected

(Continued)

Table 27.1   (Continued)

England	USA
	1980 – ALI[†] test used – a person is not responsible for criminal conduct if he lacks substantial capacity to appreciate the criminality of his conduct
	1981 – Estelle v. Smith[29] – Smith indicted for murder arising from armed robbery. Considered competent to stand trial. Death sentence considered as viewed as dangerous in the future. Death sentence commuted as a constitutional error in psychiatric testimony at the penalty phase
	1982 – Hinckley NGRI[*] following attempted assassination of President Regan
1983 – Mental Health Act[30] – required psychiatrists to establish treatment or prevention of deterioration	
	1984 – Bonnie rule – defendant should be found NGRI[*] if as a result of mental disease or defect he was unable to appreciate the wrongfulness of his conduct at the time of the offence.
	1992 – Medina v. California[31] – concerned with whether Medina was tried and sentenced to death whilst being unable to defend himself
	1996 – Cooper v. Oklahoma – concerned with whether Cooper was competent to understand proceedings and inform his defence council. The court concerned with fairness, accuracy and dignity of the trial process. Cooper charged with brutal killing of 86-year-old man
2007 – Mental Health Act[32] – more community focused.	

Notes: [*]NGRI: not guilty by reason of insanity. [†]ALI: American Law Institute.

may well be but guilty he most assuredly was'. The common law judges were requested to clarify the defence of insanity and report to the House of Lords. After due deliberation they offered their opinions, which are now know as the McNaughtan rules, and stated that it had to be proved that 'at the time of the committing of the act, the party accused was labouring under such a defect of reason, from disease of the mind, as not to know the nature and quality of the act he was doing; or if he did know it, that he did not know he was doing what was wrong'.[3] Daniel McNaughtan was held at Bethlem until Broadmoor was built and then transferred there until his death in 1865.

In one form or another the McNaughtan rules remain today in many legal systems but have been controversial, provoking intense debate. Given the science of the time, the 'disease of the mind' is a legal concept referring to defects of cognition arising internally and not through ingestion of external substances such as drugs or alcohol. However, arguments arose about the relation between the 'disease' and the 'defect of cognition', as in terms of cause and effect it is only an assumed relationship (see Chapter 17). A point that is hotly debated today. Furthermore, in referring to the 'nature and quality of the act' this focuses on the physical aspect of the act and its consequences, that is, differentiating between cutting a persons throat rather than their hair. The cognitive ability to reason that the former is wrong refers to a legal statement rather than a moral position. The basis of many arguments refer to the point that some mentally disordered offenders may well know that what they are doing is both legally and morally wrong but are simply unable to control themselves. This led to the adoption of a volitional test in the form of an 'irresistible impulse' criterion in Alabama in 1887, which spread to further American states and some British courts. However, as Blackburn[3] observes 'the problem with "irresistible impulse" notion is that it is never logically possible to distinguish inability to resist and "impulse" from simple unwillingness'.

Arguments and debate continued with several developments in legal and psychiatric thinking. In New Hampshire in 1870 a new test was devised which did not focus on cognitive or volitional aspects but required that the act was 'the product of mental illness', which clearly located this in the domain of psychiatrists' expertise. This rise in the medical model focused attention more closely on the causal relationship between crime and mental disorder, which continues today. Concerns with legal and medical semantics drew attention to the fact that a 'not guilty by reason of insanity' (NGRI) verdict was actually an acquittal but which invariably led to detention in secure psychiatric provision. Thus, in England, from 1883 to 1964 this was changed to 'guilty but insane'. The American Law Institute (ALI) developed a further test which was widely used by 1980. This states that 'a person is not responsible for criminal conduct if at the time of such conduct as a result of mental disease or defect he lacks substantial capacity to appreciate the criminality of his conduct or to conform his conduct to the requirements of law'.[3] The ALI test embraces cognitive, volitional and affective components to knowledge of right and wrong (legal principle) and was employed in the trial of John Hinckley who shot at President Reagan in 1982. Hinckley received an NGRI verdict which caused public concern similar to Hadfield and McNaughtan. Finally the American Psychiatric Association in 1983 recommended the Bonnie rule, which suggests that a person should be found NGRI if 'as a result of mental disease or defect he was unable to appreciate the wrongfulness of his conduct at the time of the offence'. The Bonnie rule was adopted in federal courts in 1984 despite concerns with the ability of psychiatrists to reliably judge a person's cognitive and volitional controls.

Incompetence to stand trial

The difficulties referring to whether a person is guilty or not guilty and who is considered insane focus on whether the act was committed by that person (guilty) or whether they are culpable for that act (not guilty). A person who does not know that what he is doing is wrong may be considered guilty but not culpable. The problem here is the ability of psychiatrists to accurately establish the person's culpability for their actions. In dealing with a person's ability to understand right and wrong it may be that their 'disability' or 'disease' of the mind may well incapacitate their ability to follow the court proceedings, instruct their defence council or challenge evidence and in these cases we are concerned with their incompetence to stand trial. The terms 'unfit to plead' and 'under disability such that it would constitute a bar to his being tried' are used in England in the Criminal Procedures (Insanity) Act of 1964,[7] whilst 'insane in bar of trial' is employed in Scotland.[3] In the United States they are concerned with 'competence to stand trial' and use the term 'unfit to stand trial' as a common description. They also use 'competence to proceed with adjudication' and 'fitness to stand trial' but the terms can be used interchangeably. Although these pleas are more common than an insanity defence they tend to be unsuccessful with Kerr and Roth[8] reporting 11 per cent successful in America and Grubin reporting 2 per cent in England.[9] Scotland, on the other hand, uses it more frequently.[3] This situation has remained largely the same in more recent times.[10] In all cases it is the defendant's ability to engage with the court proceedings that lie at the heart of the incompetency, or competency, to stand trial issue.[10]

The importance of the assessment of incompetence to stand trial is that the defendant may likely be subject to detention in secure psychiatric facilities, which may be for many years and even life. In America it usually results in an adjournment of the trial for a period to see if the defendant's mental condition improves so that they become competent to stand trial. However, if they are deemed 'unrestorable incompetent' a special trial may result to establish the facts and judicial discretion may find a 'not guilty' verdict with a disposal to psychiatric facilities. Despite the journey their destination is long-term psychiatric detention.

Whilst there may be 'clear-cut' cases where a person is incompetent to stand trial there are many others that are less so and the state of psychiatric and psychological science to evaluate the issues involved is not well developed. Having received the psychiatric evaluations it is the judge that must decide, and an example of such deliberations may suffice to show the humanness of such decisions. A trial judge concluded:

> my shirt sleeves opinion of Mr. Cooper is that he's not normal. Now, to say he's not competent is something else. I think it's going to take smarter people than me to make a decision here. I'm going to say that I don't believe he has carried the burden by clear and convincing evidence of his incompetency and I'm going to say we're going to trial.[11]

Thus, we can see that the judgement is very much a human one; although based on an honest attempt to weigh the evidence accordingly, it is fundamentally a *judgement*. If everyone in the theatre of the court plays a honest card then we can at least claim to have done our best within the limitations of our science. However, in the assessment of the incompetence to stand trial we have to deal with a further issue; that of malingering.[12]

A number of people who are brought before the law and are referred for psychiatric evaluation are found to be malingering. Whilst some perceive that it is in their best interests to feign a mental disorder others will attempt to hide the disorder and feign sanity. Malingering refers to the former in which a person will engage in bizarre and unusual behaviour in an attempt to convince the judge, jurors or barristers that they are insane. It is said that in at least 10 per cent of cases referred for psychiatric evaluation an attempt is made to feign mental problems.[13-15] Malingering has been a long-standing problem as can be seen in the following quote: 'does the mental impairment of the prisoner's mind, if such there be, whatever it is, disable him … from fairly presenting his defense, whatever it may be, and make it unjust to go on with his trial at this time, or is he feigning to be in that condition'.[16] The rationale for such malingering is psychologically complex[17] and whilst we can see its utility in avoiding capital punishment or life sentences given that in the United Kingdom and in the United States indeterminate psychiatric detention may merely be different forms of 'life sentences'.[18] Furthermore, in the United States if a court considers that a defendant is malingering the judge can pronounce a 'sentence enhancement' to extend the imprisonment as a deterrent.

Diminished responsibility

In England, following Scotland, the 1957 Homicide Act provided the conditions for a person to be found not guilty of murder but guilty of manslaughter due to their having a diminished responsibility, if 'he was suffering from such abnormality of mind (whether arising from a condition of arrested or retarded development of mind or any inherent causes or induced by disease or injury) as substantially impaired his mental responsibility for his acts and omissions in doing or being party to the killing'.[19] This Act, along with the abolition of capital punishment (de facto) in 1965, has reduced the number of insanity defence pleas. However, what constitutes diminished responsibility has been open to interpretation and debate. The first point to note is that the abnormality of mind within this Act goes well beyond the 'defect of reason' referred to in the McNaughtan rules. The 'substantial impairment' is both gross and wide and can incorporate almost any or all mental states, including those of omission and failure to resist an impulse. Lord Parker[20] defined an 'abnormality of mind' as 'a state of mind so different from that of ordinary human beings that the reasonable man would term it abnormal'. However, this is less than helpful in any clinical sense and must restrict itself to a concept in law or a concept of morality.[21,22] The question is whether a person is responsible for their acts and whether degrees of responsibility (greater or lesser) should be confined to murder and not other offences.[23]

To answer the foregoing we need to discuss in a plea of diminished responsibility just exactly what is diminished. Responsibility for one's actions assumes a relationship between the functioning processes of the mind and the physical actions of the body, and when the former malfunctions the person may engage in behaviour that breaks moral and legal codes. This ambiguous relationship, pivoting on 'responsibility', assumes that it is a psychological faculty amenable to psychiatric evaluation, which allows psychiatrists to pronounce on 'ultimate issues' and 'provides psychiatrist's charter at trial'.[23] Peter Sutcliffe, the so-called Yorkshire Ripper, who killed 13 women, was considered to be suffering from paranoid schizophrenia by both prosecution and defence psychiatrists. Yet, despite the plea of diminished responsibility the jury rejected this and the judge sentenced Sutcliffe to life imprisonment following a verdict of murder. In a relatively short space of time Sutcliffe was transferred from prison to a high-security psychiatric hospital where he remains today.

A plea of diminished responsibility has been successful in a number of cases including reactive depression, premenstrual tension, psychoses and personality disorder.[3] However, it does not 'necessarily lead to more lenient disposal, and only about a third of males found guilty of manslaughter under Section 2 have received a hospital order in recent years, possibly reflecting an increased tendency of psychiatrists to argue that psychopaths are untreatable'.[3] It should also be noted that women employ psychiatric defences such as diminished responsibility to a greater degree than men[23,24] and diminished responsibility has been a successful plea in infanticide. However, it has also been noted that this pathologizes women as abnormal and mad whilst men are perceived as normal and bad[23] and hence the higher ratios of women to men in high-security psychiatric hospitals and the higher ratios of men to women in prison. Thus, diminished responsibility for women may well be more of a case of 'who they are rather than what they have done'.[23] This reinforces the tension between the legal and moral aspects of diminished responsibility and the assumed psychological clinical aspect.

Conclusion

There has been a long-standing consideration regarding people who are viewed as insane and who are facing adjudication in courts of law, from early Roman times to the present day. These concerns are based on an assumed relationship between a person's mental state and a criminal act. Degrees of responsibility, or culpability, for a person's wrongdoing has undergone many changes throughout our history, usually in response to a particularly heinous crime that has caught professional, political and media attention. Laws, rules and adjudications have led to changes by which defendants are evaluated for competency to stand trial and their extent of diminished responsibility. This is likely to continue as psychiatry and law fuse together in the form of medical jurisprudence and deal with issues of human rights, fairness, justice and dignity. This forms the basis of a just society, which centres on the moral values relating to how the vulnerable in society are treated.

Notes

1   Eastman, N. (2000) Psycho-legal studies as an interface discipline. In: J. McGuire, T. Mason and A. O'Kane (Eds.) *Behaviour, Crime and Legal Processes*. Chichester: Wiley.
2   Buckland, W.W. (2007) *A Text-Book of Roman Law: From Augustus to Justinian*. Cambridge: Cambridge University Press.
3   Blackburn, R. (1993) *Psychology of Criminal Conduct: Theory, Research & Practice*. Chichester: Wiley.
4   HMSO (1744) *The Vagrancy Act*. London: HMSO.
5   Foucault, M. (1978) About the concept of the 'Dangerous Individual' in 19th century legal psychiatry. *International Journal of Law and Psychiatry* 1 (1): 1–18.
6   Mason, T. (2006) An archaeology of the psychopath. In: T. Mason (Ed.) *Forensic Psychiatry: Influences of Evil*. Totowa, NJ: Humana Press.
7   HMSO (1964) *Criminal Procedures (Insanity) Act*. London: HMSO.
8   Kerr, C.A. and Roth, J.H. (1986) Populations, practices and problems in forensic psychiatric facilities. *Annals of the American Academy of Political and Social Science* 484: 127–43.
9   Grubin, D.H. (1991) Unfit to plead in England and Wales, 1976–1988: a survey. *British Journal of Psychiatry* 158: 540–48.
10 Buchanan, A. (2006) Competency to stand trial and the seriousness of the charge. *Journal of the American Academy of Psychiatry and Law* 34 (4): 458–65.
11 Cooper v. Oklahoma (1996) 517 U.S. 348.
12 Jackson, R.L., Rogers, R. and Sewell, K.W. (2005) Forensic applications of the Miller forensic assessment of symptoms tests: screening for feigned disorders in competency to stand trial evaluations. *Law and Human Behavior* 29 (2): 199–210.
13 Rogers, R. and Sewell, K.W. (1994) Explanatory models of malingering: a prototypical analysis. *Law and Human Behavior* 18: 543–52.
14 Gothard, S., Rogers, R. and Sewell, K.W. (1995) Feigning incompetency to stand trial: an investigation of the Georgia Court Competency Test. *Law and Human Behavior* 19: 363–73.
15 Brockman, J.E. and Chamberlain, J.R. (2007) Commitment following a finding of not guilty by reason of insanity. *Journal of the American Academy of Psychiatry and Law* 35 (2): 268–69.
16 United States v. Chisolm (1906) 149 F. 284 (C.C.S.D. Ala. 1906).
17 Gudjonsson, G. (2002) *The Psychology of Interrogations and Confessions: A Handbook*. Chichester: Wiley Blackwell.
18 Mason, T. (1999) The psychiatric 'Supermax'?: Long-term high-security psychiatric services. *International Journal of Law and Psychiatry* 22 (2): 155–66.
19 HMSO (1957) *The Homicide Act*. London: HMSO.
20 Parker, C.J. (1960) R v. Byrne. 2 QB 396 at 403.
21 Butler Committee (1975) *The Butler Committee on Mentally Abnormal Offenders*. London: HMSO.
22 Mayman, D.M. and Guyer, M. (2008) Not guilty by reason of insanity defense. *Journal of the American Academy of Psychiatry and Law* 36 (1): 143–5.
23 Peay, J. (1994) Mentally disordered offenders. In: M. Maguire, R. Morgan and R. Reiner (Eds.) *The Oxford Handbook of Criminology*. London: Clarendon Press. pp. 1119–60.
24 Walklate, S. (2005) *Criminology: The Basics*. London: Routledge.
25 King v. Pritchard (1836) 173 Eng. Rep. 135 (1836).
26 Durham v. US (1954) 214 F.2d 862 (1954).
27 HMSO (1959) *The Mental Health Act*. London: HMSO.
28 Drope v. Missouri (1975) 420 U.S. 162 (1975).
29 Estelle v. Smith (1981) 451 U.S. 454 (1981).
30 HMSO (1983) *The Mental Health Act*. London: HMSO.
31 Medina v. California (1992) 505 U.S. 437 (1992).
32 HMSO (2007) *The Mental Health Act*. London: HMSO.

Section 5 – Ethical dilemmas

Phil Barker

The law exists to contain and control people. In so doing it can, however, provide a means to reassure people of their freedom. The primary purpose of much mental health law appears to be focused on control: especially providing a legal basis for ensuring that people are 'cared for' or 'treated', whether or not they desire this. In that sense, mental health law has little interest in assuring the freedoms of the 'mentally ill'. This is, however, a crude picture. The finer detail shows the efforts made within the broad legislation, to ensure that aspects of freedom are maintained. However, in the final analysis not much has changed since the first such laws were framed over 150 years ago. Few people can avoid some version of 'involuntary commitment' (or 'sectioning') if someone decides that this is in *their* 'best interests' or to the benefit of society.

There are, however, major differences between the forms of mental health legislation developed in Scotland, compared with Ireland and England. The Scots emphasis on an underpinning set of 'ethical principles' illustrates the possibility for developing legislation, which – at least – takes account of human rights. This may be unsurprising, given the part played by Scots philosophers in the Enlightenment. However, it seems unlikely that John Stuart Mill, author of *On Liberty*, would offer much applause for the current England and Wales mental health legislation.

Without doubt, the most significant human right is that of self-determination. The advanced directive offers a good example of how people can exert some control over their lives. However, as with most psychiatric situations, it is not watertight, and 'expert opinion' can override efforts at self-determination.

1   *Whose best interests does coercion serve?* A wide range of coercive practices has been used throughout psychiatric history, mainly to contain people who were 'socially disruptive'. Today, the rationale for coercion relates primarily to the management of people who are 'at risk to self or others'.

> How do you reconcile the use of coercion with your professional ethical standards?
> To what extent will the risk of coercion deter people from seeking help?
> In the final analysis, is not all mental health legislation designed to appease society, rather than act in a person's best interests?

2   *Free to be unhealthy?* People with heart disease, cancer or other life-threatening conditions are under no obligation to accept treatment. People can and frequently do die as a result of discontinuing treatment or from the long-term effects of 'unhealthy lifestyles'.

>   How do you justify enforced care or treatment *only* for people with psychiatric disorders?
>
>   By focusing attention on the enforcement of certain kinds of treatment – such as taking medication – do you run the risk of failing to help people deal with the problems they experience in other areas of everyday life?

3   *Free to dissent?* Mental health legislation legitimises the use of coercive practices by mental health professions – especially nurses.

>   In what situations might observance of such laws result in a compromise of your professional ethical standards?
>
>   If you believe that the enactment of some aspect of mental health legislation is not in the person's best interests, what action should you take, to maintain your own ethical practice?

4   *Perpetuating stigma?* Although there is much more openness about 'mental health problems', people with more 'serious psychiatric disorders' continue to believe that they are stigmatised.

>   Does any form of mental health legislation, which legitimises coercion, ultimately reinforce the age-old stereotypes, which lie at the heart of psychiatric stigma?
>
>   If people can determine the kind of care and treatment they will receive, will this reinforce their standing as an autonomous person and reduce stigma?
>
>   Should people be free to deny themselves access to any treatment (however life-saving it may be considered) if they so wish, through an advance directive?

Section 6
The ideological context

Section preface

Phil Barker

Although psychiatry long harboured ambitions to be recognised as a 'science', this remains unfulfilled. Today, 'mental health' is clearly an *institution*, complete with its own methods, customs and practices, if not also formal ceremonies. It has the support of the law and a public presence, if no longer in the form of the intimidating asylum, then signposted through a wealth of 'therapeutic services' and 'therapeutic settings'.

Contemporary mental health is also an *ideology*, in the sense that it embraces a specific set of beliefs – about 'mental illness' or 'psychiatric disorder' – that provide a rationale for developing 'mental health services', training 'mental health professionals' and invoking 'mental health laws'. All these depend, ultimately, on the psychiatric diagnosis, which may in time be revised, to become a 'mental health status', should political correctness survive.

Section 6 begins by considering some of the recent *talk about recovery*. Where once 'madness' was seen as 'incurable', now it is widely accepted that people can and do 'recover', but may need a different kind of support if this is to come to fruition.

The key ethical conflict, which has threaded its way through this book, involves the debate over whether or not anyone can be said to be in his/her 'right mind'. Are our notions of *individuality* and *autonomy* real or merely *illusion*?

Finally, we try to close the circle, by returning to some of the key ethical themes that have been explored throughout the book. Ultimately, the challenge for everyone involves *thinking ethically* and *behaving morally*. Assuming that science has little or nothing to offer the ethical enterprise, where might we draw inspiration from? What are the enduring themes that might support the further development of mental health ethics?

28 Talking about recovery

Poppy Buchanan-Barker

The end of the age of madness

In my home town in the early 1950s, the few people who had 'nervous breakdowns' usually were dispatched to a 'mental hospital' 40 miles away. Few thought of them as 'psychiatric patients' and no one had any idea what kind of 'psychiatric treatment' they received. Some disappeared for months while others were never seen or heard of again.

In my small town in lowland Scotland there was a mix of Irish, Scots and English. It also had one man who came from the Caribbean. You could say it was something of a multicultural society. I have no idea what it must have been like to be the *only* 'non-white' person in a small Scottish town, but my memory is that 'Charlie' was just 'Charlie'. Maybe people were more respectful or welcoming back then. They accepted Charlie, respectfully, as just another member of the community. I never apologise for believing that I grew up in a special place; maybe that was part of some 'Golden Age'.

Our town was also home to a man whose difference was something of a cause for celebration. He was one of the people who had 'disappeared' to the mental hospital. However, on his return, he lived quietly, in a quiet street, and worked quietly in the local industry. He was, however, far from ordinary. He dressed always in black: trousers, waistcoat, jacket and Stetson. He would tie the handlebars of his bike to the rail outside the local pub, as if tethering his horse. He was the 'Sheriff', complete with a silver badge. He would tilt his Stetson as I passed him on my way to school and at Christmas would entertain the children at the social club, with a dazzling display of his 'six-shooters'. Visiting my hometown recently, I discovered that he had died of old age and was buried in the local cemetery. His workmates had collected money to dedicate a special tombstone: to 'The Sheriff'.

It is easy to romanticise childhood memories but mine appears genuine. People who knew him as a fellow worker or neighbour said, 'He was odd, but harmless... he was good company'. I now realise that people like the 'Sheriff' were not actually expected to 'recover' and, not surprisingly, most of them didn't. The 'Sheriff' probably waxed and waned like most people do. After the 'rough times' he probably 'got going again', pretty much like everybody else. What was the big deal? If we had never invented psychiatry, the 'Sheriff' would have been just another 'celebrity', who had his 'rough patches'. Like most of today's celebrities, the 'Sheriff' was famous for just *being* the 'Sheriff'. The only difference is that someone locked him up for it.

Living in an age of recovery

Fifty years ago, most people who were 'mentally ill' were expected to be 'disabled' for life. In that sense, the 'Sheriff' appeared to be an exception. Perhaps, living in a small, supportive, respectful, accommodating community proved to be the best kind of 'treatment' for whatever it was that made him 'different'.

Today we live in a new age of 'recovery'; an idea that has come to dominate mental health services in many Western countries. However, people still squabble about what, *exactly*, recovery means; and most importantly, *who* is it for? This, we might call the *politics* of recovery.

Talk about 'recovery' in the mental health field began in the 1970s and had become a 'buzzword' by the beginning of the twenty-first century[1]: an 'idea whose time has come'.[2] However, it is a very old idea, first used by groups like *Alcoholics Anonymous* (AA) over 70 years ago,[3] when 'alcoholism' was thought to be a life-long 'disease' (see Chapter 18). Indeed, *AA* not only believed this too, but also believed that people could recover *despite* the 'disease'. Such optimism found an echo 40 years ago in the principles of 'normalisation', in the disability field.[4] People like Wolfensberger believed that however 'disabled' people might be, they could still live a full, meaningful life, providing that others 'treated' them respectfully – accepting them for 'who' they were – and supporting them accordingly. Maybe the people in my small town had an intuitive feel for that sort of philosophy. Treating people in a respectful, considerate manner is hardly 'rocket science'.

It is worth asking why the idea of recovery – or 'normalisation' – took so long to find its way into psychiatric thinking. Maybe it had something to do with medicine's narrow understanding of recovery, long associated with 'cure'. Or maybe it was because 'recovery' was something that 'patients' tended to do on their own[5]: sometimes in defiance of medical opinion. In the same vein, ideas like 'normalisation' were unashamedly social in nature; having little need for medical technology. Perhaps psychiatry *is* caught in a time warp, as one psychiatrist observed:

> Psychiatrists like to think that they have moved beyond simple medical models but, insofar as they continue to focus on the treatment of *episodes of illness* as the main thrust for intervention, they remain firmly attached to that model.[6]

All this talk about recovery seemed to scare some psychiatrists into thinking that their authority might be under threat. If 'patients' could organise their own recovery – do it 'on their own', as Judi Chamberlin[7] famously said over 30 years ago – where would this leave psychiatric medicine? Such anxieties seemed to fuel the 'wake-up call' issued by a group of senior British psychiatrists in 2008; urging their colleagues to 're-establish biomedicine at the heart of contemporary psychiatric practice'. This group found much of the talk about 'service-users', 'mental health' and 'well-being', a bit unnerving. Instead, they wanted to revive terms like 'patient' and 'mental illness': reminders of 'who' was doing 'what' to 'whom' and 'why'.[8] If anyone needed a reminder that 'psychiatry' and 'mental health' are two, very distinct political camps, this was it.

The 'Sheriff' always seemed just like another 'man' to me. If people recover any single *thing* during their 'recovery', it must be their identity as a *person*. This emphasis on the 'personal' is vital. *My* recovery might bear comparison to that of other people, but ultimately it can only be *my* recovery. That is part and parcel of what it means to be a person. As Anne Helm wrote:

> Recovery is not a destination, but the journeying task of making sense of life itself, and I ask the reader to accept the universality of the task. We are all in recovery. There are no *patients* to seek recovery for, no *nurses* to map the waterways and guide the boats on the voyage. We are all fellow wayfarers, who can share experiences and insights from our own lives, thereby facilitating each other's progress.[9]

Recovery: from the personal to the political

People have been talking about recovery in mental health for almost 40 years but 'what' recovery actually *means* remains unclear.[10] In this 'evidence-based' world, there is a big emphasis on so-called *outcomes*[11] – like 'good quality of life despite the continued presence of psychiatric symptoms'.[12] However, what actually *needs to happen* to enable recovery seems to escape most people.

Like most things in psychiatry, talk about 'recovery' is riddled with jargon or waffle. For example, recovery is a 'non-linear lived experience' involving both 'self-discovery' and 'transformation', culminating in an understanding that symptoms of illness are not definitive of one's 'self-identity'.[13] Ordinary people tend to think more about ordinary things like *hope, connection* or *healing*.[14] Simple ideas like self-help, mutual-support, self-determination, resilience, choice, justice, taking responsibility, community involvement and an emphasis on one's existing skills or other 'personal assets' appear also to be important.[15,16]

Recovery also appears to mean different things in different countries. In the United States, the idea emerged from the civil rights movement of the 1960s and 1970s, where taking charge of a life that had either gone out of control or was controlled by others was all-important. The *American Declaration of Independence* reinforced this emphasis on self-determination. Other countries, like New Zealand, took a different tack, emphasising cross-cultural dialogue; giving more emphasis to ideas like social support.

However, despite these philosophical differences, by the beginning of the twenty-first century, 'recovery' had been picked up by most Western countries: New Zealand,[17] Australia,[18] England,[19] Scotland[20] and Ireland[21] as well as the United States. However, many of these government-based policies were no more than 'paper plans' for some 'recovery-focused' future.

Recovery of 'what' by 'whom'?

Only a few people now think about recovery in terms of getting a cure for 'mental illness'. Since Thomas Szasz first drew attention to the 'myth of "mental illness"' 50 years ago,[22] it has become increasingly obvious that when people become 'ill at ease' with themselves or others, or appear 'ill-fitted' for the challenges that life offers, the 'illness' we are referring to is only metaphorical. Not surprisingly, much of the talk about 'recovery' echoes Szasz by challenging the idea that some 'disease' is involved.[23] However, if people have only been 'sick' in a metaphorical sense, *what*, then, are they recovering from?

Sally Clay survived a 40-year-long experience of psychiatric 'care and treatment' and is well aware of how ideas like 'recovery' can be used as political weapons. Over a decade ago she wrote: 'Recovery is the latest buzz word in the mental health field. For the last year or so, I have been labelled 'recovered from mental illness.'[24]

After being invited to discuss her 'recovery' with psychiatrists in 'Recovery Dialogues facilitated by the New York State Office of Mental Health', Sally realised that these discussions had paid no attention to:

> . . . the nature of mental illness itself. . . . If we are recovered, what is it that we have recovered from? If we are well now and were sick before, what is it that we have recovered to? . . . The psychiatrists in our dialogue become visibly uneasy when the subject

arises, and they divert the discussion to less threatening lines of thought. 'Coping mechanisms' are just such a diversion, an attempt to regard the depth of madness as something that can be simply 'coped' with.[25]

Sally was among the first to appreciate that *her* personal efforts to deal with problems that *she* had encountered in *her* life could be hijacked by psychiatry, becoming just another piece of its political capital. Recovery had become just the latest psychiatric/mental health *game*.

Radical recovery: getting going again

Much of the academic talk about recovery seems unnecessarily complicated, but complicating matters, or giving simple ideas complex names, is probably what academics do best. However, taking a dip into any dictionary will help to bring us back to earth. Recovery may mean all sorts of things, but at heart the meanings are all much the same:

* taking (something) back again into one's hands, or *re-possessing*;
* regaining *possession* of something that has been lost;
* winning back *ground* that has been *lost* (for example, in battle);
* *finding* something the second time around;
* *bringing*, drawing or winning back (a person) to friendship;
* *regaining* a right to (something);
* *making up* for loss or damage to oneself;
* *getting over* a loss or misfortune.

All these definitions emphasise the *action* that needs to happen for a person to realise something. So, people talk about regaining their right to be viewed and treated as a *person*; getting over the damage done to our reputations or self-confidence; making up for lost time; regaining the ground that they seem to have lost, in the incessant battle with time and life itself. In short, recovery seems to mean repossessing, or reclaiming, one's life; in an effort to live it, again, as best as one can.

In my view all recovery involves *getting going again*.

This is rarely easy and reminds me of how we reclaim land that has been submerged by the sea. As long as it is beneath the water, it is of no use to us. However, if we can drain it, with great effort, we can bring it back to be part of the 'mainland' again.[26] This seems to be a fitting metaphor for what people need to do, perhaps with help, in reclaiming their lives from the depths of despair, or some 'defeat' that life has inflicted upon them.

In my view, the very first step in any recovery must be *reclamation*: taking back ownership of *my* life, *my* identity, *my* story.

The ethics of recovery

People like Sally Clay can tell powerful stories about how they 'recovered' from specific *life* situations. How they reclaimed the story of their lives, which are far richer and far more revealing than any of the 'clinical histories' offered by psychiatry. Those stories tell of *problems* that grew over time *in* their lives, and which were personally *meaningful*; rather than from anything remotely like an 'illness' of the body with its accompanying 'symptoms'. To know *what* exactly Sally 'recovered' and what was its *meaning*, we would have to ask Sally; and be prepared to listen, carefully.

I have been fortunate never to have been 'committed' to a psychiatric hospital, like Sally Clay. However, I have experienced many difficult situations in the course of my life, and expect that fate will have more such 'situations' in store for me. All generated problems which affected the living of my life. Some of these I talk about and others I keep to myself. But, all such *problems in living* remind us that weakness and vulnerability, and the unpredictability of life, is something we all have in common. Harry Stack Sullivan said, 'we are all more simply human than otherwise'. In Scotland we say, 'we are a' Jock Tamson's bairns[27]'. We are all, pretty much, the same under the skin. If we need a specific set of ethical principles for the mental health field, this idea would form the basis of my *first ethical principle.*

- Recognise that recovery is something we *all* need to do, at some point in our lives. If 'we are all the same under the skin', recovery *cannot* be peculiar to people who have been cast as 'psychiatric patients'. To suggest otherwise is to maintain the myth that 'mentally ill' persons are some kind of aliens – and that 'we' are somehow perfect.

Some will say that psychiatric 'service users' or mental health 'consumers' *are* different, because they need special help. This idea is full of prejudice and is deeply patronising. It has always been clear to me that people who experience great problems in living do not experience such problems every moment of the day, every day of their lives. They flow in and out of such difficulties. However, when I think about the kind of problems people experience *and* seem to endure, I often wonder: 'why do they not appear much worse?' Clearly, lots of people bring to bear some resilience, stoicism or creativity when they have to face up to some problem. These belong uniquely to them. This was something that Wolfensberger thought he saw, even in people who were grossly physically and perhaps intellectually 'handicapped'. This, in turn, forms the basis of my *second ethical principle*:

- Help people to be self-supporting, if they ask for such help. Stop working so hard to 'solve' others' problems: they already have everything they need to do whatever they need to do to get going again in their lives. However, they will only do this when the time is right for them.

We also need to remember that, however much we might appear to share experiences, I can never *know* someone else's experience. The actual personal experience of others will always remain, to a large extent, a mystery to me. However, if I pay careful attention to what they tell me, I might learn a little of what that experience entailed; how it affected the person; and especially what it appears to *mean*.[28] This appears to be no more than common sense, but may be more like 'uncommon sense'.[29] This forms the basis of my *third ethical principle*:

- Remember that every person is a mystery. Never assume that you can know other people, unless they are willing to let you into their mystery.

Regrettably, people talk about 'patients'…

- The personal has always been political. Give up all the foolish talk about 'patients', 'clients', 'consumers' or 'service users' and choose only to relate to unique, individual *persons*.

Of course, some people will choose to define themselves as a 'service user' or a 'patient'. This is their prerogative. However, if they do, you might find their motives interesting, if not intriguing. Hopefully, you will be left wondering: 'OK, but *who*, exactly, are they?'

Some 'psychiatric survivors' or 'experts by experience' develop careers as 'advocates' or 'peer-support workers.' I always expected such people to be even keener than I am, for favouring the personal *as* political. Regrettably, I still hear such people talking about 'my clients' or 'a client of mine': a most unfortunate echo of slave-ownership that was long modelled by psychiatric professionals. 'Patients' and 'clients' are, by definition, vulnerable people, who are in some way dependent on someone else. For someone to *be* their own person, others must treat them as if they *are* that person.

I did consider calling this chapter the 'concept of recovery', but realised that I might be trying too hard to impress. A concept is just an 'idea' or a 'notion' that becomes more real, the more we talk about it. So, I decided to dump all talk of 'concepts' and just focus on talk, which is the nub of the issue. Recovery becomes real, the more we talk about it; give examples of it; try to communicate our 'ideas' and 'notions' about it. This forms the basis of my *final ethical principle*:

- Talk in the kind of ordinary language that is meaningful to the person you are talking to.

The problems in living that people experience are always ordinary, since they emerge from the ordinary circumstances of their lives. People talk about those problems in much the same way they talk about the weather or sport or anything else. The great psychiatric conjuring trick involves turning those simple, straightforward accounts into some kind of psychobabble. The *language* of psychiatry, psychology and psychotherapy usually involves turning simple, straightforward stories into exotic-sounding concepts. They only *sound* exotic, because they are liberally sprinkled with bits of Latin or Greek. Like all conjuring tricks, we have been deceived by cleverness.

Regrettably, some professionals still hanker for 'educating patients' or their families: teaching them how to use the psychiatric gobbledegook. Usually this nonsense is called 'psycho-education'. George Orwell famously said, 'never use a long word, where a short one will do'. Orwell believed that all 'fiddling' with the English language damaged our capacity to communicate effectively. As such, it was inherently political.[30] Fortunately, Orwell did not live to experience much of the linguistic nightmare that became twenty-first century psychiatry and psychology.

Conclusion

As I have said, the story of 'recovery' is new. It is a story that has been hidden, especially by those who had something to gain from suppressing it. Professional pessimism and reliance on outmoded ideas have proven to be the biggest hurdles.[31] People can 'get going again' with a little self-belief and a lot of social support.[32,33]

As a social worker and counsellor I have never been that interested in research 'evidence': what 'works' is so often either obvious, or particular to the situation, and the idea of 'researching' it seemed pointless. I was always more interested in finding out how I might be helpful to someone, who asks for my help. When people ask 'what is the evidence for "recovery" there appears to be plenty around, and it has been there for quite some time. However, it also seems obvious that what we are calling 'recovery' *today* has more to do with a mind-set, or philosophy, than science. As Henry Ford famously said, 'Whether you believe you can or believe you can't you're right'. No matter how serious the problems, some believe (or can come to believe) that they *can* recover: this inspires them to set about creating the sort of conditions that might help it happen.[34] Those who sit around waiting to be given some 'proof' might have a long wait. In the meantime, nothing much changes.

Perhaps I should add one more ethical principle before ending.

- Recovery must be seen as everybody's business.

Notes

1 Craig TKJ. Recovery: say what you mean and mean what you say. *Journal of Mental Health* 2008: 17(2), 125–8.

2 Shepherd G, Boardman J and Slade M. *Making Recovery a Reality*. London: Sainsbury Centre for Mental Health, 2008.

3 Frank D. *The Annotated AA Handbook: A Companion to the Big Book*. Fort Lee, NJ: Barricade Books, 1996.

4 Wolfensberger W. *The Principle of Normalization in Human Services*. Toronto: National Institute on Mental Retardation, 1972.

5 Chamberlin J. *On Our Own: Patient Controlled Alternatives to the Mental Health System*. New York, NY: Hawthorn Books, 1978.

6 Whitwell D. The myth of recovery from mental illness. *Psychiatric Bulletin* 1999: 23, 621–2 (emphasis added).

7 Chamberlin J. The medical model and harm. In: P Barker, P Campbell and B Davidson (Eds.) *From the Ashes of Experience*. London: Whurr, 1999, pp. 170–6.

8 Craddock N, Antebi D, Attenburrow MJ, Bailey A, Carson A, Cowen P et al. Wake-up call for British psychiatry. *British Journal of Psychiatry* 2008: 193, 6–9.

9 Helm A. Recovery and reclamation: a pilgrimage in understanding who and what we are. In: P Barker (Ed.) *Psychiatric and Mental Health Nursing: The Craft of Caring*. London: Arnold, 2003, p. 50 (Chapter 8).

10 Davidson L, O'Connell M, Tondora J, Styron T and Kangas K. The top ten concerns about recovery encountered in mental health system transformation. *Psychiatric Services* 2006: 57, 640–5.

11 Onken SJ, Dumont MJ, Ridgway P, Dornan DH and Ralph RO. A national study of consumer perspectives on what helps and what hinders recovery. Paper presented to the conference of the International Association of Psychosocial Rehabilitation, June 10, 2004. Vancouver, British Columbia, Canada.

12 Deegan P. Recovery: the experience of rehabilitation. *Psychosocial Rehabilitation Journal* 1988: 11(4), 11.

13 Davidson L, Sells D, Sangster S and O'Connell M. Qualitative studies of recovery: what can we learn from the person? In: Ralph RO and Corrigan PW (Eds.) *Recovery in Mental Illness*. Washington, DC: American Psychological Association, 2005, pp. 147–71.

14 Jacobson H and Greenley D. What is recovery? A conceptual model and explication. *Psychiatric Services* 2001: 52(4), 482–5.

15 Ministry of Health. *Te Kōkiri: The Mental Health and Addiction Action Plan 2006–2015*. Wellington, New Zealand: Ministry of Health, 2006.

16 Ohio Mental Health Commission. *Changing Lives: Ohio's Action Agenda for Mental Health*. Columbus, OH: Ohio Mental Health Commission, 2001.

17 Mental Health Commission of New Zealand. *Recovery Competencies for New Zealand Mental Health Workers*. Wellington, New Zealand: MHC, 2001.

18 Rickwood D. Recovery in Australia: slowly but surely. *Australian e-Journal for the Advancement of Mental Health (AeJAMH)* 2004: 3(1), 1–3.

19 Repper J. Adjusting the focus of mental health nursing: incorporating service users' experiences of recovery. *Journal of Mental Health* 2000: 9(6), 575–87.

20 Scottish Executive. *Rights, Relationships and Recovery – The Report of the National Review of Mental Health Nursing in Scotland.* Edinburgh: Scottish Executive, 2006.

21 Mental Health Commission. *A Vision for a Recovery Model in Irish Mental Health Services: Discussion Paper.* Dublin, Ireland: MHC, 2006.

22 Szasz TS. The myth of mental illness. *American Psychologist* 1960: 15(February), 113–18.

23 Deegan P. Recovery as a journey of the heart. *Psychiatric Rehabilitation Journal* 1996: 11, 11–19.

24 Clay S. Madness and reality. In: P Barker, P Campbell and B Davidson (Eds.) *From the Ashes of Experience: Reflections on Madness, Survival and Growth.* London: Whurr, 1999, p. 26 (Chapter 2).

25 Clay ibid. pp. 26–7.

26 Buchanan-Barker P. Beyond recovery. In: P Barker (Ed.) *Psychiatric and Mental Health Nursing: The Craft of Caring.* London: Arnold, 2009.

27 'We are all John Thomson's children'. Attributed to an Edinburgh minister in the mid-nineteenth century called John Thomson, who referred to his parishioners as 'my bairns'.

28 Barker P and Buchanan-Barker P. *The Tidal Model: A Guide for Mental Health Professionals.* London, Brunner-Routledge, 2005.

29 Buchanan-Barker P. Uncommon sense: the tidal model of mental health recovery. *Mental Health Nursing* 2004: 23(1), 12–15.

30 http://www.orwell.ru/library/essays/politics/english/e_polit (accessed 22/02/10).

31 Harding C. Empirical correction of seven myths about schizophrenia with implications for treatment. *Acta Psychiatrica Scandinavica: Supplementum* 1994: 384, 140–6.

32 Mosher L. Non-hospital, non-drug interventions with first-episode psychosis. In: J Read, LR Mosher and RP Bentall (Eds.) *Models of Madness: Psychological, Social and Biological Approaches to Schizophrenia.* London: Routledge, 2004.

33 Warner R. *Recovery from Schizophrenia: Psychiatry and Political Economy* (2nd ed.). New York, NY: Routledge and Kegan Paul, 1994.

34 Fisher D. Hope, humanity and voice in recovery from mental illness. In: P Barker, P Campbell and B Davidson (Eds.) *From the Ashes of Experience: Reflections on Madness Survival and Growth.* London: Whurr, 1999, pp. 127–33.

29 Illusion, individuality and autonomy

Craig Newnes

There can be no such thing as mental illness. The reasons for this are multiple but the simplest is that 'mental' – as an entity – doesn't exist in the material sense. If something has no material existence 'it' cannot be ill, wayward, disturbed or any other qualified state. People are said to be distressed when they display a host of different reactions and conduct. Each display is codified within a social rubric familiar to anyone sharing cultural norms with the so-called distressed person. Invariably such displays are physical – from weeping to laughing. Accompanying such displays may be a statement from the person concerning something we conceive as an internal world – what they are thinking, words meant to convey their feelings and so on. This conception of an internal world includes the notion that there is a 'mental' world, presumed to consist of thoughts and feelings to which, via words, we have access. Social norms dictate which aspects of this mental world are to be considered desirable and, via a sleight of hand to which few are privy, 'normal'.

Normality so defined excludes common states of being and limits what can be expressed or stated. It is thus 'normal' to fear someone with a gun but 'abnormal' to fear someone who points a banana at you, unless he/she does it in the socially determined 'threatening' way. It can be said to be normal to think you are a creature of flesh and bone but abnormal to say that you are capable of transmitting your spiritual essence across mountain tops. To cry and wail at the death of a loved one will be seen as normal unless the conduct is deemed 'excessive'. This will then be re-normalized via investigation by another person (often designated an expert) who probes your past and discovers 'reasons' for your 'mental distress'. From there it is a short step to claim that all such distress is explicable if only you search hard enough and thus represent problems in living rather than an illness. Once again, however, an appeal to socially sanctioned norms is being made; the 'explanation' follows a simple formula along the lines:

> Most people would find X difficult and many would express their reaction to X in a variety of ways. Your way, Y, is not socially acceptable though easily understood as a reaction to X.

In the majority of cases, classified under the rubric 'neurotic', the person's conduct is not acceptable to themselves either. In such a way, violence to self and others, hearing voices that no one else seems to hear, feeling overwhelmed, fear and a host of other modes of expression can be justified via expert analysis.

Such analysis carefully neglects to mention that numerous other people experiencing X do not express themselves via Y. At this point a new dimension of explanation emerges: people are genetically vulnerable to expressing X via Y, others have a brain-biochemical imbalance that makes Y inevitable, yet others have a 'world-view' or attributional set which, when disrupted by X, leads to Y. The explanations are as varied as the practitioners available who claim to ameliorate human distress.

Coding conduct

Psychiatric and psychological science differ from genuine science in at least two key respects. First, both involve theories which cannot be refuted.[1] As people claiming to be scientists, members of both professions, are bound to follow certain guidelines in relation to their theory and practice. One such is that any scientific theory must be open to refutation. In fact the theories employed by psychiatry and psychology involve untestable hypotheses which can neither be proven nor refuted. A standard hypothesis in psychiatry – one that justifies the use of human subjects as pharmaceutical company guinea pigs – is the notion that so-called psychiatric diseases are due to brain malfunction, often rooted in biochemical imbalances. As humans are individually unique in their metabolisms any such theory would require knowledge of the biochemical balance before the onset of the diagnosed disease. We don't yet have a way of determining the full biochemical constitution of any given person's brain. We cannot therefore know what a balanced brain looks like biochemically. The inferred imbalance in a diagnosed individual comes from limited, often self-reported, information about the person's modes of expression and conduct – all external signs. No brain or blood test is given before diagnosing schizophrenia, depression or the majority of diagnoses possible (the newest *Diagnostic and Statistical Manual of the American Psychiatric Association* promises in excess of 500 such diagnoses) (see Chapter 11). Psychiatric professionals offer neither pre-morbid nor post-treatment physical tests to support their diagnoses.

Psychology fares no better. In claiming that unwanted or upsetting conduct is due to childhood trauma, unconscious drives, the economic climate or whatever, psychologists fail to explain why the conduct is inevitable nor – in the case of drive theory – can they prove the existence of such drives (see Chapter 7).

The second key departure from science in both psychiatry and psychology – arising directly from the failure to provide a refutable explanation – is the inability of either profession to say, 'We were wrong. We shall drop that theory'. Instead, people are treated *as if* the underlying theory is correct but the evidence not quite available yet. Thus some forms of psychological practice involve interminable searches for evidence of, say, hostility towards one's parents, faulty thinking, repressed desires or behavioural reinforcers, when such evidence is not to be found. As with the brain-biochemical theories, the existence of such causative factors is inferred from the person's reported conduct. The whole scenario is further complicated by the simple fact that people lie – especially to professionals who they may only meet a few times.

There is nothing new about so-called explanations for human conduct which invoke obscure causes. Mankind moves through phases where the dominant discourse can be spiritual or physical. Excavations from ancient Egypt reveal score of skulls where the person had undergone trepanning, a more or less surgical procedure involving drilling holes into the skull to release evil spirits. The dominant discourse of the era saw such treatment as beneficial as, though the person died, the spirit was able to move into a beneficent afterlife. Such procedures established a common thread in medical interventions to this day; a certain mortality rate is inevitable when physicians are involved. Such an ethos underpins devastating actions in the world of psychiatry like electrocution (termed electro-convulsive therapy) where death rates range from 1:100,000 to 5:100,000 (see Chapter 14). Or the cult of drug treatment for so-called illnesses such as schizophrenia (see Chapter 15); it has been estimated that millions of people worldwide have been left with irreversible brain damage (tardive dyskinesia), after drug treatment (from neuroleptics to lithium) for entirely fictitious illnesses like 'schizophrenia' and 'manic depression'.

Schizophrenia is fictitious (as an entity) in the way that the king of France is fictitious but the term gains credence from attributions made to it; Bertrand Russell famously claimed that the existence of anything could be suggested through adjectives used to describe the object of concern. Ergo, 'The king of France is bald' would lead one to assume (1) there is a king of France and (2) he has no hair. The familiar descriptor (baldness) subtly implies the existence of that being described (a king). But what if the statement was made any time from 1793 onwards when the king of France had lost his head and no successor was to follow? The term schizophrenia falls into the same domain of illusion. Statements can be made about attributes of schizophrenia (delusions, hallucinations, etc.). Such statements imply there is an external reality to schizophrenia even though what is actually being said is, 'I believe one can realistically describe people as schizophrenic and in order to do so those people must conduct themselves in the following ways'. As a belief, such a statement is, of course, questionable. But, implicit in the statement is the idea that the statement can refer to a real, externally verifiable, entity. In short, statements about any psychiatric diagnoses are just that – statements (definitions). It is no accident that diagnoses tend to use archaic language – often Greek or Latin – as such language obscures that what is being described is not an external, verifiable reality but merely a medical or psychological definition of the word (depression, schizophrenia, autism, etc.) being used.

Such definitions serve to obfuscate the tautology within explanations of conduct based on the identification, through classification of conduct, of so-called disorders.

This labelling-as-causation tautology can be seen in the recent book, *Why Kids Kill* where author and psychologist Peter Langman analyses various school shootings in the United States.[2] After dismissing simplistic (though sensible) explanations along the lines, 'Children get hold of guns easily in the US so there are more shootings', he categorizes ten shooters as psychopathic, psychotic or traumatized. He then gives the categorization as the *cause* of the behaviour. For example, Eric Harris (one of the two murderers in the Columbine High School shootings) is said to be psychopathic because he displays X, Y and Z. His murderous rampage is then said to be *caused* by his psychopathy. Curiously, Langman fails to come to a more obvious conclusion (in modernist terms) from his categorization table. Here, his research has revealed that the two killers labelled psychopathic had fathers who used guns and all three of the killers labelled traumatized had fathers who used guns illegally – including one who was involved in a hostage-taking crime. Langman fails (in modernist mode) to draw any causal link between parental gun use – an *obsession* according to the author in one case – and gun violence perpetrated by their offspring.

Clinical Psychology as accomplice

Clinical Psychology has been a major contributor and benefactor in the modernist smokescreen concerning distress and diagnosis. Combining physical causal explanation with an equally obscurantist 'psychological model' has proven profitable for the profession (see Chapter 7). The gloss of science is provided by a fixation with classification that shores up and expands psychiatry's own endeavours. Thus, a person's conduct will be classified and coded via observation and testing and, if required, explanations will then be proffered which might combine any number of physical, personal and environmental causes. A typical example could be the use of the Beck Depression Inventory which marks a person as 'depressed'. Suggested reasons for the diagnosis can include genetic pre-disposition, 'faulty' cognitions, brain-biochemical imbalance, unconscious drives, early childhood experience, recent trauma, unemployment and so on. Again, no effort is made to reason that millions of people would not receive such a diagnosis after experiencing similar life events and – of course – no physical evidence is forthcoming to substantiate the genetic or biochemical hypotheses. Psychologists might appeal to the idea that a 'combination' of factors is necessary to produce conduct that is classifiable as deviant or abnormal. Such analyses are coded way of saying, 'All sorts of things make us who we are and I'll keep throwing factors into the pot until you ask me to stop'. These multifactorial analyses cloud the whole endeavour in more expert-led obfuscation and give no verifiable weighting to any particular-stated 'cause'.

An example in the field of psychology is the expansion of cognitive neuropsychology. Here, memories, thoughts and feelings are said to be rooted in brain (dys)function. At a recent seminar, I asked a senior neuropsychologist where in the brain *love* was to be found. He confidently responded that research indicated limbic involvement. He remained unfazed – though a little surprised – when I asked others present to define 'love' and received five different responses. To ask the neuropsychologist where 'abnormal' love was to be found would have been a step too far. Love is, of course, a word that like any other means different things to different people. For neuropsychologists apparently the lack of consensus on the word's meaning presents no difficulty in locating love in the limbic system. All words used to describe emotional or physical states are idiopathic – unique to the individual. A consensus on a word's meaning is a social phenomenon; we nod, smile, shake our heads, say, 'Yes' and 'No' and so on. The social ritual is constrained by certain rules and power hierarchies which mean we cannot know whether actual agreement is taking place – nor can we know that a person's report on their presumed internal state is accurate. Psychologists act as if this presents no problem. It is not hard to see why psychologists, in general, operate within the same rules and assumptions of their given cultural Zeitgeist and, when reporting their own internal states, are no more able to do so accurately than anyone else. The difference, however, is that professional psychologists are rewarded for their expert status and have a vested interest in maintaining a status quo that has elevated them to a position of seers, advice givers and professional comfort givers.

Clinical psychologists should not be seen as operating in bad faith. Many take for granted that there is an internal world that can be accurately described and assume that links between our conduct and various brain functions have been proven. Similarly, many work in multi-disciplinary teams where the expression of doubt in any shared model of the causes of conduct – be it the idea of madness, brain-biochemical imbalance or the parlous condition of modern housing estates – is socially undesirable and a slight on colleagues. All will have been inducted, from their undergraduate years on, into the modern obsession with the importance of the brain and numerous psychological theories based on so-called human attributes like personality, cognitive sets and the like. There are exceptions to this rule and a small cadre of professional psychologists take very seriously indeed notions of social construction. But it hardly matters – they still take an income from a social framework which declares them experts and, by comparison with the numbers in the majority (there are more than 100,000 clinical psychologists trained in the individualistic modernist framework in the United States alone) their constituency barely raises a voice. In this respect, Clinical Psychology remains firmly embedded in the professional elitism through which paternalism flows.

Failure to speak out at multidisciplinary meetings is only part of the sorry story. Though trained in research methodology clinical psychologists tend to research subjects who have been psychiatrically diagnosed or psychologically labelled and apply a myriad of therapies that are wholly individualistic at their core – 'Think this and you'll feel different', 'Keep a stress diary and it will help', 'Tell me your dreams and I'll explain them' and so on. In this way, psychologists maintain their position of privilege and switch to the latest fashionable discourse to stay one step ahead. In UK psychology this has meant a movement from the 'Scientist-practitioner' position to the 'Reflective-practitioner' position. The profession doesn't seem to spot the irony that seeing a non-reflective practitioner would be dangerous indeed. Nor do most clinical psychologists have sufficient grounding in economics, history or philosophy to make sense of the term 'self-reflective'. When asked at a recent seminar which paradigm she preferred for reflection a bemused female student responded, 'I just write my thoughts down', thus demonstrating no awareness that such thoughts could hardly be original and were themselves shaped by the same cultural, historical, political and economic framework in which we all find ourselves. Who knows what she would have made of Sartre's position that the self cannot adequately describe the self as it cannot describe the part that is describing.[3]

In any case, it seems unlikely that the thoughts of a well-paid, car-owning white, female, doctoral professional in her mid-twenties would be helpful to an old guy who had waited 30 minutes for a delayed bus to get to the therapy session; though these thoughts would have been dutifully recorded and later reviewed as a contributing factor in the student's qualification. In much the same way the student would have kept notes on what the pensioner had said and attempted some kind of analysis of what was troubling the patient. These notes would have disappeared into the system to be re-read, re-interpreted or lost by another professional.

The gaze

Foucault[4] termed the way in which professionals discipline themselves and others through coding conduct as the *gaze*. Through observation of those less powerful than themselves, professionals – particularly those in the so-called mental health professions – define abnormality and, by default, normality. As willing servants of psychiatry clinical and educational psychologists thus perform a powerful social function. They are the guardians of what is to be considered normal. Clinical psychologists have thus contributed both to the labelling as deviant of numberless persons over the last century and, in many cases, their destruction at the hands of so-called mental health services. It follows that so-called mental health services do not serve people, at least not those they claim to serve – rather, they observe, label and persecute in the name of a normality governed by those with power (see Chapters 23–25). Those lucky enough to avoid state-subsidized services have seen psychological practitioners on a fee-paying basis to enter into any number (500 plus at the last count) of so-called therapies (see Chapter 8). Indeed, there remains a drive in Britain to promote Cognitive Behaviour Therapy (or funnier still, *Mindfulness*-based CBT – imagine having an 'unmindful' therapist) as the latest panacea despite the reality that thoughts, feelings and behaviour are entirely different – rather than mutually influencing – modalities and, again, the therapy is based on the assumption of an internal world that can be accurately conveyed to others through speech.

Clinical Psychology, as a normalizing profession is the tip of a vast psychological iceberg. Educational psychologists run tests on perfectly ordinary, if annoying, children and diagnose them with attention deficit hyperactivity disorder. Military psychologists are involved in devising interrogation techniques (as if it takes an expert to understand that isolating and blindfolding someone will frighten them) and occupational psychologists make all sorts of claims which justify exploitation of workers by management. Did you ever wonder why there are sweets at supermarket check-outs? It's because industry psychologists 'discovered' the power of nagging and supermarket chiefs were advised to place delectables at check-outs so busy and harassed parents would be sure to pay up when children grabbed a handful.

The nature of responsibility

A patient on a psychiatric acute admissions ward secretes a knife in her room so that she can cut herself; when the knife is found all her personal possessions are confiscated to prevent her from self-harming. When she becomes distressed, the staff say she must learn to take responsibility.

The phrase 'taking responsibility' is often used in such situations but the concept of responsibility nests within two assumptions: the idea that persons (and their various characteristics) are continuous and the related notion that people can be meaningfully described in terms of stable (and internal) attributes.

Assumed continuity (of the self, personhood, memory, day-to-day life and so on) is given within much philosophical discourse.[5] To fundamentally change someone's circumstances through incarceration or psychiatric admission is not seen as affecting this essential continuity. Even when direct physical damage is sustained by an individual that damage is made sense of (by the individual and others) by reference to the ways in which the individual's continuous personal characteristics have been affected or interrupted. Damasio[6,7] sees these as an aspect of extended consciousness (his term) that he calls the autobiographical self. We do not easily admit to major personality change (selves are seen as, more or less, intact across time and place). We almost never consider the possibility that the changed person is so different as to make the notion of taking responsibility for previous action the equivalent of being responsible for someone *else*. What might psychology look like in a world where the self was not assumed to be continuous? Therapy would be irrelevant as people would not need to be accountable for the self they were seen to be yesterday. Sadness or fear would be met with assertions that there is no need to face saddening or fearful events or relationships from one day to the next; parenthood, marriage and friendship would have to face the lack of commitment inherent in the notion of the discontinuous self. I suspect there would be anarchy. Certainly, the prison system and psychiatric system would struggle to exist if the idea of contingent behaviour was made irrelevant by the loss of any individual accountability for that same behaviour across time.

At least one novelist, Carol Shields,[8] has no difficulty in challenging the assumption of continuous personhood. She opens *The Box Garden* thus: '… we change hourly or even from one minute to the next, our entire cycle of being altered, our whole selves shaken with the violence of change' (p. 1).

Such a position is rare indeed in the numberless texts on counselling, self-improvement and the more academically inclined psychology end of the market.

Further, I would challenge the view that responsibility is an individual attribute. An alternative position is essentially Strawsonian[9]; that you cannot separate something called responsibility from the various attitudes and responses from which we infer that someone is responsible (Strawson's 'reactive attitudes'). This position owes much to Ryle[10]: see, for example, his discussion of other mental predicates, such as 'understanding', as public displays. Responses such as guilt, shame, pride, indignation and so on are subject to change as contexts change. Even allowing that persons are continuous across time, these attitudes will surely change with circumstances; such as admission to a psychiatric ward. To expect someone's sense of responsibility and display of what would typically be described as responsible conduct to remain undiminished or unaltered seems to expect too much.

Psychiatric staff are, implicitly, taking a position that emotions do not affect will, and thus, responsibility. For the psychiatric system, one can be responsible or otherwise, however one feels (arguments for and against this position can be found in Sabini and Silver[11]; and such arguments take up much of Oakley[12]). Emotional reaction to, for example, being sectioned under the Mental Health Act is not seen as relevant to responsibility and moral culpability. People who are upset after being sectioned under the Act are thus still urged to 'take responsibility' even though their legal accountability for their actions has been suspended (see Chapters 23–25).

If the mental health professionals involved in the (fictional) example given above were to be asked what they had meant by taking responsibility they are likely to have talked about accepting the consequences of actions, feeling sorry and trying to find more constructive ways of solving problems. They tacitly assume that the person is still *capable* of these things despite their admission to hospital or other changed circumstances. Such capabilities are seen (conveniently) to be continuous.

Even within the definition typically used by mental health professionals, it is entirely possible that someone could engage in self-harm and similar behaviours and yet still be described as acting responsibly. When someone self-harms, it seems possible that they have found a behaviour that provides a singularly powerful solution to the problem of expressing or coping with overwhelming feelings.[13] They may also be prepared to accept the consequences, such as loss of blood, permanent scarring and even alienation from others. It is only when they come in to contact with a system that attempts to control their behaviour that its consequences become unacceptable. This is because the psychiatric response, through removing power and control, creates 'the very circumstances that are likely to have led to the need to self injure'.[14]

There may also be times when violence represents a solution whose consequences are acceptable both to the individual and also to a wider society, in particular in resistance to oppression. For a soldier being tortured in a prisoner of war camp or a member of an oppressed minority, the consequences of violent resistance may be aversive but they may accept them, given the already aversive conditions of their life. Their resistance may also be approved or even applauded by the rest of their society or culture of origin. For many users of psychiatric services the experience is one of oppression and violent resistance may be the result.[15]

In order to be judged to have taken responsibility then, what service users must do is simply what the system wants. Although they may not be legally responsible for their behaviour, they can take responsibility for it by engaging with the system, through taking medication or participating in therapy, to prevent it happening again. The subtext of the phrase taking responsibility is thus 'do what I as the more powerful person expect of you'. The apparent desire to get someone to take responsibility (or doing what they are told) may be more about conformity or punishment than helping them to lead a more fulfilling life.

There has been a recent move towards adopting a so-called recovery-based approach within mental health services, with an associated emphasis on self-management of distress. This can be seen as a welcome move towards allowing individuals in distress to use the strategies that are most acceptable to them, to take back control from mental health professionals and to genuinely take responsibility for their lives. The Royal College of Psychiatrists' press release endorsing the 'recovery ethos' identifies a guiding principle as 'therapeutic risk taking to promote personal responsibility'[16] (see also, 'A common purpose: Recovery in future mental health services'[17]).

Such a position continues to suggest that the experiences and behaviour of people in distress are socially unacceptable and need to be controlled[18]; this time, however, people must control themselves. Self-management thus, again, represents an internalization of social control (see also Rose[19]). It seems ironic that, in industry, the best kind of management is a hands-off approach, allowing workers autonomy and space for creativity. Despite using the business argot, the self-management implied by psychologists and others is a far more authoritarian affair.[20]

Responsibility, power and autonomy

In psychiatry the recovery approach situates the cause of distress, and the focus for action, within the individual. Smail[21] argues that concepts like responsibility that are used to describe the internal psychological operations of individuals, and thus provide proximal explanations for individual distress, function to divert attention from the way in which distress is created by the operation of power in the social environment. It is thus impossible for someone to take responsibility for addressing their distress, as its origins are beyond the limit of their power. For people sectioned under the Mental Health Act the position becomes untenable; their 'Get out of jail free' card[22] has been played, they are deemed to lack responsibility and, in consequence, hospitalized. They are then frequently urged to 'be more responsible', criticized for not 'taking responsibility' and so on. Beresford and Hopton argue that rather than a recovery model what is needed is 'a rights-based' approach, involving policy changes to provide the support, public attitudes and access to allow service users to live the lives they choose.[23]

In the example given there is a tacit assumption that the processes of admission and incarceration do not affect an individual's ability to learn (or practice taking responsibility as defined by the prison or psychiatric systems). Thus, living in entirely new ways (alongside those diagnosed as mad, being labelled, having one's day ordered by sometimes invisible authority figures and rule makers who one has not chosen) is not seen as *changing* the person or at least only as having socially desirable consequences. The extraordinary lack of power now experienced by incarcerated individuals is likely to mean that the new system will impact on them in both intended and unintended ways. How does one protest about ward rounds, prison warders and hospital food? 'Going on the blanket' during the dirty protests at the Maze prison is but one example. Self-harm may well seem a powerful means of protest – and an entirely responsible means – if contrasted with a little-used suggestion box or barely visible complaints procedure. If the consequences of actions are some reduction in privileges, this is likely to feel insignificant to the already experienced loss of freedom and autonomy.

If those in power have some control in the system (for example, as psychologists working on in-patient wards), then recognition of Strawson's point is vital: if we expect people to take responsibility we must make the experience of their new environments as conducive to familiar 'reactive attitudes' as possible. Adults used to being treated *as* adults must receive the same in their new surroundings. Condescension, criticism and worse will not provoke responses construed as 'responsible'. Simply telling people to be more responsible won't help at all.

To take this argument further, so-called services cannot offer autonomy to those they serve if that autonomy has already been removed by the assumptions inherent in current conceptions of mental illness. These include the idea that distress, if displayed in certain ways, is an indication of the loss of will on the part of the person – and without will there can be no autonomy.

As stated earlier, I am not suggesting that those working as mental health professionals are doing so in bad faith. They share the same assumptions (there can be an internal expressible world, and that world consists of thoughts and feelings conveyable though word or deed, etc.)

as the people they are paid to help. Further, those in charge, though fostering such assumptions through self-interest, work within pretty much the same understanding of what it is to be human. It is too much to hope that human service professionals will simply close down their services and do something genuinely useful – plumbing comes to mind. They might, however, step back a little from the arrogance that comes with certainty, grant that people conducting themselves in disturbing ways have a right to do so and leave them alone for a while.

Notes

1 Popper, K. (1963). *Conjectures and Refutations: The Growth of Scientific Knowledge.* London: Routledge and Kegan Paul.

2 Langman, P. (2009). *Why Kids Kill. Inside the Minds of School Shooters.* New York, NY: Palgrave Macmillan.

3 Sartre, J.P. (1943/1963). Being and nothingness – an essay on phenomenological ontology. New York, NY: Gallimard.

4 Foucault, M. (1963). *Naissance de la clinique* (The birth of the clinic). Paris: Presses Universitaires de France.

5 Murdoch, I. (1992). *Metaphysics as a Guide to Morals.* Harmondsworth: Penguin.

6 Damasio, A. (2000). *The Feeling of What Happens.* London: Vintage.

7 Damasio, A. (2004). *Looking for Spinoza.* London: Vintage.

8 Shields, C. (1977). *The Box Garden.* London: Fourth Estate.

9 Watson, G. (1987). Responsibility and the limits of evil. In: F. Schoeman (Ed.) *Responsibility, Character and the Emotions.* Cambridge: Cambridge University Press.

10 Ryle, G. (1949). *The Concept of Mind.* London: Hutchinson.

11 Sabini, J. and Silver, M. (1987). Emotions, responsibility and character. In: F. Schoeman (Ed.) *Responsibility, Character and the Emotions.* Cambridge: Cambridge University Press.

12 Oakley, J. (1992). *Morality and the Emotions.* London: Routledge.

13 Babiker, G. and Arnold, L. (1997). *The Language of Injury: Comprehending Self-mutilation.* Leicester: BPS Books.

14 Johnstone, L. (1997). Self-injury and the psychiatric response. *Feminism and Psychology*, 7, 421–6, 425.

15 Coleman, R. (1999). Hearing voices and political oppression. In: C. Newnes, G. Holmes and C. Dunn (Eds.) *This Is Madness: A Critical Look at Psychiatry and the Future of Mental Health Services.* Ross-on-Wye: PCCS Books, pp. 149–63.

16 Royal College of Psychiatrists (2004). Council report 'Rehabilitation and recovery now' points to new direction in service provision. Retrieved March 26, 2004 from the World Wide Web: http://www.rcpsych.ac.uk/press/preleases/pr/pr_513.htm.

17 Care Services Improvement Partnership, Royal College of Psychiatrists and Social Care Institute for Excellence (2007). A common purpose: Recovery in future mental health services. London: CSIP, RCPsych SCIE. http://www.scie.org.uk.

18 Beresford, P. and Hopton, J. (2003). Recovery or independent living? *Openmind*, 124, 16.

19 Rose, N. (1999). *Governing the Soul.* London: Routledge.

20 Baker, E. and Newnes, C. (2005). What do we mean when we ask people to take responsibility? *Forensic Psychology Update*, 80, 23–7.

21 Smail, D. (1993). *The Origins of Unhappiness.* London: Robinson.

22 Holmes, G., Newnes, C. and Dunn, C. (2001). Continuing madness. In: C. Newnes, G. Holmes and C. Dunn (Eds.) *This is Madness Too: Critical Perspectives on Mental Health Services.* Ross-on-Wye: PCCS Books.

23 Beresford and Hopton op. cit.

30 Ethics: the elephant in the room

Phil Barker

The devil is in the detail

Each contributor to this book has addressed a slightly different theme or topic. Arguably, all have wrestled with the same, single issue: 'what right do we have to force people to change the way they behave?' Or, in a more general sense, we might need to ask, 'what right do we have to even begin to think about changing the way people *are*, as persons?' This question could be framed, philosophically, as an issue concerning *autonomy* (see Chapter 1). However, there is no need to consult the dictionary, far less the great philosophers, to understand the central importance of 'self-determination' or 'self-government' in everyday life. Few people do not jealously guard their autonomy. Most express a wish to live their lives in peace – pursuing what they consider to be important or worthwhile – ultimately proud to have done it 'my way'. It comes as no surprise that '*My way*' is such a popular anthem choice at funerals.[1]

In protecting their autonomy people are resisting the idea that they should, necessarily, have to do it someone else's way. However, ultimately, this is top of the psychiatric agenda. Psychiatry, many aspects of psychology and most forms of psychotherapy have defined certain ways of living as 'normal', 'healthy' or 'adaptive'. Almost every psychiatric principle is rooted in such assumptions. Moreover, if people do not elect to pursue a style of living that is 'healthy', normal or 'adaptive', most psychiatric professionals believe that they *should* have the power to make such people 'see reason'. The moral imperative (*should*) is clear-cut (however 'wrong' it might be to others). However, the idea that anyone might 'make' someone see reason makes no sense. People might be encouraged to explore their current understanding of their relationship to the wider world. They might even be encouraged to examine critically the values on which they base those understandings. In the final analysis, they might be encouraged to develop further their awareness of possible conflicts between what they 'believe' and their rationale for 'believing' it. However, *forcing* (or making) someone to embrace a different form of 'sense', 'reason' or 'understanding' is the agenda of 'brainwashing' and totalitarianism, however much we might cloak it in the language of care and compassion. It requires us to deny, completely, the independent status of the 'person' – another idea that has been addressed in many of the preceding chapters.

It is one thing to talk of 'people' as some kind of social mass, within which 'individuals' make up the 'people' and so the social mass. It is quite another thing to talk of 'persons'. This requires us to think of 'individuals' not as units of society but much as we think of our own unique selves. Viewed from that perspective, persons are in constant flux –swimming in the tide of life – mysteries that largely defy explanation. The world would be an easier place to manage were it not for the reflections thrown up by the notion of 'persons'.

At the age of 19, Eric Blair, who had long harboured a fascination with the 'Orient', joined the Indian Imperial Police and was posted to Burma. Despite his youth, he was given considerable responsibility for the security of hundreds of thousands of people, including those people who were in jail. Five years later, after contracting a tropical fever, he returned to England and began to consider becoming a writer under the pen-name of *George Orwell*. His early writings reflected his life in Burma and sketched many of the humanitarian concerns that were to become the hallmark of his later, more famous, works. In one essay, he recalled the thoughts that ran through his head as he watched a condemned man step 'slightly aside to avoid a puddle', on his way to the gallows:

> It is curious, but till that moment I had never realised what it means to destroy a healthy, conscious man. When I saw the prisoner step aside to avoid the puddle I saw the mystery, the unspeakable wrongness, of cutting a life short when it is in full tide. This man was not dying, he was alive just as we are alive. All the organs of his body were working – bowels digesting food, skin renewing itself, nails growing, tissues forming – all toiling away in solemn foolery. His nails would still be growing when he stood on the drop, when he was falling through the air with a tenth of a second to live. His eyes saw the yellow gravel and the grey walls, and his brain still remembered, foresaw, reasoned – even about puddles. He and we were a party of men walking together, seeing, hearing, feeling, understanding the same world; and in two minutes, with a sudden snap, one of us would be gone – one mind less, one world less.[2]

Whether or not Orwell actually witnessed a hanging has long been debated, but is largely irrelevant. Orwell was writing about an idea, not an event. The idea that persons can, so easily, become insensitive to extinguishing another human life must have dawned on him at some point. His essay begins to explore the grey territory of the 'personal' issues, which such an act entails.

Psychiatry, psychology and many psychotherapies have cultivated the notion that persons can be explained. Their behaviour can be linked to one or more past events in their lives; or can be attributed to the influence of drugs, brain chemicals, their diet, the moon or the weather. All this seems fanciful. It might be possible to generate a plausible theory as to why someone did this or that, but theory is not explanation. Persons are enigmas – perhaps even to themselves – or at least this is my personal conclusion. The rich complexity of *who I am* and the countless events and circumstances that are part of my *becoming* render 'me' inscrutable. If one thinks about it, one realises that one can be an outsider in one's own life. The sheer complexity of our personal stories means that explaining ourselves – even to ourselves – becomes near impossible. The devil is always very much in the detail.

Is resistance futile?

Most people will have some experience of being an 'outsider' or 'odd one out'. Social groups are driven by genuine consensus, where they are not driven by the power of a single personality and will actively 'exclude' anyone who does not 'fit in' or conform to the group mentality. The English coined the phrase 'being sent to Coventry' to describe the ostracism of an individual, by the group. In its original sense, the group's action rendered the person a *non-person*.

Although democracy is almost universally understood, it has no single accepted definition. That said most definitions accept that any meaningful democracy should act as an equalising force within society, where efforts are made to determine what is in the best interests of all the people whilst respecting the rights of individuals to hold different views. At least in principle, within effective democracies people should be free – if not also actively 'empowered' – to *seek, receive, hold* and *express* views that might be in direct contrast to that of the consensus.[3]

Such ideas have always presented a problem for medicine, which has long had a significant authoritarian bias, as a profession. The day of the doctor being viewed as a 'god' may be waning but many people still expect the physician to know everything; and many physicians, tempted by such a prospect, find it difficult to accept that 'patients' might embrace dissenting views.

Conformity is highly prized in medical circles, hence the enduring popularity of the term 'compliance'. Although several 'politically correct' alternatives have been proposed – such as adherence or concordance – these mean much the same thing: obeying, sticking to or agreeing with some medical decision regarding 'necessary' treatment (see Chapter 15). If 'patients' acquiesce to medical authority they will be seen as 'good patients'. Any challenge to that authority risks the medical equivalent of ostracism: being labelled a 'bad patient'.

The late American mental health activist, Judi Chamberlin,[4] had the experience of being committed to a State mental hospital in her early twenties. Following a miscarriage she recalled that:

> I plunged into a depression so extreme that I was unable to function. I stayed in bed crying, day after day, not bathing, barely eating and unable to believe the fact that the baby was no longer within me, was not to be born.[5]

Her experience was, of course, full of personal meaning, however disturbing her behaviour might have appeared to others around her. However, psychiatric professionals showed little interest in her distress and were concerned only to manage it and contain it with drugs. Over time she recalled that:

> I was transformed from a person who was suffering a real loss to a person whose grief was a 'symptom'. I then became a patient, a person who needed drugs to control the symptom, and belonged in a hospital because of the degree and intensity of my illness. I then was further transformed into an involuntary patient, medically and legally assumed to be unable to define or act in my own interests. By this time, the cause of my original pain had long since been forgotten…I was simply a 'psychotic', a 'schizophrenic', someone whose beliefs and feelings did not matter.[6]

Judi Chamberlin's first experience of psychiatry was many years ago. This might lead us to ask:

- To what extent is the situation any different today?
- Is it still possible for people to lose their identity as a 'person' in their transformation into a 'patient'?
- To what extent are today's 'mental health services' still focused on the 'treatment' of some abstract 'illness' (a 'psychosis' or 'schizophrenia') rather than addressing the all too real problems in living, which give rise to the person's distress?
- More importantly, if people do not 'comply' with the directions of the professionals, do they still risk being branded as a 'bad patient'?

Judi Chamberlin recalled that when she had tried to express her anger in hospital, she was either drugged or secluded, so she turned to the American Civil Liberties Union for support.

However, when she asked for help in fighting for her freedom, she discovered that freedom was not something that 'mental patients' deserved. But she knew that freedom was the key, and that if she was not to be 'given' her civil rights, she would need to work out a way to get them for herself. Much later she reflected on her time in psychiatric care:

> Well, I've been a good patient, and I've been a bad patient, and believe me, being a good patient helps to get you out of the hospital, but being a bad patient helps to get you back to real life.[7]

This raises the question of what, exactly, is the *purpose* of 'mental health care' or 'psychiatric treatment'? Is it to assist, or otherwise enable, people to do whatever is necessary to get on with their lives? Or is it to shape the thinking or 'mind set' of the 'patient', so that they will be 'realistic' and 'reasonable': in effect, so that 'they' will become like 'us'?

Today, the idea that people might 'recover' from some 'mental breakdown' is enjoying something of a renaissance (see Chapter 28). Does this mean that all the energy of all the people in the mental health system is now focused on helping people to 'recover': to get back to real life? Judi Chamberlin, for one, doubted that mainstream mental health services would ever embrace such an ethic. She recognised that, however much people might *say* that they wanted only the best for 'their patients', offers of support often came at a price:

> One of the reasons I believe I was able to escape the role of chronic patient that had been predicted for me was that I was able to leave the surveillance and control of the mental health system when I left the state hospital. Today, that's called 'falling through the cracks.' While I agree that it's important to help people avoid hunger and homelessness, such help must not come at too high a price. Help that comes with unwanted strings – 'We'll give you housing if you take medication,' 'We'll sign your SSI papers if you go to the day program' – is help that is paid for in imprisoned spirits and stifled dreams. We should not be surprised that some people won't sell their souls so cheaply.[8]

Did Judi Chamberlin 'find herself'? Did she 're-discover herself' after her 'breakdown'? Did she 're-build herself' through her long journey as a mental health 'activist'? I have no idea, but I very much doubt it. These represent all the things that mental health professionals think the 'patient' *should* do; or which are the necessary components of *rehabilitation*. What little I know of Judi Chamberlin personally, tells me that she did none of these things. Instead, if she was here today, she might say, 'I did it my way'. She wouldn't sell her soul. Resistance was very much part of that 'way'.[9]

Still flying around the cuckoo's nest?

Almost 50 years ago Ken Kesey's novel, *One Flew Over the Cuckoo's Nest*[10] enjoyed widespread critical acclaim after its publication. This was overshadowed, regrettably, by acclaim for the film, in which Jack Nicholson brought Kesey's main protagonist, Randle P McMurphy to life, in 1975. Ever since, the film has been a popular part of educational programmes for mental health professionals, who are encouraged to view '*Cuckoo's Nest*' as a history lesson: this is how things were; now things are so much better.

Kesey used his experience of working as a psychiatric aide in Menlo Park Veterans Administration hospital in California in 1961, to set the scene for his novel. The target of his critique was not so much psychiatry as the hypocrisy, cruelty and enforced conformity of American life in the early 1960s. Of course, the psychiatric ward in *Cuckoo's Nest* was a reflection of contemporary social values, in much the same way that such wards are today (see Chapter 16). Not surprisingly, McMurphy's battles with the power-mad 'Big Nurse' Ratched were over hypocrisy, cruelty and enforced conformity. The enduring unreasonableness of the psychiatric system deprived all the 'patients' of their 'inalienable rights'; reducing them to the level of children in the process. McMurphy's troublemaking mission was to liberate, or at least breathe a little life into, the cowed inmates, who Big Nurse seemed to dominate so easily. From this perspective, the book's theme is a simple one: *the abuse of power.*

However, *Cuckoo's Nest* can also be read as a Christian allegory, dealing with good and evil. McMurphy represents 'good' in the form of a powerful Western hero, who puts his life on the line for the downtrodden patients around him. The 'evil' is a sickness in the American consciousness, which 'Big Chief' Bromden, the novel's narrator, calls 'the combine'. So Big Nurse isn't evil, but neither is the government nor the police. Instead, the pervasive influence of the 'machinery' of society at large (the 'combine'), controls and manipulates the actors, like puppets. 'Big Chief' Bromden describes the ward as appearing, on the surface, to be a place of order and purposeful activity. In reality it is a grotesque world of tortured individuals who are: 'like puppets, mechanical puppets in one of those Punch and Judy acts where it's supposed to be funny to see the puppet beat up by the Devil and swallowed headfirst by a smiling alligator'.[11]

The control exercised by staff – whether nurses or aides – appears to be delivered gently, with a 'caring' attitude. Nurse Ratched may appear to control the patients with rigid routines, pills, the log book (where patients are expected to 'report' any disturbing talk or actions they have witnessed) and Group Therapy, where she requires everyone to 'undress emotionally', as part of their 'treatment'. She also has Electro-Shock Therapy and other punishments that are 'muscle-flexing masquerading as socially instructive correction'.[12] But all these represent her concern for her 'patients'. As Big Nurse calmly reminds the group:

> At some time – perhaps in your childhood – you may have been allowed to get away with flouting the rules of society. When you broke a rule you knew it. You wanted to be dealt with, *needed* it, but the punishment did not come. That foolish lenience on the part of your parents may have been the germ that grew into your present illness. I tell you this hoping you will understand that it is *entirely for your own good* that we enforce discipline and order.[13]

Many things may have changed since Kesey first worked as a psychiatric aide 50 years ago. However, one thing which remains unchanged is the concern to do things in the *patients' best interests,* (whether or not they want this), which drives most mental health professionals.

Many detect a deeper theme in Kesey's novel, which 'resonates with the deep cello tones of mythology'.[14] Whatever her expressed motives, Big Nurse is a dangerous presence. Her enduring practice of developing highly destructive dependency relationships with the patients in her care echoes the 'terrible mother' figure of Jungian lore. The risk of fostering dependency remains a key ethical problem for all mental health professionals. Others saw the novel as replete with all sorts of mythological imagery, viewing McMurphy as: 'The evolving hero, the fool as mentor, the psychopathic savior, the cosmic Christ, the Grail Knight, the comic strip Lone Ranger.'[15]

For Porter, the mental ward in *Cuckoo's Nest* could be viewed as the waste land with Nurse Ratched representing:

> the waste land elements of mechanization, heartless efficiency, fear, guilt, hopelessness, and sterility, and she uses these qualities in the prolonged stultification of the inmates. McMurphy enters the waste land, conquers Big Nurse at least temporarily, cures Bromden, the ailing Fisher King,[16] and restores life to the waste land by giving the men confidence, laughter, love and self-respect.[17]

McMurphy eventually pays for his heroism with his life, but in the process, he experiences the realisation of knowing 'who' he really is. The novel is about the transformation of 'my way' into the Tao of RP McMurphy: 'From this point of view the hero is symbolical of that divine creative and redemptive image which is hidden within us all, only waiting to be known and rendered into life.'[18]

What relevance has this 1960s novel to any critical consideration of mental health ethics in the twenty-first century? Kesey revealed some years later that the character of McMurphy was 'fictional, (but) inspired by the tragic longing of real men I worked with on the ward (the psychiatric ward at Menlo Park Veterans Administration hospital)'.[19] In Porter's view, Kesey 'as a humane novelist created his heroic fictive protagonist from the real needs of actual men debilitated by the formidable strengths of the external world and by their own frailties'.[20] This is the link between Kesey's 'fictional', but all too 'real' characters, their predicaments and the predicaments of both 'patients' and 'staff' in today's mental health services. If people in mental health services today – whether women or men – *suffer* from anything, they suffer from the formidable effects of living; and their sense that they are too frail to deal with them. The language of psychiatry has been modified greatly in those 50 years (see Chapter 11), but what remains unchanged are the 'patients'' experiences of problems in living, which are translated into much the same kinds of 'illnesses', although the 'explanations' for their onset might well have changed.

The professional purpose of the staff in *Cuckoo's Nest* was to save the patients from their illness, if not also from themselves. By contrast, the hero figure – McMurphy – harboured no such ambition. He sought neither to *save* his fellow inmates; nor to 'fix' their problems; nor to change the nature of the oppressive regime that contained them. However, he did model a *way* by which they might deal with them both.

The central theme of *Cuckoo's Nest* is the *absurd*: the disparity between human aspiration, on the one hand; and the level of actual achievement that 'reality' appears to allow, on the other. We discover the 'absurd' when we set out to find meaning in our lives, only to discover that the world is, essentially, meaningless. Typically, people respond to this in three ways. They commit suicide; or they engage in some 'leap of faith', attaching themselves to something, which they believe exists beyond the absurd (such as religious faith); or they accept the absurd. Albert Camus believed that the absurd could inspire heroic resistance, if not also an actual spiritual transcendence.[21] For David Galloway the absurd: '… becomes a way of affirming the resources of the human spirit, of exalting sacrifice and suffering, of ennobling the man capable of sustaining the vital opposition between intention and reality'.[22]

This appears to be a modern update on the Stoic philosophy of Epictetus (see Chapter 1) from over 2,000 years ago: difficult circumstances do not so much ennoble a person, as reveal him.

As the hero develops within McMurphy he shifts from self-protection and survival, to being willing to sacrifice his life in an effort to restore life to others. This becomes the testimony of his heroic values: freedom, dignity, pride, love and courage. All these involve imposing some kind of *human significance* on the absurd. Indeed, the final message of *Cuckoo's Nest* is that something can always be done about absurdity.

As people like Judi Chamberlin showed, it is always *possible* to gather one's resources, and to begin to rebuild a life, that appears to have been devastated – doing it 'my way'. She realised that she could not look to psychiatry for much help to do this re-building, but instead needed to look to others, who were in much the same boat as herself; and who understood the human nature of her predicament. Not surprisingly, she named the book that she wrote, based on her experience of re-building, *On Our Own*.[23]

Living in the shadow of 1984

Cuckoo's Nest owed much to the influence of George Orwell, who over 60 years ago published his most famous novel, *1984*. Just after the end of the Second World War, in 1948, Orwell had retreated to Jura, off the coast of Scotland, to complete his manuscript – 'The Last Man in Europe'. A combination of the weather, misfortune, his dogged dedication to hard work and smoking probably exacerbated the tuberculosis that soon would kill him. Many critics have suggested that his bleak vision of the future could be attributed to his experience of fading health, if not also his vision of approaching death and the bleak landscape of Jura. This seems a little unfair. As I noted earlier, Orwell never shirked responsibility in his writing and had been cultivating his concern over the 'future of humanity' since his early twenties.

Although some critics and commentators have been keen to slim down its central message, *1984* is nothing less than Orwell's final rage against totalitarianism. As Orwell himself admitted, all his serious work, since he had returned from the Spanish Civil War, had been 'written, directly or indirectly, against totalitarianism'.[24] Russian Communism may have been Orwell's main target in *1984*, but had he lived, he would doubtless have still been raging against the abuse of power that is at the heart of everything from genocide to censorship: an abuse that he depicted as the image of 'a boot stamping on a human face – forever'.

However, what does a critique of totalitarianism have to do with mental health care and treatment? The simple answer is that any kind of power can be abused. The more powerful people become, the greater is the risk that their powerful influence will be corrupting in nature.[25] Soviet psychiatry became infamous for its use of psychiatric drugs, and ECT to control or contain political 'dissidents'.[26] However, psychiatry has been used in almost every country around the world as a means of controlling 'dissident voices'. Ken Kesey's 'Big Nurse' is merely an echo of Orwell's Big Brother who, in turn, was the personification of the faceless image of oppression that lay at the heart of totalitarianism.

However, like *Cuckoo's Nest* the plot of *1984* might conceal a more subtle message, or at least beg a more unsettling question. Fifty years ago, in an afterword to *1984*, the psychoanalyst and humanistic philosopher *Erich Fromm* suggested that *1984* asked, 'Can human nature be changed in such a way that man will forget his longing for freedom, for dignity, for integrity, for love–that is to say, can man forget he is human?'[27] This question takes us to the heart of the matter concerning all things psychiatric.

In *1984*, the dissident protagonist, Winston Smith, falls in love with the like-minded Julia. Eventually they both betray one another, after interrogation by Party officials. However, during their love affair Winston buys a paperweight in an old junk-shop. It is symbol of the fragile world that Winston and Julia have made for each other. It also symbolises the past, as Winston tries to remember the days before the Party. The paperweight symbolises his dream of freedom and his need to make a connection with the past, which has been ruined by the Party. The paperweight reminds Winston that the Party cannot control people's memories: 'It's a little chunk of history they've forgotten to alter. It's a message from a hundred years ago, if one knew how to read it'. For Winston the paperweight is like the room that they share, from time to time. The coral inside the paperweight represented himself and Julia, fixed for all eternity, at its heart. He remembers that, ultimately, he is human.

Unlike *Cuckoo' Nest*, there is to be no redemption for Winston Smith, who submits to Big Brother and ends the novel as an alcoholic wreck, awaiting execution. He has finally accepted the Party's depiction of life, to the extent that he celebrates news of a victory over Eurasia. At long last, 'he had won the victory over himself. He loved Big Brother'.

The fate of Winston Smith seems to tell us that 'resistance is futile'. Or does it? The Party will always win in the end. We should wise up and cooperate. Perhaps? Orwell's Party could be any oppressor – from a playground bully to a political juggernaut. Orwell was never a man to mince his words. Taking on authority is always fraught with danger. Like Winston Smith and McMurphy, you might lose your life in the process. The question is simple: should we resist, collude or keep silent? Or should we jealously hold on to our humanity?

The elephant in the room

Without intending any disrespect, all the authors in this book – myself included – have all *conjured* with the notion of mental health ethics. I use the expression 'conjure' intentionally. Much of what passes for 'ethics' in the traditional 'psychiatric' or contemporary 'mental health' field involves bureaucratic or terminological 'sleight of hand': some form of linguistic 'trickery'. People may mean what they say but do not always say what they mean.

Much attention has been paid to language and terminology – whether in lay, 'clinical' or legal senses. However, much if not all the available legal and professional ethical guidance balances on the pin-head concept of 'mental illness' (or its many contemporary euphemisms). Despite the absence of anything resembling the kind of scientific validation considered so vital in our ever-so scientific age, the concept of 'mental illness' is embraced, employed and reified by all sections of the community. We have built great economic empires upon this idea, which provides a professional way of life for millions of people. Others use the idea as a way of explaining the inexplicable: especially *why* people kill themselves or others. Many others use it, however, unconsciously, as a way of opting out of life and the active living of it. Largely due to the continuing influence of psychoanalysis, the assumed link between 'mental illness' and creativity continues to prove seductive to arts programmes, film makers and others, keen to romanticise madness, or to incorporate it within some socio-political agenda. It is for this final reason that I chose to close the book by drawing on the aesthetic appreciation of madness, good and evil and right and wrong, which has long been central to great literature.[28]

The excerpts I have chosen remind us that there are no easy answers to the moral challenges thrown down in life. Textbook ethics may offer some comfort, but little resolution. Edison is reputed to have said that 'genius is one per cent inspiration and 99 per cent perspiration'. The same may be true of ethics. It involves making tough decisions. It often results in fractured relationships. The 'moral' person is often seen as a 'pain in the ass'. It is hard work. It is always easier to go along with the crowd; keep your head down; avoid conflict; be popular.

The ethical path is a difficult path, which can make for a lonely journey. You tell yourself that you would be a fool to take that path; but perhaps you could not live with yourself, if you took any other. Ethics – and ethical decision-making – is never less than *personal*. It is what I believe; all the reasons for believing it; and all the necessary moral actions that flow from it. Ultimately, the decisions I took were *my* decisions. In the lines of the song: 'When there was doubt, I ate it up and spit it out. I faced it all and I stood tall'.[29] However corny Sinatra and his many imitators made it sound, this is the anthem of all who could say, *I did it my way*.

It has become a cliché, but it remains a beautiful paradox. There is an elephant in the room and *everyone* pretends it is not there.[30] The elephant *is* the ethical dilemma in mental health. It trumpets – 'do you not see me; do you not hear me; why are you ignoring me?' Not only do most people *know* that the elephant is there, they *hear* her calling and they understand the message. However, for one professional, financial, prestigious or self-aggrandising reason or another, they turn a deaf ear and a blind eye.

If there is any single problem with mental health ethics it does not lie *only* with those who promote, justify or enthusiastically engage in coercion. Neither does it lie *only* with those who promulgate the lunatic language of 'madness', 'sanity', 'personal growth' or 'mental wellbeing'; nor *only* with those who generate, popularise or otherwise publicise mythical ideas, as a means of obtaining a research grant or gaining publication in a prestigious journal. Neither does the problem lie *only* with those who patronise people with so-called mental health problems, in the blinkered belief that they are, in some, sense lesser humans. Instead, the problem lies with those of us who *know*, however intuitively, or from careful study, that there is a *right* way to treat our fellow women and men but, for whatever reason, *avoid* acting on that knowledge in our everyday lives.

The iconic struggle for civil rights in America echoed all the other struggles for the human rights – the right to 'be' – down the ages. Lest we fear to 'speak out'; lest we fear 'blowing the whistle'; lest we fear the 'trouble' we might make and the 'trouble' it might cause us, or our families; lest we fear that it is 'all common sense, anyway'– we might recall one voice from the struggle for civil rights.

> We will have to repent in this generation not merely for the hateful words and actions of the bad people but for the appalling silence of the good people.[31]
>
> (Martin Luther King)

Notes

1 http://www.guardian.co.uk/uk/2005/nov/17/arts.artsnews1.
2 Orwell G. 'A Hanging' (first published 1931). Available in full at: http://www.orwell.ru/library/articles/hanging/english/e_hanging.
3 This is most commonly understood as the principle of 'freedom of speech' or 'freedom of expression', which derives from John Stuart Mill's theory of liberty. See Puddephatt A. *Freedom of Expression: The Essentials of Human Rights.* London: Hodder Arnold, 2005.
4 Barker P. and Buchanan-Barker P. Obituary, *British Journal of Wellbeing* 2010, 1(1), p. 42.
5 Chamberlin J. The medical model and harm. In: P Barker, P Campbell and B Davidson (Eds.) *From the Ashes of Experience: Reflections on Madness, Survival and Growth.* London: Whurr, 1999, p. 171.

6 Chamberlin ibid. p. 173.
7 Chamberlin J. Confessions of a non-compliant patient. http://www.power2u.org/articles/recovery/confessions.html.
8 Chamberlin ibid.
9 The 'way' is the metaphor for the spiritual journey in a wide range of secular and religious philosophies – from Taoism to Christianity and beyond.
10 Kesey K. *One Flew Over the Cuckoo's Nest*. New York, NY: Viking Press, 1962.
11 Kesey ibid., p. 37.
12 Porter MG. *One Flew Over the Cuckoo's Nest: Rising to Heroism* Boston, MA: Twayne Publishers, 1989, p. 51.
13 Kesey op. cit., p. 171.
14 Porter op. cit., p. 85.
15 Hunt JW. Introduction to 'Perspectives on a Cuckoo's Nest: A Symposium on Ken Kesey', *Lex et Scientia* 1977, 13(1 and 2), p. 7.
16 The king in Arthurian legend who, wounded in the legs, can do little more than fish.
17 Porter op. cit., p. 85.
18 Campbell J. *The Hero with a Thousand Faces*. Princeton, NJ: Princeton University Press, 1972, p. 39.
19 Kesey K. *Kesey's Garage Sale*. New York, NY: Viking Press, 1973, p. 7.
20 Porter op. cit., p. 13.
21 Camus A. The Myth of Sisyphus. http://www.nyu.edu/classes/keefer/hell/camus.html.
22 Galloway D. *The Absurd Hero in American Fiction: Updike, Styron, Bellow, Salinger*. Austin, TX: University of Texas Press, 1981, p. xiii.
23 Chamberlin J. *On Our Own*. London: Mind, 1988.
24 http://www.orwell.ru/library/essays/wiw/english/e_wiw.
25 Lord Acton famously said, 'Power corrupts: Absolute power corrupts absolutely', http://www.mcadamreport.org/Acton.html (accessed 10/04/10).
26 Bloch S and Reddaway P. *Soviet Psychiatric Abuse: The Shadow Over World Psychiatry*. London: Victor Gollancz, 1984.
27 Orwell G. *(Afterword by E Fromm) 1984*. New York, NY: Signet Classics, New American Library, 1961.
28 Booker C. *The Seven Basic Plots: Why We Tell Stories*. London: Continuum, 2004.
29 http://en.wikipedia.org/wiki/My_Way_%28song%29 (accessed 12/04/10).
30 Despite claims that this phrase is American in origin, it was popularised by the Irish writer Bernard MacLaverty, who referred to the 'Troubles' in Northern Ireland as like 'having an elephant in your living room'. He had also used the idea in a children's story in the 1970s.
31 'Letter from Birmingham Jail' (April 16th, 1963). In: King ML (Ed.) *Why We Can't Wait*. New York, NY: Signet Classic, 2000.

Section 6 – Ethical dilemmas

Phil Barker

Any ideology is *either* a set of ideas that reflect the social needs and aspirations of one person, a group or a whole society, *or* a set of doctrines that form the basis of an economic, political or other system. The *ideology* of mental health is clearly all of these things, but most people relate to it in one particular way.

- *Intellectually*, the mental health ideology provides us with a way to think about 'what' mental health *is* and how we should relate to it.
- *Economically*, it provides many people with a source of income based on their 'contribution' to the field, whether they be a care-worker or shareholder in a pharmaceutical company.
- *Politically*, it provides governments with a rationale for framing legislation, aimed at containing sections of the community, who might be seen as 'problematic'.
- *Emotionally*, it helps provides comfort and reassurance to people who are distressed by aspects of their own lives or by others.
- *Socially*, it provides a means for containing groups of people; establishing 'pecking orders', shaping the structure of our 'class' system, such as the mad and the sane; the successful and the failures and the powerful and the incompetent.
- *Aspirationally*, it provides us with 'goals' and 'objectives': seeking to become more socially competent, less anxious, with greater self-esteem or a 'better' self-image.

As with most ideologies, this is merely the tip of the iceberg. It is already clear, however, that this ideology is so central to our lives that few of us could live without it. The question is not, perhaps, *could* we live without, but *should* we?

For people like my father, whom I introduced in the Preface, all this would be 'double-Dutch', which shows how far we have come – or how low we have fallen – in a couple of generations. For people like him – and there are still many of them around – life was something that one lived with; it was not an enemy to conquer; nor a devil to outwit. However, he was a man who believed very much in being 'his own man', rather than seeking to be a company man, a man of the people or any of the other illusory ways of being a 'better person'. He already was the best person he could be and the challenge was to live up to that, whatever life threw at him.

This was not a fate peculiar to my father or people like him. Rather, it seems to be the challenge that everyone faces. All children are born near perfect, even when they might appear to be blemished in some way. They only become difficult, damaged, awkward or otherwise troubled, as they begin to encounter the world and the various problems it has in store for them. The moral journey begins, almost as soon as we can walk and talk and start to make sense of what is 'me' and 'not me'. For some people – perhaps many people – this difficult business of working out how to play the game of life dogs their every footstep. For some people, the only way they can deal with it is to pretend it is not there, or to make up stories about it; or to deceive themselves into thinking it is not what it is or they are not what they are. We call such people 'crazy' or 'deluded' or 'personality disordered', but we could, just as easily call them 'mental health professionals'. They too *can* have a great capacity for self-deception, for ego-inflation, for self-aggrandisement, for failing to spot the obvious and for persistently failing to learn from experience.

However, as Albert Camus might have said if he was still with us: there is no need to despair. The situation may be desperate but it is not serious.[1] Or if my father was listening in, he would likely say, 'There's nothing else for it'. He had never heard of Samuel Beckett, but he was paraphrasing the final lines of Beckett's *The Unnamable*[2]: 'I can't go on; You must go on; I'll go on'.

However, going on, in this absurd manner, becomes a moral undertaking. It always was, we simply were not as aware of that fact, as we are now.

To conclude I suggest some of the ethical dilemmas that appear to have dogged the whole book and which might represent the key ethical dilemmas of all things 'psychiatric' or 'mental health'.

- *What if 'mental illness' is real?* As several authors have observed, there is no disputing the fact that people experience all manner of distress and discomfort, some of which becomes extremely distressing or disturbing to those around them. The question seems not to be 'what' shall we call this; far less 'what' has caused it – the answers to which might be as vague and abstract as the notion of 'mental illness' itself.

The obvious question seems to be, 'what shall we do now?' This is the key moral question – both for the person, whose moral dilemma this is, and for anyone who cares to offer a helping hand.

- *What if people want to be contained, sectioned, take psychiatric drugs or otherwise be changed by psychiatric means?* Freedom has long been the most jealously fought for human value. Indeed, today, governments of all political complexions appear keen to liberate all sorts of people from all manner of tyrannies. The question begged here is 'do people want to be free?' Or perhaps, 'how free should they be, to be in chains (however metaphorical)?' In my personal view, people should be free to ask for anything to be done for them or to them by other people – but only within the context of a consenting, contractual, relationship. People are free to pay others to beat them, in the name of sado-masochism; to have their bodies mutilated, in the name of cosmetic surgery or body art; so they should, in principle, be free to have electro-convulsive therapy (ECT), to take psychotropic drugs, experience the latest 'therapy' or to have psychosurgery.

The question is, would you be willing to *do* this to them, as part of a *professional* service?

- *What if people can't survive without help?* One need not experience a minor disaster – whether a leaking roof or being locked out one's house – to realise that no-one can survive without help; at least not for long. Good Samaritans are on most street corners almost anywhere in the world. If they are in short supply, one can always pay a builder or locksmith to bail us out. Tragedy – whether trivial or catastrophic is an everyday matter. The issue lies in how we 'frame' such tragedies: how do we interpret them and eventually respond to them. Historically, psychiatry, psychology and psychotherapy translated the tragedies of everyday life into forms of 'mental illness', 'personality defects' or 'self-esteem issues'.

The question is, how do we respond to people who appear to need or want our help? How do we 'frame' the help that we offer? And what message does this give about ourselves to the person we are helping?

- *What if people clearly need help but won't accept help?* This is the toughest question for any professional to answer, since how they answer it risks putting their professional standing on the line. People can and do choose to die (by rejecting life-saving treatment) while others are forcibly prevented from doing so, in the name of life-saving psychiatric treatment. The various legal, theoretical, professional and philosophical arguments for removing (however temporarily) a person's liberty have been covered in detail throughout the book. None of these answer the question posed, which is, should people have the right to deny themselves 'help'?

Or rather, the question is, what right do I have to deny their right to reject my offer of help or that of anyone else?

Many of these dilemmas seriously risk disturbing the professional calm of contemporary mental health services. They may even appear to challenge the philosophical basis on which many professions are established. However, such questions – along with the various other questions begged by other authors throughout the book – need to be asked, if a genuine form of mental health ethics is to develop, and if mental health professionals are to practice ethically, in an ever-changing world.

Notes

1 Saying attributed to an Austrian general. Greenberg, P. Quotes of the week. *Jewish World Review*, August 3, 1998.
2 Beckett, S. *Three Novels: Molloy, Malone Dies, the Unnamable.* New York, NY: Grove Press, 1994.

Index

Note: Page numbers in **bold** refer to illustrations.

Pierce, Charles S. 16
Pilgrim, David 99, 102, 103
Pinel, Philippe 58, 73–4, 161
Pinfold, V. 94
Pink, Graham 53
placebo effect 76–7, 183–4
Plato 8, 9, 11, 52, 260, 319
P/MH nurses *see* psychiatric/mental health
  (P/MH) nurses
policy 43, 53, 77, 152, 171, 191, 200; addiction
  215, 224–5, 226; children/young people
  229, 240; deinstitutionalisation 89–90;
  discriminatory 251; international 288;
  makers 83; nursing 198, 283; older people
  239, 240, 241; organisational 85, 94, 121,
  198, 199, 201, 301; political 77, 82;
  recovery 333, 346; reform 276; and suicide
  261, 262; spiritual care 124
political: agenda 59, 61, 62, 140, 276, 355;
  attitudes 7, 219, 261; authority 15; control
  85, 95; correctness 17, 57, 62, 138, 329,
  350; dilemmas 280; dissidence 255, 354;
  factors 4, 14, 101, 206, 261, 276; ideology
  103; imperative 98; language 335–6; policy
  77, 82; power relations 61, 318; problems 9,
  101; rights 232, 236; systems 358
politics 65, 336, 342, 355, 358; and coercion
  159; of diagnosis 23, 101, 140, 144, 145,
  190, 255; of difference 255; of recovery 82,
  332, 333, 334
politicisation 57, 61–2, 65
Popper, Karl 18, 19
Porter, Roy 24, 55, 180
positivism 159, 253
post-modernism 14–15, 16, 41, 159–60
post-traumatic stress disorder (PTSD) 59, 144
Powell, Enoch 251
power 73, 126–7, 141, 190, 200, 280, 283, 343,
  345, 346–7; abuse of 77–8, 352, 354
powers of detention 56, 277
practical ethics 21, 23, 32, 42, 51, 243; *see also*
  applied ethics
pragmatism 16, 70, 159, 161–2
prediction *see* prognoses
prejudice 35, 54, 85, 109, 256, 269, 288, 355
prescribing 40, 76, 103, 138, 180–1, 185–6
Priebe, S. 56
Prilleltensky, I. 163–4
primary care workers/services 103, 230, **231**, 241
principled autonomy 151–2, 153, 154
principles approach-based ethics 199, 200
prison 207–9, 211, 212, 216, 217, 236, 241,
  257, 275, 323, 346; *see also* imprisonment
prisoners 23, 34, 206, 208, 275, 322
privacy 19, 22, 84, 232, 233, 237, 313
Private Lunatic Asylums (Amendment) Act 1842
  286

professional: accountability 126, 186, 191, 212,
  236; allegiance 133–4; authority 53, 55, 69,
  71, 77–8, 86, 90, 111–12, 350; autonomy
  91, 98, 134, 154–5, 277; behaviour 3, 72,
  73, 77, 81–2, 156, 174, 256 (*see also*
  professional conduct); choice 81, 86–7, 103,
  165; competence 82, 118, **120**, 121, 186;
  conduct 86, 107–8, 115, 118, 242; culture
  82, 87, 119, **120**, 150, 154, 163, 164–5,
  202, 303, 342; duty 133 (*see also* duty of
  care; obligations); education 118, **120**, 201,
  202, 283, 351; identity 81–2, 98, 154, 283;
  integrity 84, 118, **120**, 121, 122, 126, 133,
  281; knowledge 69, 91, 99, 108, 124, 128;
  philosophy 69, 109, 133, 202, 360; purpose
  149, 155–6, 157, 351, 353; relationships
  77–8, 82, 87, 94, 109, 134, 137, 149–58,
  190, 243–4, 256, 283; responsibility 69, 73,
  84, 86–7, 102, 133, 134, 174, 230, 242,
  256; standards 118, **120**, 121, 242 (*see also*
  standard(s) of care); values 24, 82, 90, 202,
  242, 246, 300; *see also* named professionals
professionalism 62, 149–50
professionalisation 150, 190
prognoses 142, 209, 210–12, 318
prohibition: alcohol 220; drugs 216–18, 223,
  224, 226
promise-keeping 20
Protagoras 15
protection 22, 84, 118, 119, **120**, 232, 287, 288, 289
psyche 38, 70, 106, 129
psychiatric: diagnosis 32, 62, 76–7, 101, 104,
  137, 139–48, 229, 263–4, 329, 341 (*see also*
  diagnosis); 'disorder' 4, 46, 61, 70, 109, 139,
  140–2, 190, 191, 195, 229, 326, 329; drugs
  58, 73, 138, 141, 145, 172, 180–2, 183–4,
  191, 209, 341, 354, 359 (*see also* medication);
  ethics 7, 31–50, 51 (*see also* psychiatry
  ethics); medicine 24, 76–7, 190, 332 (*see also*
  medicine); survivors 49n87, 58, 60, 64n42,
  83, 97, 104, 172, 336 (*see also* recovery); will
  273, 306
psychiatric advance directives (PADs) *see* advance
  directives
psychiatric/mental health (P/MH) nurses 262,
  265, 266
psychiatrists 24–5, 32, 51–2, 53, 69, 71–9, 92,
  332; and addiction 225; and advance
  directives 309; autonomy 277; and
  children/young people 230, **231**; and
  detention 288, 289; and diagnosis (*see*
  psychiatric diagnosis); and diminished
  responsibility 318, **320**, 321, 323; and ECT
  170–1, 172; and involuntary admission 290;
  and older people 239; and recovery 332,
  333–4; and restraint 159, 160–1; *see also*
  psychiatry

UNCRC *see* United Nations Convention on the Rights of the Child
United Kingdom *see* UK
United Nations Convention on the Rights of the Child (UNCRC) 232, 233, 237
United Nations Principles on the Protection of Persons with Mental Illness and for the Improvement of Mental Health Care (1991) 287
United States *see* USA
Unmasking Medicine (Kennedy) 23
USA 37, 72, 109, 206, 216, 342; addiction 218, 223, 225, 226; advance directives 306, 307, 310, 311; competence to stand trial 321–2; CTO 94; dangerousness 210, 212; dementia 239; diagnosis 142–3, 147n1; ECT 171, 175, 177n1; insanity defence **319–20**; legislation 222, 306, 310; lobotomy 44; moral philosophy 16, 23; prohibition 220; racism 251, 255; recovery 333; schizophrenia 60; school shootings 341; suicide 264
utilitarianism 12, 21, 39, 42, 199, 200

Vagrancy Act 1744 318, **319**
validation 181, 355
validity 159–60, 161–2, 163–4
values 5, 20, 78, 90, 159–60, 184–5, 199, 200; -based decision-making 201, 232; -based practice 103, 122, 201–2, 243, 296, 300, 301, 304; ethical/moral 6, 26, 242, 324; family 7; personal 6, 24, 82, 109, 202, 223–4, 242, 246, **263**, 304, 348, 354; professional 24, 82, 90, 202, 242, 246, 300; social 7–8, 17, 41, 90, 242, 250, 280, 352; universal 200, 201
van Praag, H.M. 264
veracity 22, 84
violence 102, 128, 199, 206–7, 211, 217, 226, 339, 345; against children 232; categorisation 164; by children 341; legislation 278; management 153, 162–6, 210
virtue ethics 9, 17, 18, 19, 199, 200, 219, 242
voluntary admission 56, 72, 293–4
vulnerability 60, 73, 84, 90, 100, 108, 118, 156, 205, 297, 301, 303–4, 335, 336; older people 172, 242, 244, 246; professional 53, 164; women 172, 205; young people 232

vulnerability-stress model 100

Wales 60, 91, 160, 208, 275–85, 286, 306, 307, 310, 312
Walsh, Paul 53
Wardhaugh, J. 163
Warren, Mary Anne 38, 39
Webster, G. 86
Weisstub, D.N. 260
welfare 5, 7, 18, 19, 21, 22, 103, 118, 119–20, **120**, 275; *see also* child welfare
wellbeing 116–17, 122, 137, 144, 155, 199, 200, 291, 332, 356; older people 241, 293; spiritual 125, 126, 127; young people 228–9, 230, 237
Wells, J. 292
Werth, J.L. 262, **263**, 266–7
West Dunbartonshire Literary Project 103
whistle-blowing 52–3, 62, 65–6
Whitaker, Robert 24–5, 145
White, S.M. 292
Whitehead, Alfred North 8
WHO *see* World Health Organisation
Why Kids Kill: Inside the Minds of School Shooters (Langman) 341
Wiesel, Elie 5
Wilding, P. 163
Wilkinson, R. 102
Williams, Bernard 15
Williams, N. 154
Willis, Francis 71, 72, 74
Winston, M. 306
Wolfensberger, W. 332, 335
Wollstonecraft, Mary 36
women 18, 23, 34–5, 36, 153–4, 261; and diminished responsibility 323; and ECT 172; and forensic care 205, 210
Woodbridge K. 202
Woolf, Virginia 43
World Health Organisation 60–1, 72, 102, 124, 142, 143, 239, 243
World Psychiatric Association 239
Wrigley, M. 293–4

young people 173, 195, 228–38, 270, 278, 290, 341
youth *see* young people

Zeno 10

Lightning Source UK Ltd.
Milton Keynes UK
UKOW020616150513

210668UK00008B/84/P